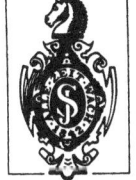

Springer-Verlag France S.A.R.L

Proceedings of the 3rd International Congress on
Neo-Adjuvant Chemotherapy

Edited by :

P. Banzet, J.F. Holland, D. Khayat, M. Weil

Springer-Verlag France S.A.R.L

Professeur P. Banzet
Hôpital Saint-Louis
1, avenue Vellefaux
75475 Paris Cedex 10, France

Professor J.F. Holland
The Mount Sinai Medical Center
1 G. Levy Place
New York
NY 10029-6574, USA

Professeur D. Khayat
Service d'Oncologie Médicale
Hôpital Pitié-Salpétrière
Pavillon Jacquart
47, boulevard de l'Hôpital
75651 Paris Cedex 13, France

Docteur M. Weil
Hôpital Pitié-Salpétrière
Pavillon Jacquart
47, boulevard de l'Hôpital
75651 Paris Cedex 13, France

© Springer-Verlag France 1991

Originally published by Springer-Verlag Paris Berlin Heidelberg London New York · Tokyo Barcelona Budapest in 1991

ISBN 978-2-8178-0784-3   ISBN 978-2-8178-0782-9 (eBook)
DOI 10.1007/978-2-8178-0782-9

2918/3917/543210 — Printed on acid-free paper.

Contents

UROLOGY

BREAST

GASTRO-INTESTINAL TUMORS

LOCO-REGIONAL

ESOPHAGUS

GYNECOLOGY

HIGH-DOSE CHEMOTHERAPY

RADIO-CHEMOTHERAPY

PEDIATRIC TUMORS

BONE AND SOFT TISSUE SARCOMAS

HEMATOSARCOMAS

PHARMACOKINETIC

Contents

NEW DRUGS

LUNG

SPECIAL LECTURES

Foreword

This book includes some selected presentations given at the 3rd International Congress on Neo-Adjuvant Chemotherapy which was held in Paris from February 6th to February 9th, 1991.

It was attended by over 2000 physicians from around the world and by 700 nurses. Its organisation was saddened by the untimely death of Professor Claude Jacquillat on October 12th, 1990. It was further complicated in January and February 1991 by the gulf events which led some guests to cancel their participation. However with the outstanding help of the two presidents chosen by Claude Jacquillat before his death, Pierre Banzet from Paris and James F. Holland from New York, the organizers could set up an exciting meeting confirming the impact of neo-adjuvant chemotherapy on relatively new indications such as non-small lung cancers, bladder cancer, esophagal cancer, cervix cancer, etc...

It is noteworthy that a contradictory debate on primary chemotherapy in non-small lung cancer turned into a consensus conference.

In breast cancer, the downstaging induced by primary chemotherapy is acknowledged by all and the conviction that Jacquillat defended so heartily that breast preservation should be proposed to all patients with breast cancer whatever their tumour size is shared now by more and more people.

A special emphasis was given to new drugs, new combination, new access (locoregional therapy) and new developments such as that of growth factors and of interleukin 2.

But the cost of these therapeutic advances cannot be ignored and this topic was discussed at a round table gathering economists and physicians.

The developments of modern medical oncology should imply as often as possible ambulatory treatment and modern devices such as implantable ports, ambulatory pumps, make it feasible in more and more patients. Therefore more and more nurses should be familiar with such managements : an educational program for nurses during the congress was attended by a large audience and met a frank success.

The organisation of this congress was made possible solely due to the generous financial support of many sponsors and of pharmaceutical firms which participation at this meeting was very active.

We would like to express our utmost gratitude to all the sponsors and to extend our deep thanks to those who shared with us the scientific and material organisation of the congress ; the members of the scientific committee and the administrative staff.

Finally the success of the congress should be ascribed to all the participants who came from all continents despite difficult circumstances.

Their participations was an invaluable tribute to the memory of Claude Jacquillat to whom the congress and this book are dedicated.

The first Claude Jacquillat Memorial Lecture : Chemotherapy of cancer

J.F. Holland

The steady improvement in cancer therapeutics that has occurred in the period after World War II is the fruit of laboratory and clinical research. Neither discipline could have produced the improvements alone. Claude Jacquillat was a leader in clinical research, a man whose intimate knowledge of human disease led him to recognize the areas where treatment was insufficient or ineffectual, and this recognition provoked him to find new solutions. Because he saw the same problems that confronted every oncologist, but with a different vision, he was able to formulate solutions they had not seen. We Americans come from a young nation. When older civilizations, Claude Jacquillat's among them, were enjoying high levels of cultural achievement in architecture, music, art, literature, science, and medicine, American frontiersmen were pushing westward to discover the vast wealth in land and resources of our new country. The most important man on the pioneer voyage was the trailblazer ; he chopped small chips from the trees he passed, to indicate the best route for the settlers and wagons that followed. Claude served such a role in cancer research, blazing trails that many others would follow. Once a path is chosen, repetitive travel converts it into a highway, but choosing the path is the critical creative step. Highways that lead nowhere are not nearly so valuable as a single trail that leads in the right direction. Only the best scouts can identify the right path to discover the secret places. The ramparts that defend the unknown are criss-crossed by networks of highways leading nowhere that follow trails blazed by lesser men than Jacquillat.

Creativity in research is of the essence. Creativity is centrifugal, probing new concepts at the intellectual periphery, rather than congregating at the center where it is safer, but far less likely to lead to discovery. Creativity leads to interchange of new approaches, hybrid ideas, new flowering from new seed, in short : cross pollination. Creativity is auto-inhibitable, when vaulting leaps of the imagination fall of their own weight by tests of reality. Great creative minds recognize their own faults quickly and move on, swiftly blazing another better way. In research, as in biological evolution, survival of the fittest describes the eventual outcome of ideas.

Although we mourn the loss of Claude, we celebrate his major contributions, of which I shall describe only three. The first is this Congress of neo-adjuvant Chemotherapy, which stands as testimony to his commitment to professional education and scientific discourse, and the trail which has become the highway of neo-adjuvant chemotherapy that he, and a very few others, served to blaze. His second contribution was in the field of childhood leukemia. To appreciate its significance, we must return to the late 1950's and 1960's, for an overview of leukemia research.

Two great observations sprang from animal research on leukemia that dealt with the reasons for success and failure of treatment. Two kinds of resistance

exist : biochemical and kinetic. Those leukemic cells that are not responsive
to azaguanine led to death in mice bearing leukemia ; those not responsive
to Amethopterin (the original name for Methotrexate), led to death from biochemical resistance. In combination, there is much longer survival and, indeed,
animals who were cured. This classic experiment of Lloyd Law, that biochemical resistance can be an explanation for failure, is the biochemical rationale
for combination chemotherapy (Fig. 1).

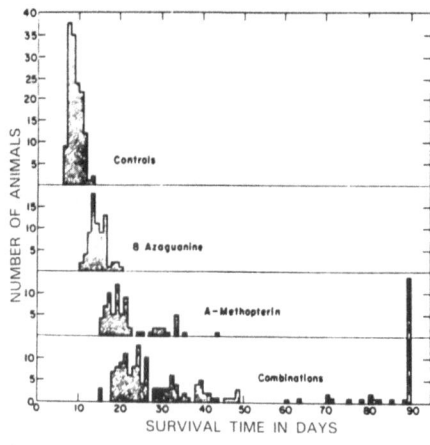

1

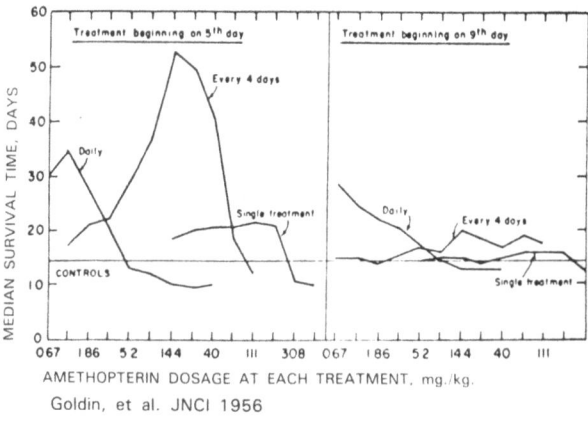

2

Fig. 1. Combination chemotherapy of leukemia L-1210 in a classic experiment of Lloyd
Law

Fig. 2. The importance of tumor size, drug dose and drug schedule using methotrexate
for the chemotherapy of leukemia L-1210

The second classic experiment was conducted by Abraham Goldin, in which kinetic resistance is the clear explanation. Animals with advanced leukemia treated on the ninth day after transplantation had no effective therapeutic outcome from using Amethopterin (Methotrexate). Identical animals treated earlier in the disease, five days after tumor transplant, were indeed much more therapeutically responsive, and differences are appreciable in the schedule of drugs (Fig. 2). Thus, there is kinetic resistance, as well as biochemical resistance. We tested this kinetic concept in children with leukemia back in the late 1950's and early '60's using the higt-dose twice-a-week regimen, which Goldin had shown was superior in mice with early leukemia, and the low-dose daily regimen which was characteristic of the time. Children to be treated in the Cancer and Leukemia Group B (CALGB) were randomized between the two treatment schedules. The drug was relatively inactive, and only 20 % of children reached remission on either schedule. This low effectiveness was similar to the result in mice with advanced disease. The leukemic children also had kinetic resistance. Insufficient numbers reached the second randomization to test the effect on « early disease ». Then we learned how to use Vincristine and Prednisone, two drugs which could induce remission, thus returning the child to the equivalent of the early mouse leukemia. In this circumstance, the high-dose twice-weekly Methotrexate wes significantly superior to the daily administration. This is shown in Figure 3, a composite of CALGB results that was made sometime in 1966. The median survival, in the report of Tivey, et al, of children with leukemia who were untreated is marked with T. The first combination chemotherapy experiment (58), which was based on the concept of biochemical resistance is shown. The treatment using intensive twice-weekly methotrexate (65 striped), is compared to daily Methotrexate (unlabeled line), both treatments allocated at random after Vincristine and Prednisone induction. This demonstrated that kinetic resistance had occurred in man, predicted by the results in mice.

In Figure 4, three separate experiments are compared, all of which start with Vincristine and Prednisone induction. In the early '60's, children were treated in CALGB with Vincristine and Prednisone, and were then observed untreated until the time of relapse. The unmaintained remission time is a method to quantify the residual burden of leukemic cells ; Vincristine and Prednisone alone led to short unmaintained remission time. Freireich and Frei at the National Cancer Institute described the four-drug simultaneous combination VAMP (Vincristine, Prednisone, Amethopterin (methotrexate), and Mercaptopurine), which was aimed at biochemical resistance ; it led to a significant advantage. At the same time, CALGB looked at Vincristine and Prednisone induction followed by single short courses of Methotrexate, 6-Mercaptopurine, Cyclophosphamide, and Carmustine, giving the drugs in sequence. The results are at least as good as the simultaneous combination. Biochemical resistance and kinetic resistance co-exist in human cancer.

We next organized a study based upon the curative impact of Methotrexate for choriocarcinoma in that the drug was given in five-day intensive courses. Vincristine and Prednisone induction was followed by 3 courses of intensive Methotrexate. This strategy was aimed at kinetic resistance. There was a major anti-leukemic effect, but we realized that we had treated for too short a period

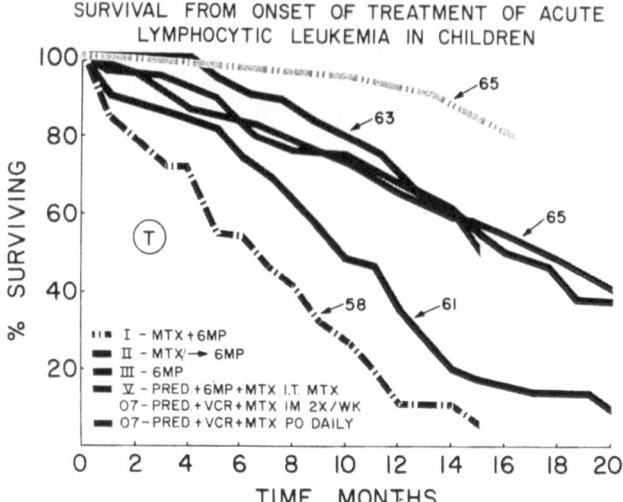

Fig. 3. Successive early protocols of the acute leukemia group B. Protocols I, II, III and V begun in 1958, 1961, 1963, and 1965 respectively. Protocol 07 test of Goldin's experimental design (see fig. 2). In 1965, striped line represents vincristine and prednisone (VP), followed by twice-weekly methotrexate. The unlabeled line (ending at 15 monts) represents VP followed by daily methotrexate. T, with a circle around it, represents the median survival of children with acute leukemia who are not treated, as reported in the literature survey of Tivey

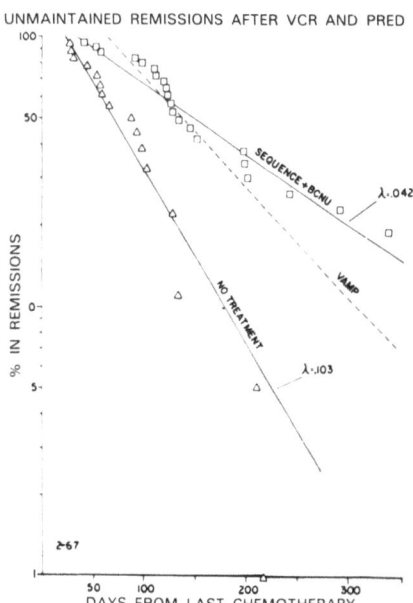

Fig. 4. Unmaintained remissions after vincristine and prednisone (VP) induction. The VP was given silmultaneously in the VAMP combination treatment of Freirich, Karon, and Frei. The sequence consisted of VP, methotrexate, 6-mercaptopurine, cyclophosphamide, and caramustine

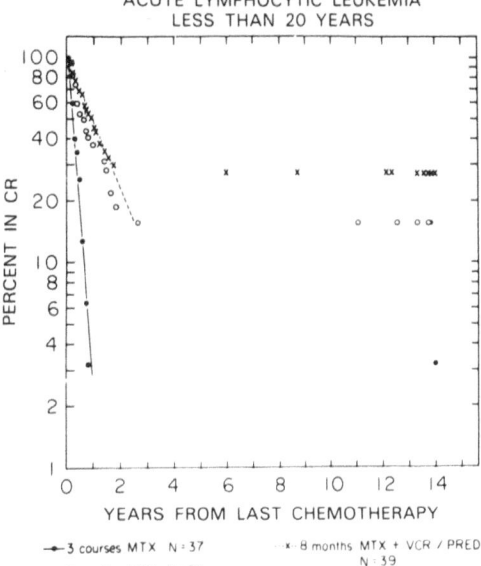

Fig. 5. Unmaintained remissions after VP induction on 5-day courses of methotrexate is shown. No further treatment was given. The failure slopes are shown at left. Those off the line are without evidence of disease when last seen. Two patients in the MXT = VCR/PRED arm were lost at 6 and 9 years, still in complete remission

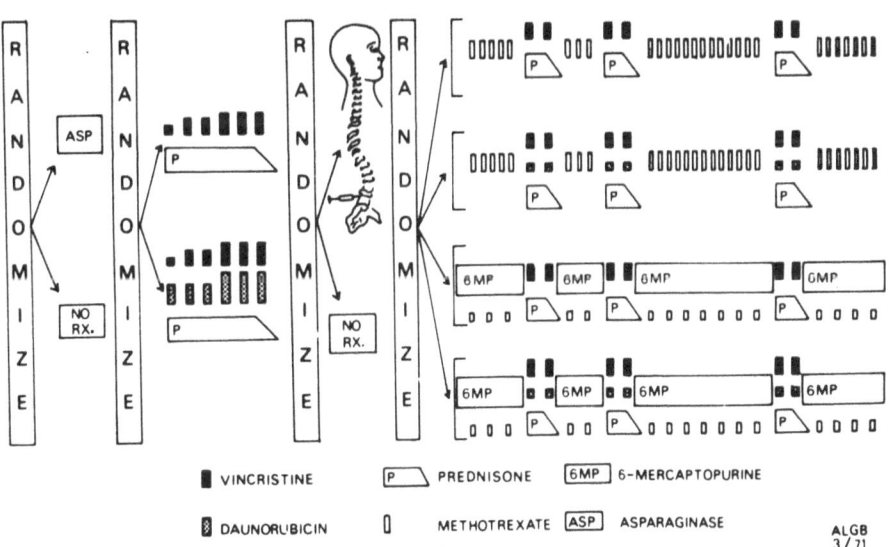

Fig. 6. Schema of ALGB Protocol 6801. Five randomizations gave 32 separate arms, of which the best was not asparaginase, vincristine, prednisone induction, intrathecal methotrexate, 6-mercaptopurine plus methotrexate maintenance with vincristine and prednisone reinforcement

of time. Had we continued to treat to the theoretical intercept of the mathematical model with the abscissa, perhaps we might have had a substantially better outcome out for 120 days. Thus, for added assurance, we treated for 240 days. This is an experiment in which Claude Jacquillat's influence was felt. Jacquillat had discovered that repetitive use of Vincristine and Prednisone during the remission phase, a treatment that he called re-induction, was useful. We tested this maneuver prospectively, because by this time Jean Bernard and his colleagues at Hopital St. Louis, Claude Jacquillat, Marise Weil, and Michel Boiron had joined the CALGB. After 3 courses of treatment with Methotrexate, 1 child was cured at 14 years. After 8 months of courses the cure rate was 16 %. After 8 months of courses plus Vincristine and Prednisone re-induction, the cure rate was 27 %. The emphasis was on eliminating kinetic resistance, rather than biochemical resistance. Thus, 25 years ago Jacquillat's influence was of great importance in pointing the way. Eventually, a study was led by Marise Weil, then still at Hopital St-Louis. This complex multifactorial study of remission maintenance compared Asparaginase or none, Vincristine and Prednisone, or Vincristine prednisone and Daunorubicin, for induction and re-induction, with random allocation for maintainance with Methotrexate or 6-Mercaptopurine plus Methotrexate, with or without intrathecal prophylaxis ; in reality 32 separate arms. The best arm was the one Jacquillat had been using in France all along, Vincristine and Prednisone induction, intrathecal prophylaxis, the combination of 6-Mercaptopurine and Methothexate together with Vincristine and Prednisone re-induction. This treatment led to a considerable improvement in the cures of leukemia. The part these two studies played in advancing the frontiers of leukemia research using Jacquillat's concepts of re-induction are shown in Figure 7.

Leukemia is a tumor with many more similarities to, than differences from, other types of cancer. One of the important methodological approaches to curing acute lymphoblastic leukemia was the ability to quantify the tumor mass. I have attempted to quantify the nomenclature of carcinomas and sarcomas. It is of great importance to recognize that a million cells cannot be seen, except at the operating table perhaps, and are not palpable ; they are not recognizable by any of the external diagnostic techniques we use. A billion cells are barely detectable. A trillion cells are massive. When we encounter clinically detectable tumors, therefore, we are dealing with cancers at a very late stage in their evolution. The kinetics of late stage growth are different from intuitive interpretation of what we see. The data presented by Laird in 1968 demonstrate Gompertzian kinetics for a whole spectrum of different transplanted tumors in rat, mouse, and rabbit (Fig. 8). The Gompertzian equation holds true for human fetal growth, and has been shown for some human cancers. When large tumors are encountered clinically, we may be seeing tumors then in their asymptotic phase. Yet, they may grow extremely rapidly in the subclinical stage. This emphasizes the potential basis for kinetic resistance, in addition to the more generally appreciated biochemical resistance.

A mathematical model derived by Norton, showed that a single combination chemotherapy for breast cancer allows for eradication of a sensitive population, but emergence of a resistant one. If an effective treatment against the sensitive cells is used for a shorter period of time, and then a different effec-

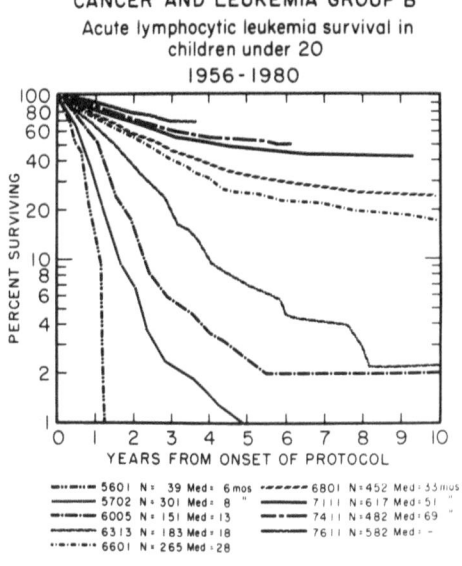

CANCER AND LEUKEMIA GROUP B
Acute lymphocytic leukemia survival in children under 20
1956-1980

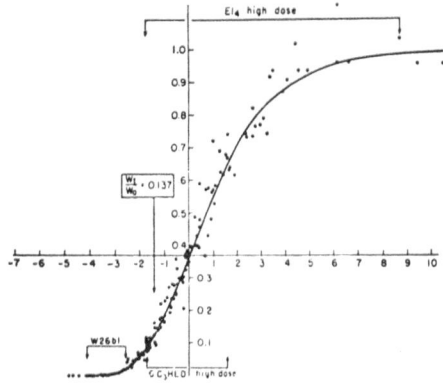

A "normalized" Gompertz plot, in which the growth data for 19 examples of 12 different tumors of the rat, mouse, and rabbit have been superimposed after adjustment of the units on the 2 axes The point of reference, at the intersection of the 2 scales, is the inflection point of the growth curve. The units on the ordinate (tumor size) are decimal fractions of the asymptotic tumor size. The unit of time on the abscissa is the time required for the doubling immediately preceding the inflection point (extending from −1 to 0 in this text-fig.).

Reproduced from *Brit J Cancer* 19 : 278-291, 1965, with permission of publishers

LAIRD, 1968

Fig. 7. Survival data in over 3,000 children with acute leukemia studied by Acute Leukemia Group B, and its successor organization CALGB, as compiled under the supervision of Oliver Glidewell, Group Biostatistician. The data from Figure 4 are incorporated in 6313 ; the data from Figure 5 are 6601 ; the results for all of Figure 6 are in 6801. Study 7611 is currently being uptated

Fig. 8. Gompertzian growth of tumors in 3 species

tive treatment is used against the emerging resistant cells, it is possible to attain cures that were not possible by the initial treatment alone. This led us, through a series of steps, to a regimen with which we now treat patients with breast cancer after surgery, an intensive program for 16 weeks (of CMFVP), a short recovery time, and an intensive program of a different drug for another 12 weeks (escalating Doxorubicin) (Fig. 9). This strategy has produced prolonged disease-free survival for premenopausal women. It is possible, using kinetic as well as biochemical approaches, to avoid resistance and to change the outcome of cancer with the drugs that we have as tools today.

The group of Jacquillat has made a major contribution to the therapy of breast cancer. Their data first published in 1986, related to women with breast cancer who were diagnosed predominantly by needle aspiration cytology. They then were treated with chemotherapy and radiotherapy, but not with surgery. These are women who did not undergo the psychic and physical trauma of surgical procedures, but whose data, even with advanced local cancer, are highly estimable at 3 years ; 87 % disease-free survival for those who had T1 and T2 tumors, 55 % disease-free survival for those who had T3 and T4 tumors. The series has been extended. This constitutes a major accomplishment of Jac-

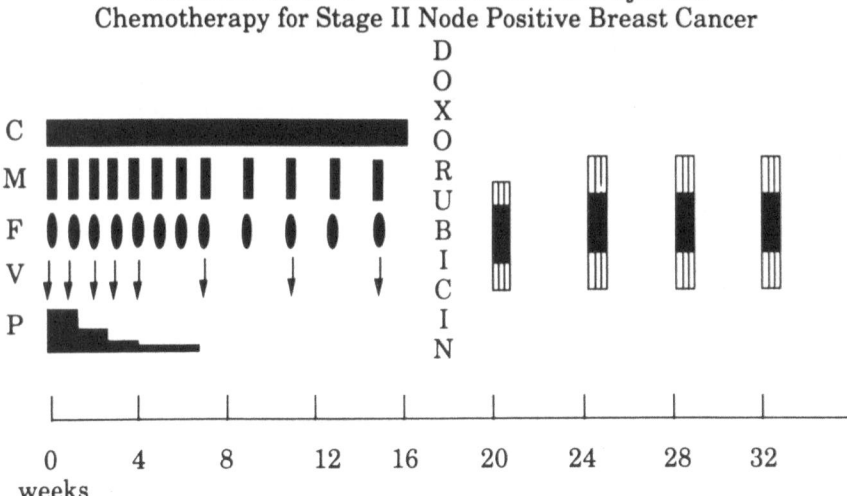

Fig. 9. Schema for adjuvant chemotherapy of breast cancer designed to affect emerging resistant clones refractory to the Cooper CMFVP regimen

quillat and his colleagues, in the simplification of the treatment of breast cancer, and its improvement by using neo-adjuvant chemotherapy, the only one of the major therapeutic modalities that addresses systemic disease. And it is, after all, extramammary disease that kills.

Considering the progress that has been made with chemotherapy, it is still more daunting to realize that we are still at the beginning of the molecular biological revolution. Oncogenes, 50 or more of them, have been discovered that mediate phenotypic tumor behavior. I believe that even more significant, however, are the tumor suppressor genes, of which the retinoblastoma gene serves as the first example. Tumor suppressor genes serve as the intracellular counterpoise to the oncogenes, controlling cellular division rates and acting as prohibitors of unrestrained cellular growth. The existence of tumor suppressor genes was first conceived and then demonstrated in retinoblastoma, where

Table 1. Characteristics of Polycytomas

Name	Cell number	Logarithmic expression	Approximate size	Comment
Polycytoma	Many	10^n	Any	"Solid tumor"
Kilocytoma	Thousand	10^3	0.001 mm³ = 1 nl	Invisible
Megacytoma	Million	10^6	1 mm³ = 1 μl	Impalpable
Gigacytoma	Billion	10^9	1 cm³ = 1 ml	Barely clinical detectable
Teracytoma	Trillion	10^{12}	1 000 cm³ = 1 liter	Massive tumor

acquired loss of a functioning gene on both chromosomes led to this extremely rare spontaneous tumor. Inherited loss or mutation of the gene on one chromosome, however, allowed a single acquired mutation of the remaining retinoblastoma gene to produce the tumor, accounting for the major difference in attack rates in sporadic and heredofamilial cases. The ultimate proof occurred when Huang and his colleagues were able to study osteosarcoma cells in culture and retinoblastoma cells xenografted in nude mice. Both lacked the retinoblastoma gene ; they were transfected with a plasmid containing the retinoblastoma gene. The osteosarcoma cells then began to produce the RB protein, changed their morphology, slowed their growth and were no longer able to grow unless attached to a surface. The gene-transplanted retinoblastoma tumor lost its tumorgenicity and lethality in the nude mouse. Thus, these investigators were able to convert the tumors back to a phenotypically more benign tissue by reintroducing a deleted tumor suppressor gene. This implies that the neoplastic state was perpetuated because it lacked the tumor suppressor gene.

There are already 12 recognized tumor suppressor genes. The retinoblastoma gene, for example, is absent or mutationally inactivated in retinoblastoma and some instances of osteosarcoma, synovial sarcoma, small cells carcinoma of the lung, and carcinoma of the breast. Perhaps the most important tumor suppressor gene yet recognized is P53, a tumor suppressor gene on chromosone 17. P53 is increased in normally proliferating cells, an in lymphocytes after a mitogenic stimulus. This represents the counterpoise, a balance that controls growth rates in proliferating cells, and after mitogenic stimuli. P53 is also increased in several transformed cell lines, but this is deceptive. In lines where it is increased, a mutant P53 gene appears to be present in abundant quantity, but the P53 protein produced by it does not exercise tumor inhibition. Of 126 miscellaneous cancers isolated fresh, none showed P53 gene product, which suggests that there was a substantial decrease in the presence of this tumor suppressor. It has subsequently been shown that P53 gene can be introduced into lung cancer lines *in vitro*, thereby eliminating their oncogenicity. This is a critical concept with high specificity for controlling the neoplastic process.

The P53 gene is about 20,000 nucleotides long, and codes for the P53 protein, which is approximately 400 aminoacids long. There are many people now working on it, but its therapeutic use as such is not yet assured.

I choose as a different example, one that has been more clearly worked out, proopiomelanocortin. Figure 10 shows the gene product as it is translated from the messenger RNA, the composition of which was specified by the gene in which resides the coding for ACTH. Proopiomelanocortin is 200 amino acids long, but ACTH is only 39 amino acids within it. When ACTH is produced by virtue of endocrine stimulation, it is synthesized as Proopiomelanocortin, and post-synthetic processing modifies it to become ACTH. Although the formula for ACTH contains 39 amino acids, the terminal 15 amino acids are not necessary for biological activity. The 24-amino acid residue is Cosyntropin, a peptide that can be made synthetically, which produces all the activities of administered ACTH (Fig. 11).

I am extremely optimistic that we can, in the course of time, learn more about the P53 gene product and other tumor suppressor gene products, and

PRO-OPIOMELANOCORTIN

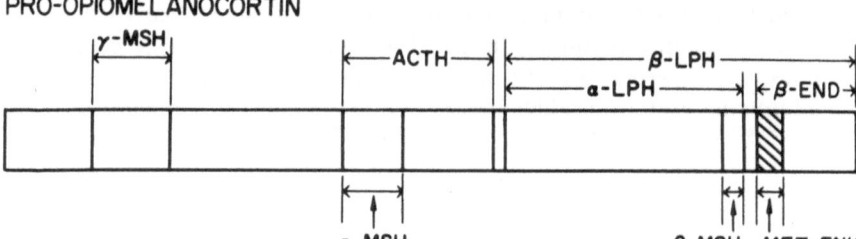

Fig. 10. Pro-opiomelanocortin, the gene product that contains ACTH and several other biologically important molecules

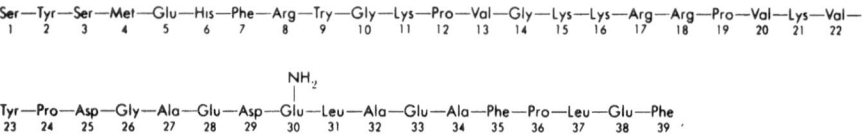

Fig. 11. The formula for ACTH. Cosyntropin, the first 24 aminoacids, convey all the hormonal activity of ACTH. This polypeptide can be synthesized

that aminoacid segments, or other small molecular configurations, will be found that impart the tumor suppressive activity of the gene products. For cancer, this will be a logical chemotherapy, using the same type of tumor inhibition that nature ordinarily uses.

In the years following the Gulf war, which everyone hopes, but no one believes, will be the last war, let us, through our professions that are concerned with medicine and health, help heal this sick world. In our original continental configuration physical reality kept the continents together. In the trailblazing research for better health, of which Claude Jacquillat was a foremost exponent, we can aspire to make meaningful contributions to mankind on every continent that will keep up together. Chemotherapeutic control of cancer can be one mechanism to accomplish this.

Head and neck

Neo-Adjuvant chemotherapy for patients with oral and oro-pharyngeal T3/T4 carcinomas

H Szpirglas, D Nizri*, JP Lacoste, A Thomas, S Godeau, L Benslama

We presented in 1987, a randomized trial for neo-adjuvant chemotherapy before radiotherapy, called INSERM [1] trial, dealing with 14 patients with oral and oro-pharyngeal T3/T4 carcinomas. Then, we concluded that chemotherapy did not rise the number of remissions achieved after radiotherapy (about 50 % in each group) ; also, that chemotherapy was predictive of the short term result, as the patients responding to chemotherapy had four times more chances to achieve remission after radiotherapy than non-responders. Unfortunately, after remission, the evolution remains the same and disappointing, with only 2 out of 114 patients who survive, one in each group.

However, surgery being the prefered treatment in our institution it allowed to select, for this trial, patients discarded by surgeons. We could think that may be our chemotherapeutic protocol called GIFA, which associates Adriamycine, Vincristine, Bleomycine and Cisplatin was not the best one with 50 % major responses compared with the 80 % or more promised with the 5FU-Cisplatin combination. So we activated our new protocol called VADS (Aero-Digestive Upper Tract), in 1987, to evaluate the neo-adjuvant chemotherapy in populations as homogeneous as possible, limited to oral and oro-pharyngeal squamous cells carcinomas, so called « advanced » tumors classified T3/T4. We did not include multiple primaries, palliative treatments and patients with any contra-indication to one of the proposed treatments.

Our first purpose was to evaluate the neo-adjuvant chemotherapy for operable patients, compared with the same experiment on non-operable patients. The second purpose was to compare surgical and radiotherapeutic treatments for operable patients which will be presented separately.

Methods and results

Our protocol VADS entered 164 patients from 1987 until 1990. They were 136 males and 28 females whose mean age was 55 years. A first stratification was decided by surgeons during the VADS committee, leading to 2 groups : 109 operable patients and 55 not operable. The age and sex of these patients interfere little in the decision. Nevertheless, there are many more T4 in the non-operable group (80/39 %) and they are bigger (about 20 % more) while the T3 are identical according to the tumor size measured on 2 diameters. In the same time, the clinical invasion of nodes is more severe for non-operable patients (36 % N3 versus 16 %) (Fig. 1). We can also notice more posterior

Département d'oncologie et stomatologie médicale (clinique de chirurgie maxillo-faciale et stomatologie Prof JM Vaillant), * Département de radiothérapie, CHU Pitié-Salpêtrière, Paris, France

T / N		N0	N1 N2	N3
OPER.109 PTS	67 T3	22	36	9
	42 T4	14	21	8
NO OPER.55 PTS	8 T3	3	3	2
	47 T4	7	22	18

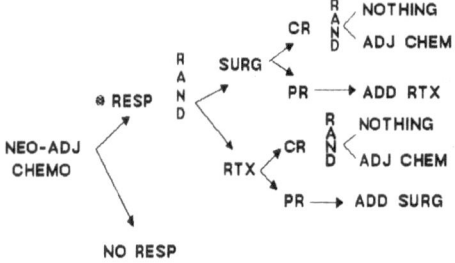

Fig. 1.

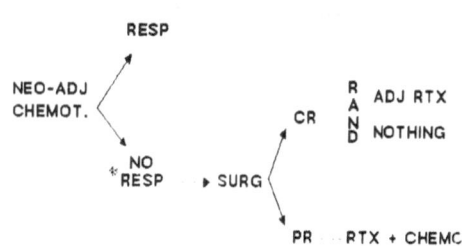

Fig. 2.

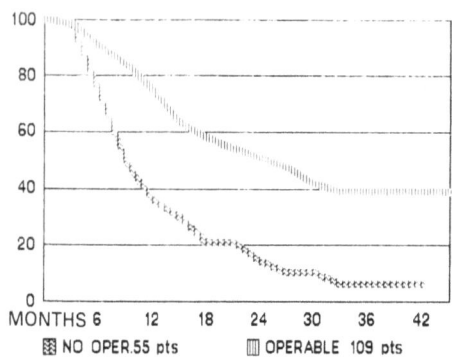

Fig. 3.

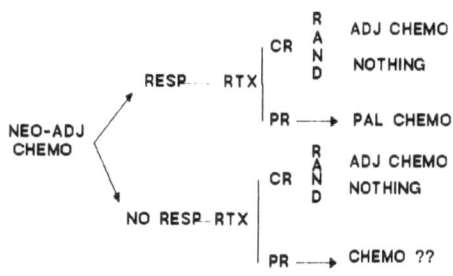

Fig. 4.

Fig. 5.

lesions, particularly on the base of the tongue, that we isolated from oropharynx because the pronostic is very different.

All patients operable (Figs. 2, 3) or not (Fig. 4) were to receive 3 courses of neo-adjuvant chemotherapy, with association of 5FU-Cisplatinum in 5 days, which had really become the reference protocol in head and neck carcinology. Therefore, the division into operable and non-operable appears clearly motivated on the survival curves of the two groups, with a 40 % difference on the long term (Fig. 5).

As first observation, the treatment was very well tolerated in both groups. In cases of no response or of tumoral progression at the second course, 15 patients were operated or irradiated without delaying any more (10 %).

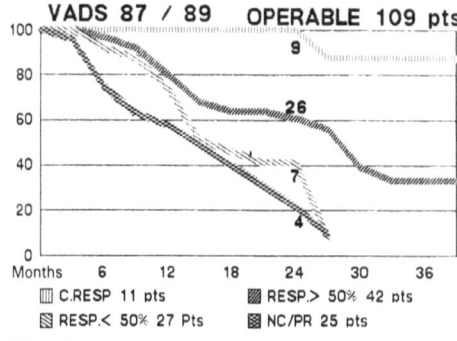

VADS 87 / 89   OPERABLE 109 pts

Months 6   12   18   24   30   36

▥ C.RESP 11 pts   ▨ RESP.> 50% 42 pts
▨ RESP.< 50% 27 Pts   ▧ NC/PR 25 pts

Fig. 6.

T. RESPONSES TO 5FU-CISPLAT.

OPERABLES 109

	1ST C/80	2nd C/76	3RD C/88
CR	0	1	11
RP>50%	9	33	39
	= 11%	= 45%	= 57%
RP<50%	52	29	21
NC/PG	18	11	14
INEV	1	2	3

Fig. 7.

T.RESPONSES TO 5FU-CISPLAT

NO OPERABLES

	1ST C/41	2nd C/35	3RD C/43
CR	0	0	2
RP>50%	4	8	12
	= 10%	= 22%	= 32%
RP<50%	25	16	23
NC/PG	12	10	6
INEV	0	1	0

Fig. 8.

The second observation shows a dramatically different response rate in the two groups, where major responses are concerned. For over 15 years, we obstinately kept considering that only a diminution of over 50 % in the size of the tumor is a response to chemotherapy. We will further see that this appreciation is still too optimistic. Decreased of a few dissociated responses on the nodes, this response rate did not reach 50 % in the operable group — though with 10 % of complete responses — and only half of this result in the non-operable group.

The actuarial survival of the 109 operable patients according to the response to neo-adjuvant chemotherapy shows that a response below 50 % makes no difference with no response at all. On the contrary, the complete responses are a first step to recovery (Fig. 6).

We arbitrarily fixed 3 neo-adjuvant courses, keeping 3 more adjuvant courses for responders. To explain this choice, we wanted to evaluate the response rates to the first, second and third courses (Figs. 7, 8) ; considering the progessive increase in response, one question remains : is the intensification of the neo-adjuvant treatment justified and how much ?

In the non-operable group, the conclusions are the same as with the INSERM protocol, the immediate results sanctioning the response to chemotherapy. All responders were irradiated and 58 % achieved remission. On the contrary, most of the non-responders could not end the radiotherapy, and only 14 % achieved remission (20 % of the irradiated).

After remission, we decided of an adjuvant treatment with 3 additional courses of 5FU-Cisplatin for responders. The short term benefit is very small and falls to nothing on the long term ; thus, we can say that a non-operable patient has 1 or 2 chances out of a 100 to reach 5 years, with or without chemotherapy.

The group considered as operable at the first consultation was thus divided into 2 grossly equivalent sub-groups : majors responders (50 pts) and non-responders (58 pts) ; the responders were randomized between surgery and radiotherapy as second treatment (separate study). On the contrary, all non-responders would have been operated.

Remission and survival show a very significant difference between responders and non-responders which lasts up to long term (Fig. 9), but, as in non-responders, a greater number could not get the planned treatment ; we compare in each group only patients who where operated. Although they all experienced the same delay before intervention due to chemotherapy, survival is still significantly much better for responders. But as some operated patients reach remission after an additional radiotherapeutic treatment, we still compare patients that were considered in remission after surgery alone. Half of the responders received an adjuvant chemotherapy with 3 more courses of 5FU-Cisplatin ; half of non-responders were irradiated. In spite of this, survival curves are still significantly different, much better for responders to neo-adjuvant chemotherapy (Fig. 10).

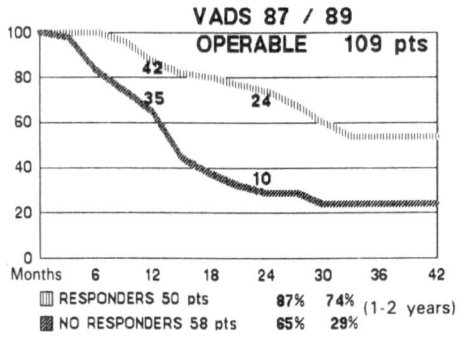

Fig. 9.

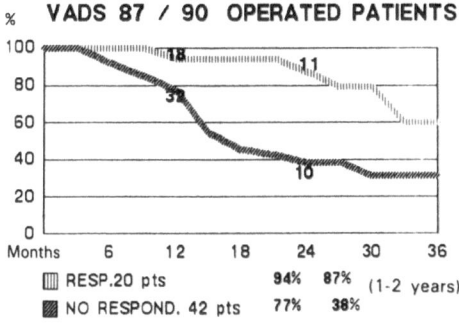

Fig. 10.

Conclusion

As a conclusion we may return to the evaluation of a response to chemotherapy and of its pronostic value. First, we may clearly distinguish between oral and other head and neck cancers. But, just as important, the estimation of a major response after 50 % decrease of the tumoral size proves us too optimistic and will lead in three directions :

— to get a better evaluation of the clinical response : but there are time, cost and patient confort restraints that limit the possible investigations ;

— to adopt one more step would be a pragmatic attitude, for instance 80 or 90 % very near to complete remission ;

— finally, to do the maximum to reach the complete remission which only can predict a good prognosis. That means increase quality, quantity and lasting of neo-adjuvant or possibly adjuvant chemotherapy.

Reference

1. Szpirglas H, Marneur M, Lacoste JP, Nizri D (1986) Chimiothérapie néo-adjuvante des cancers avancés de la cavité buccale et de l'oro-pharynx chez 208 patients. Colloque INSERM/John Libbey Eurotext Ltd, vol. 137, pp 437-445

Abstract. The disappointing result of a randomized trial for neo-adjuvant chemotherapy before radiotherapy with patients presenting an oral or oro-pharyngeal tumor (classified T3/T4) led us to start on a different trial, stratifying the recruitment of these tumors according to their apparent resectability (109 patients vs 55 non-resectable), on the only criterium of loco-regional extension. The elected protocol associated 5FU and Cisplatin on conditions widely adopted for head and neck cancers, and proposed three courses before curative treatment, radiotherapeutic or surgical. The major responses rate was very different for the tow groups, 25 % for non-resectable tumors patients versus 50 % for resectable ones. In all cases, the response to chemotherapy was predictive of the immediate therapeutic result. For non-resectable patients, 7 out of 13 responders (58 %) achieved remission versus 6 out of 42 non-responders (14 %). Among resectable patients, 69 % of responders achieved remission versus 34 % of non-responders. However, we observed the same relapse rate for patients in remission : 15 out of 33 for responders and 8 out 18 for non-responders. According to long term survival, only 1 or 2 % of non operable patients have a chance to be alive after four years, though the survival curves fall down from 50 % for operated responders to 30 % for operated non responders.

Induction chemotherapy with Cisplatin and 5-FU for squamous cell carcinoma of the head and neck. Six years experience at the Nice Cancer Center

M Schneider, F Demard, P Chauvel, A Thyss, MH Gaspard, J Santini, J Vallicioni, O Dassonville, C Caldani

The efficacy of Cisplatin-5-FU combination has been widely demonstrated in induction chemotherapy of head and neck cancers [1, 2]. We have confirmed these results a few years ago [3-5]. After a 6 years experience, the objective of this study is to evaluate the overall results and the impact of neo-adjauvant chemotherapy on disease free interval and survival in head and neck cancer patients.

Material and methods

The present data concern 406 patients (345 men, 61 women) treated at the Centre Antoine-Lacassagne from september 1983 to september 1989. Mean age was 61 (25-82). All patients had histologically confirmed squamous cell carcinoma of the head and neck. None had been treated previously or had metastatic disease.

The sites of primary tumors were as follows = 82 oral cavity (20 %), 162 oropharynx (40 %), 90 larynx (22 %), 52 hypopharynx (13 %), 10 rhinopharynx (2.5 %) and 10 facial sinuses (2.5 %).

Table 1 list patients by TNM criteria.The distribution by UICC criteria was as follows = 7 stage I (1.7 %), 74 stage II (18.6 %), 160 stage III (40.8 %), 145 stage IV (38.9 %). 79.7 % of the patients were stage III or IV.

Table 1. Patients distribution by tumor size and node involvement

	N0	N1	N2a	N2b	N2c	N3	Total
T1	7	4	2	8	2	2	25
T2	75	31	5	5	6	5	127
T3	76	54	8	16	25	13	192
T4	16	12	6	8	7	7	56
Tx	2	2	0	0	0	2	6
Total	176	103	21	37	40	29	406
	43.3 %	25.4 %	5.2 %	9.1 %	9.9 %	7.1 %	
				24.2 %			

Centre Antoine-Lacassagne, Nice, France

Chemotherapy protocol

A central venous catheter was first inserted for all patients. Treatment consisted of continuous infusion of Cisplatin : 100 mg/m^2 on day 1, followed by 5-FU 1,000 mg/m^2 from day 2 to day 6. The protocol called for 3 courses per patient. The interval between cycles was 15 days.

Drug doses were reduced 10 % for every 5 years over 70 years of age. At half cycle, the 5-FU dosage was adapted according to the half cycle AUC. Between 15,000 to 30,000 ng/ml/hr, the 5-FU dose was reduced from 70 % to 0.

Before treatment, lesions biopsies were sampled during endoscopy, under general anesthesia. Response was assessed by multiple biopsies obtained under identical conditions 10 days after the last chemotherapy course.

After completion of the induction chemotherapy, patients were given loco-regional treatment : either uni or bilateral surgical resection, sometimes completed by irradiation (65 to 75 grays) or radiotherapy alone (65 to 75 grays) to the tumor bed and 55 to 65 grays to nodal areas or, in some cases, with added nodal dissection.

Results

Response could be evaluated for 367 patients. As shown by Table 2, an objective response was obtained in 80 % of the patients. There were 44.5 % of clinical complete response (CR), 35.5 % of partial response (PR) and 20 % non response (NR). Analysis of response as a function of tumor size revealed that a CR was achieved for 77.2 % of T1, 59.3 % of T2, 37.4 % of T3 and 15.5 % of T4. Good results were obtained in all anatomic sites but the percentage of CR was particularly high for patients with lesions of the hypopharynx (59 %) ; the results seem poor for rhinopharynx but there were only 10 patients.

Table 2. Results on the primary tumors

	CCR	PR	NR
Overall response	44.5 %	35.5 %	20 %
Oral Cavity	45.8 %	33.4 %	16.8 %
Oropharynx	43.4 %	36.2 %	20.4 %
Larynx	40 %	37.4 %	22.6 %
Hypopharynx	59 %	29.5 %	11.5 %
Rhinopharynx	22.2 %	44.4 %	33.4 %
Facial Sinuses	37.5 %	50 %	12.5 %

As it is often the case, the quality of clinical response was not as good as for primary tumors. Even so, the overall response rate is high, including 27 % of CR, from 40 % for N1 to 12 % for N3.

Local control after completion of the treatment

After induction chemotherapy, 14.4 % of the patients were treated locally by surgery alone, 23.8 % by surgery followed by radiotherapy, 57.3 % by radio-therapy alone and 4.4 % by radiotherapy and node dissection.

Local control was obtained in 84.2 % of the patients after completion of the treatment (Table 3).

Table 3. Local treatment after chemotherapy

Radiotherapy	57.3 %
ND + Radiotherapy	4.4 %
Surgery + Radiotherapy	23.8 %
Surgery	14.4 %
Local control after completion of the treatment	84.2 %

Evaluation of the histologic response

One hundred and twenty six patients underwent surgery immediately after induction chemotherapy. Histologic examination revealed complete sterilization of the surgical specimen in only 7/17 patients who had been clinically classed CR but also in 9/66 patients classed PR and also in 4/43 patients who had been classed NR.

Toxicity (Table 4)

Table 4. Cisplatin - 5 Fu toxicity (1050 Cycles)

Toxicity	WHO Grade III-IV
Hematological	2.2 %
Mucositis/Diarroea	6.6 %
Venous	0.8 %
Coronary spasm in 11 patients ; 9 deaths attributable to chemotherapy	

Most of the patients experienced asthenia, nausea and vomiting. Severe venous damage has almost entirely been eliminated since a central catheter has been inserted on a routine basis. Toxicity was evaluable for 1,050 cycles. Hemato-logical toxicity (W.H.O. grade III-IV) was observed in only 2.2 % of the cycles, severe gut toxicity in 6.6 % of the cycles, and coronary spasm in 11 patients [6].

Nine deaths were attributable to chemotherapy but most of these patients had significant medical complications : alcoholic cirrhosis, myocardial infarc-tion, severe arteriosclerosis. At this time, the toxic manifestations of this treat-ment have been considerably reduced thanks to pharmacokinetic monitoring of the 5-FU-AUC on day 3 which can predict and thereby allows prevention of severe toxicity by reduction of drug dose [7].

Disease free interval and survival

At 1, 2, 3 and 5 years, the tumoral relapse rate is respectively 15 %, 24 %, 30 %, 35 %. The lymph node relapse rate is 13 %, 17 %, 19 %, 21 % ; the distant metastasis rate is 13 %, 18 %, 19 %, 53 %. A second cancer was observed at 5 years in 25 % of the patients.

The overall survival of the patients at 1, 2, 3 and 5 years is respectively 75 %, 59 %, 53 %, 42 %. Figure 1 reveals that there is a significant difference in survival in favour of patient who achieved a CR as opposed to partial and non responders. The 5 years overall survival is different according to the site of primary tumor = 60 % for larynx, 45 % for oropharynx, 32 % for oral cavity and 20 % for hypopharynx.

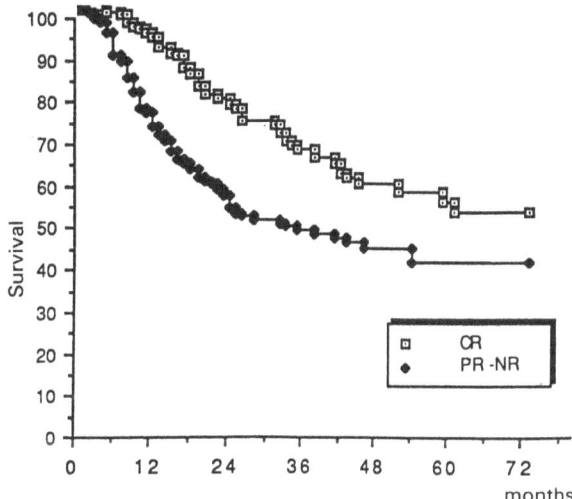

Fig. 1. Survival/Response

Conclusion

Our results confirm that 3 courses of Cisplatin-5-FU constitute one of the best induction chemotherapy regimens for head and neck cancers, but the long term results are not significantly better than those of patients treated only with locoregional treatment : surgery and/or radiotherapy. This combination chemotherapy is highly effective, improves the local control rate and allows reduction of the need for certain major surgical procedures in favor of radiotherapy, especially in primary tumors of larynx and hypopharynx were irradiation can be utilised in about 60 % of the cases, which often permits the organ conservation.

This advantage in patient comfort and functional results is very important, but when comparing with our numerous historical controls and the randomized studies in the recent litterature [8], we think there is not yet a significant improvement in whole survival and disease free survival for head and neck cancer patients treated by neo adjuvant chemotherapy.

New strategies and new control trials are thus justified and warrant immediate attention.

References

1. Al Sarraf M, Amer MH, Vaishaupayong et al (1979) A multi modality therapeutic approach for advanced previously untreated epidermoid cancer of the head and neck. Preliminary Report. Int J Radiat Oncol Biol Phys 5 : 1421-1423
2. Kish J, Drelichman A, Jacobs JR et al (1982) Clinical trial of cisplatinum and 5-Fluorouracil infusions as initial treatment for advanced squamous carcinoma of the head and neck. Cancer Treat Rep 66 : 471-474
3. Thyss A, Schneider M, Santini J, Caldani C, Vallicioni J, Chauvel P, Demard F (1986) Induction chemotherapy with cisplatinum and 5-Fluorouracil for squamous cell carcinoma of the head and neck. Br J Cancer 54 : 755-760
4. Demard F, Schneider F, Chauvel P, Ramaioli A, Vallicioni J, Santini J (1987) Chimiothérapie d'induction platine 5-Fluorouracile. Résultats actuels en cancérologie cervico faciale. Ann Oto Laryng 104 : 399-406
5. Demard F, Schneider M, Thyss A, Chauvel P, Vallicioni J, Santini J and Caldani C (1988) neo-adjuvant chemotherapy. In : Jacquillat C (ed) John Libbey Eurotext, vol. 169, pp 321-325
6. Thyss A, Falewee MN, Leborgne L, Viens P, Schneider M, Demard F (1987) Cardiotoxicité du 5-Fluorouracile. Spasme ou toxicité myocardique directe. Bull Cancer 74 : 381-385
7. Milano G, Santini J, Thyss A, Renee N, Viens P, Chauvel P, Schneider M, Demard F (1989) Optimisation par la pharmacocinétique de l'index thérapeutique du traitement CDDP-5-FU cinq jours continus. Bull Cancer 76 : 905-8
8. Shirinian MH, Zatopek NK, Lippman SM, Dimery IW and Hong WK (1990) Adjuvant therapy in head and neck cancer. In : Salmon S (ed), Philadelphia, pp 53-59

Abstract. From sept. 83 to sept. 89, 406 patients with advanced squamous cell carcinoma of the head and neck were given 3 courses of chemotherapy (Cisplatin 100 mg/m² D1 and 5-FU 1,000 mg/m² D2-D6), before any local treatment. The toxicity of this protocol was acceptable. An objective response was obtained in 80 % of primary tumors (44.5 % CR and 35.5 % PR) 27 % of CR were obtained for nodal metastasis. After induction chemotherapy, 38.2 % of the patients were treated locally by surgery alone or plus radiotherapy, and 61.7 % by radiotherapy alone or plus node dissection. Local control was obtained in 84.2 % of the patients after completion of the treatment.

At 5 years, the local recurrence rate is 35 % the distant metastasis rate is 21 %, the second cancer rate is 25 % and the patients overall survival is 42 % and is significantly longer for CR as compared to PR and NR.

Neo-Adjuvant chemotherapy for organ preservation with high dose continuous infusion of Cisplatin, 5-Fluorouracil, and Mitoguazone for head and neck cancer : a preliminary report

S Urba*, A Forastiere, G Wolf, A Thornton

Traditionally, patients with locally advanced head and neck cancer have been treated with surgery and/or radiation therapy. Recently, neo-adjuvant chemotherapy has been used in an effort to preserve organ function. We conducted a study designed to test an intensive regimen of induction chemotherapy/radiation therapy in patients with newly diagnosed disease, with feasability of organ preservation as an endpoint.

Materials and methods

Over a period of 32 months, 43 patients with advanced, resectable head and neck cancer were evaluated in the departments of otolaryngology, medical oncology, and radiation therapy at the University of Michigan, and were enrolled in a protocol of induction chemotherapy. The chemotherapy consisted of Mitoguazone (400-500 mg/m²) on days 1 and 8, Cisplatin (25-30 mg/m²/day) continuous IV infusion on days 8-12, and 5-Fluorouracil (800-1,000 mg/m²/day) continuous infusion on days 8-12. Mitoguazone was included in the regimen because of its moderate activity against head and neck cancer, as well as its reported ability to allow Ehrlich ascites tumor cells and HELA cells to accumulate in S and G2 phase. By administering the drug 7 days prior to Cisplatin and 5-FU, it was considered theoretically possible to exploit Mitoguazone's ability to synchronize cells for potentially greater tumor cell kill. Three cycles of chemotherapy were given at 28 day intervals. At the end of the third cycle, patients underwent full tumor evaluation. Those who had experienced a complete response or whose tumor had been downstaged to T1N1 went on to receive radiation therapy only. Five daily fractions per week of 180 cGy were administered, to a total dose of 6,600-7,380, depending on the extent of neck disease. Those patients whose tumor was more extensive than T1N1 at the end of all chemotherapy went on to immediate salvage surgery.

Results and survival

Forty-three patients were enrolled. 58 % had Stage IV disease, 35 % Stage III, and 7 % Stage II (piriform sinus). Sites of disease included oral cavity-14 %,

University of Michigan, Division of Oncology 1500 E. Medical Center Drive, Ann Arbor, Michigan 48109, USA
* Susan Urba, MD University of Michigan, Division of Oncology, Ann Arbor, Michigan, USA

pharynx-63 %, larynx-19 %, and sinuses-4 %. All patients had squamous cell carcinoma except one, who had adenocarcinoma of the maxillary sinus. Thirty-seven patients are evaluable for response to chemotherapy ; 4 patients died after 1 cycle of treatment before tumor could be evaluated, 1 patient was lost to follow-up, and 1 patient with metastatic disease was removed from protocol when it was discovered he had been enrolled erroneously. The response to chemotherapy was complete in 46 %, partial in 40 %, stable disease in 3 %, and progression in 11 %. 19/37 (51 %) of patients were spared all surgery, and 79 % of these remain disease-free. In addition, 7 patients (19 %) had a neck dissection only for residual disease, and were spared surgery to the primary site. Only 28 % of these patients remain disease-free, indicating that residual nodal disease implies a worse prognosis. The primary tumor sites of patients spared surgery include oral cavity, pharynx, larynx, and sinuses. Forty-two patients were evaluable for survival. At median follow-up of 21 months, the median survival is 26 months, and 60 % of all patients are still alive.

Toxicity

All 43 patients were checked for toxicity. Fifty-three percent of them received 3 cycles of chemotherapy, 21 % received 2 cycles, and 26 % tolerated only 1 cycle. There were 4 deaths after 1 cycle of treatment : 2 were due to sepsis, 1 was due to a probable pulmonary embolus, and 1 was due to tracheal bleeding (platelet count was normal at the time). Grade 3-4 granulocytopenia was experienced by 65 % of patients, grade 3-4 thrombocytopenia by 30 % of patients, and 11 % of patients had to be removed from the study because of renal toxicity.

Discussion and conclusions

The complete response rate of this chemotherapy regimen was promising, but the toxicity was substantial. The survival data were not significantly different from the estimated 2-year survival of 50 % attained by a historical control group of 152 patients from our institution with Stage III/IV cancer treated with surgery and radiation. Our data suggest that it is possible to achieve organ preservation at a variety of sites of head and neck cancer, but we emphasize that this must be investigated more intensively in a prospective, randomized trial, designed to evaluate induction chemotherapy versus surgery/radiation, in particular sites and stages of head and neck cancer.

Significance of tumour site in assessing survival benefit of Neo-Adjuvant chemotherapy in advanced head and neck cancer : a lack of survival advantage in patients with oral cavity tumours despite achieving a high clinical complete remission rate after local therapy

BT Hill* and LA Price

The role of chemotherapy in the multidisciplinary treatment of advanced head and neck cancer remains to be defined. Results from uncontrolled adjuvant studies integrating chemotherapy with local therapies have indicated that high response rates to initial chemotherapy and high complete remission rates are achievable, as reviewed recently [1]. Both of these factors appear to predict for improved survival. Data from our large series of 208 patients revealed that primary tumour site is a significant predictive factor for response to treatment and survival [2]. Subset analyses of 50 patients with oral cavity tumours, however, indicate that all patients responding to initial Schedule A chemotherapy and/or achieving a final complete remission after local therapy do not automatically have improved survival.

Patients and methods

Fifty patients with advanced, histologically-proven previously untreated epidermoid carcinoma of the oral cavity were eligible for these retrospective analyses. Thirty-five patients were male and 15 female. The age range was 27-80 years (median 60). Ten patients had stage IV and 27 stage III disease. The 13 patients with stage II tumours (T2N0) were considered « bad risk » because of extension to an adjacent site or involvement of two sites. The study design involved patients receiving 2 courses of Price-Hill Schedule A as initial treatment on days 1 and 14. Details of the protocol containing Vincristine, 5-Fluorouracil, Methotrexate and Bleomycin, given over 24 hours, with Hydrocortisone followed by a Folinic acid rescue have been published [2]. On day 28, patients were assessed for chemotherapy response and « curative » local treatment was initiated. Thirty-three percent of patients had radiotherapy only (total dose of 65 Gy) as detailed earlier [3]. Thirty-one percent of patients had similar radiotherapy to a total dose of only 40 Gy and then went on to surgery, whilst 16 % had surgery only and the remaining 20 % had surgery followed by post-operative radiotherapy. Five patients failed to complete local therapy. Standard definitions of response and statistical analyses were used [2].

* Imperial Cancer Research Fund Laboratories, London WC2A 3PX and 111 Harley Street, London WC1N 1DG, UK

Results

Forty patients (80 %) responded (at least a partial response) to two courses of initial Schedule A chemotherapy. By logistic regression analyses, none of the following factors affected significantly the response to initial chemotherapy ; stage, N status, T classification, sex, age or histologic grade. Provided the standard medical precautions were always observed, the toxicity associated with Schedule A chemotherapy was minimal. Sixty-six percent of patients had no side affects at all. In the remaining 10 patients there were 2 incidences of mucositis, 7 of nausea and vomiting and 6 of partial alopecia. These symptoms were all described as mild. There were no treatment-related deaths and patient compliance to Schedule A chemotherapy was 100 %.

After local therapy, the final complete remission rate was 76 %. By logistic regression analyses, none of the factors analysed, including the type of local therapy used, significantly affected this rate. Furthermore, the final complete remission rate for chemotherapy responders was not significantly higher than that achieved by chemotherapy non-responders (p = 0.22).

Median survival was 21 months for all patients, 22 months for chemotherapy responders and 30 months for patients achieving a final complete remission. These figures are significantly lower than those obtained analysing the whole series of 208 patients, where all patients had a median survival figure of 30 months, all chemotherapy responders 40 months and those achieving a final complete remission 71 months (Fig. 1).

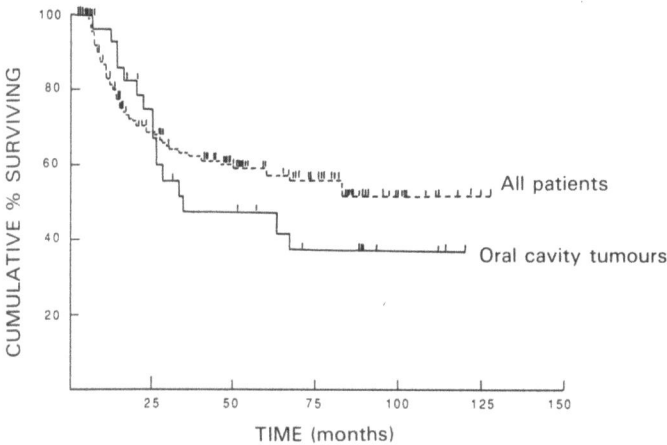

Fig. 1. Actuarial survival analyses for the overall group of 208 patients [2] versus the subgroup with oral cavity tumours

Discussion and conclusion

These data provide evidence of a lack of survival advantage in patients with oral cavity tumours treated with Schedule A chemotherapy prior to definitive local therapy, despite their high clinical complete remission rate. This result highlights the fact that achievement of a complete remission does not automatically result in a durable survial period and emphasizes the need for randomised trials, with sufficient patient numbers, to identify optimal strategies in tumours at specific sites within the head and neck region.

References

1. Hill BT, Price LA (1990) The role of adjuvant chemotherapy in the treatment of advanced head and neck cancer. Acta Oncol 29 : 695-703
2. Hill BT, Price LA, Mac Rae K (1986) Importance of primary site in assessing chemotherapy response and 7-year survival data in advanced squamous-cell carcinoma of the head and neck treated with initial combination chemotherapy without cisplatin. J Clin Oncol 4 : 1340-1347
3. Price LA, MacRae K, Hill BT (1983) Integration of safe initial combination chemotherapy (without cisplatin) with a high response rate and local therapy for untreated stage III and IV epidermoid cancer of the head and neck : 5-year data. Cancer Treat Rep 67 : 535-539

Abstract. Multivariate analysis of 208 patients with advanced previously untreated epidermoid cancers of the head and neck, receiving Price-Hill Schedule A neo-adjuvant chemotherapy, revealed significant survival differences for patients with tumours at specific sites. Patients with oral cavity lesions, despite achieving a high clinical complete remission rate after local therapy, had significantly lower survival figures (p = 0.0014) than those with carcinoma of the larynx, nasopharynx and oropharynx.

Preservation of the larynx following Neo-Adjuvant chemotherapy. A preliminary report

O Laccourreye, V Bassot, M Menard, D Brasnu, H Laccourreye

Local treatment in case of squamous cell carcinoma of the larynx frequently leads to a total laryngectomy. This preliminary report suggests that neo-adjuvant chemotherapy may allow for preservation of the larynx in selected cases.

Materials and methods

Two hundred and seventy-seven patients presenting with a squamous cell carcinoma of the larynx were treated at our institution utilizing a preoperative chemotherapy regimen from 1980 through 1988 (Table 1). Staging was performed according to the 1987 UICC. Staging System (Table 2). Following chemotherapy, either a partial laryngectomy (128 patients) or a total laryngectomy (149 patients) was initially planned. Table 3 presents local treatment modifications following neo-adjuvant chemotherapy. The initially planned local treatment was modified in 27.8 % (77/277) of cases. Patients were followed up at least 3 years or until death occurred. Twenty patients were lost to follow up. Stastitical comparison was performed utilizing the Chi square test.

Table 1. UICC Staging system 277 patients

	N0	N1	N2	N3
T1	16	2	1	2
T2	74	7	2	3
T3	87	19	14	5
T4	27	5	8	4

Results

Out of 277 patients, 6 (2.1 %) died related to chemotherapy complications. Modification of the initially planned treatment was statistically more due to happen if the patient was a female ; the tumor was staged as T3 or T4, the chemotherapy regimen performed was the regimen B, the clinical response to chemotherapy was over 50 % and the local surgery planned was a total laryngectomy. Survival in our series did not vary if the initial of surgical local treat-

Hôpital Laennec, Université Paris V, Paris, France

Table 2. Chemotherapy regimen performed : 277 patients

	Regimen A	Regimen B
PATIENTS (number)	103	174
PRODUCTS		
Cisplatin	bolus injection	continuous I.V
5 Fluorouracil	continuous I.V	continuous I.V
Bleomycin	bolus injection	—
POSOLOGY (mg/m²/day)		
Cisplatin	20	25
5 Fluorouracil	1 000	1 000
Bleomycin	15	—
COURSE (duration)	4 days	6 days
COURSES (number)		
< 3	9 (8.7 %)	4 (2.3 %)
3 to 5	93 (90.3 %)	152 (87.4 %)
> 5	1 (1 %)	18 (10.3 %)

Table 3. Local treatment initially planned versus local treatment performed following neo-adjuvant chemotherapy

■ : local treatment initially planned
□ : local treatment performed
LT : total laryngectomy
LP : partial laryngectomy
RT : radiotherapy
CH: exclusive chemotherapy

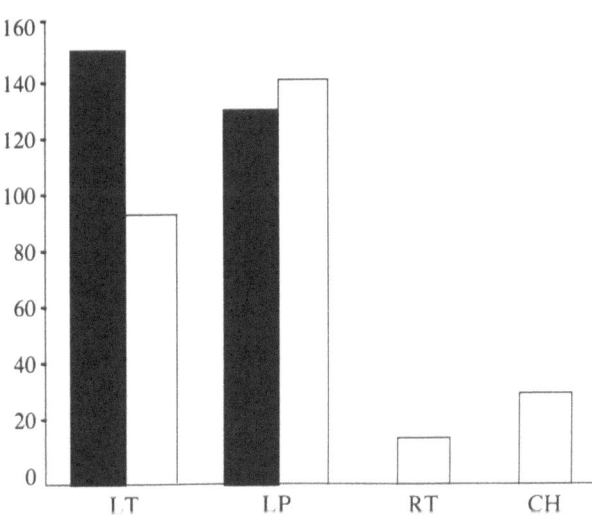

ment was performed or not. Out of 149 patients in whom a total laryngectomy was initially planned, 52 had their local treatment modified (23 partial laryngectomy, 14 laryngeal radiotherapy and 15 exclusive chemotherapy were performed). Local recurrence among those 52 patients was statistically less frequent if a partial laryngectomy was performed (Table 4) (Chi square test p = 0.0000). Overall preservation of the larynx was achieved in 26.4 % of patients (37/149) in whom a total laryngectomy was initially planned. Out of 128 patients in whom a partial laryngectomy was initially planned, 16 had their local treatment modified (2 total laryngectomy, 2 laryngeal radiotherapy and 12 exclusive chemotherapy were performed). Overall, 3.1 % of patients (4/128), in whom a partial laryngectomy was intially planned, had a total laryngectomy performed.

Table 4. Local Recurrence Rates, 52 patients

Local Treatment	Local Recurrence
Partial Laryngectomy	4.3 % (1/23)
Laryngeal Radiotherapy	57.2 % (8/14)
Exclusive Chemotherapy	46.7 % (7/15)

Discussion and conclusion

This preliminary report is the first presentation of a large series of patients with a laryngeal carcinoma in whom neo-adjuvant chemotherapy allowed for modification of the initially planned local surgical procedure. Our analysis underscores that preoperative chemotherapy allowed for preservation of the larynx in 26.4 % (37/149) of patients in whom a total laryngectomy was initially planned. Modification of the local treatment did not reduce survival in our series even though 2.1 % of patients (6/277) died from chemotherapy related complications. Once modification of the surgical procedure has been elicited, our report underscores that partial laryngectomy yields a statistically better local control rate (p = 0.0000) than does laryngeal radiotherapy or exclusive chemotherapy. Further prospective studies are under way at our institution in order to confirm such figures.

References

1. Brasnu D, Menard M, Fabre A, Bassot V, Janot F, Jacquillat C et Laccourreye H (1988) Cancers inopérables des voies aérodigestives supérieures. Intérêt de la chimiothérapie : 185 observations. Press Med 17 : 1067-1070
2. Brasnu D, Fabre A, Menard M, Bassot V, Janot F et Laccourreye H (1988) Analysis of Survival after Induction Chemotherapy in Pyriform Sinus Carcinoma. Head and neck Surg 10 : 396-401

3. Brasnu D, Laccourreye H (1990) Combination Therapy in T3 Supraglottic Cancer. Head and Neck Cancer. Decker BC Inc. Publishers 2 : 120-123
4. Demard F, Chauvel P, Santini J, Vallicioni A et coll (1990) Response to Chemotherapy as Justification for Modification of the Therapeutic Strategy for Pharyngolaryngeal Carcinomas. Head and Neck 12 : 225-231
5. Laccourreye H, Bonfils P, Brasnu D, Menard M et coll (1988) Chimiothérapie et Chirurgie Partielle dans les épithéliomas du Pharyngolarynx. Ann Otolaryngol Chir Cervico-fac 105 : 409-414

Abstract. Two hundred seventy-seven patients presenting with a well differentiated squamous cell carcinoma of the larynx were treated with preoperative Cisplatin and 5-Fluorouracil at our institution from 1980 through 1988. The initially planned laryngeal surgery was modified in 27.8 % (77/277) of cases following chemotherapy. This present report analyzed reasons for modification of surgery. Local control rates and survival are presented. Modifications of the initially planned local treatment allowed for preservation of the larynx in 24.8 % (37/149) of patients in whom a total laryngectomy was initially planned.

Selection of radiocurable head and neck cancers by Neo-Adjuvant chemotherapy response

JM Deneufbourg

In spite of advantages observed in treated patients over historical controls and notwithstanding increasing efficiency of protocols, the benefit of neo-adjuvant chemotherapy is still much discussed. Up to now, randomized trials have been unsuccessful to prove a better survival, and the results of recently performed meta-analysis are pessimistic.

Accumulating arguments support a role in optimization of treatment strategy, not only from the point of view of tumour control, but also of quality of life.

Patients

Two hundred and sixty-one patients (213 males and 48 females) were enrolled consecutively without any case selection e.g. for age 26 to 91, mean 61 (20 % > 70), for Karnofsky index (90 in 21 % of cases, 80 in 47 %, $\leqslant$ 70 in 32 %), for life expectancy and other criteria. They were all recently diagnosed and previously untreated. Most tumours were locally advanced (23 % stage III and 53 % stage IV). Predominant sites were oropharynx (92), larynx (59), oral cavity (54) and hypopharynx (39). Histology essentially consisted of squamous cell carcinoma (254) with various degrees of differentiation.

Neo-Adjuvant chemotherapy

One hundred and fifty-nine patients received Bleomycin (10 mg), Etoposide (100 mg) and Cisplatin (15 mg) given 6 times over a 3 weeks period (days 1, 3, 5 and 15, 17, 19). Fluorouracil (250 mg) has been added in 58 cases and Ifosfamide in 44 others with 3 additional injections (days 29, 31, 33). This out-patient treatment is administred in a 3 hours perfusion of 1 liter normal saline and does not require hyperhydration nor forced diuresis.

A significant response was obtained in 70 % of cases (11 % CR + 59 % PR). Primary tumours proved more sensitive than lymph nodes (80 % of response against 65 %). A major response, defined as a three quarters reduction of tumour, occured among 26 % of patients.

Owing to the low doses, side-effects were minimal : digestive intolerance (15 % grade 3), mild leukopenia (5 % grade 3 and 1 % grade 4), reversible alopecia (13 % grade 3). Compliance amounted to 99 % and dose intensity has been optimal (80-100) among 87 % of the patients.

Oncology-radiotherapy department, University hospital, B 4000 Sart Tilman, Liège, Belgium

Chemotherapy response and radiation effect

One hundred and eighty-one patients were treated by exclusive radiotherapy given to full dose (63 Grays equivalent-TDF 103) with unchanged tolerance. Chemotherapy response predicts radiation effect : 81 % of disease complete regression are obtained in chemotherapy responders as opposed to 37 % in chemotherapy non responders ($p < 0.0001$). The same discrepancy is observed for primary tumours (94 % and 52 % with $p < 0.0001$) as well as for nodes (64 % and 33 % with $p < 0.01$). The correlation is highly significant when the degree of chemotherapy response defined as major (76 % to 100 %), intermediate (51 % to 75 %) and minor (0 % to 50 %) is considered. A gradient of disease clearance by radiotherapy is observed for patients taken as a whole (94 % ; 69 % ; 37 % with $p < 0.001$), for tumours (100 % ; 91 % ; 52 % with $p < 0.001$) and also for nodes (84 % ; 53 % ; 33 % with $p < 0.01$).

The predictive value of chemotherapy is observed for the various stages of primary tumours. Major responders are all controlled whatever their stage (T1 = 14/14 ; T2 = 21/21 ; T3 = 24/24 ; T4 = 15/15).

Intermediate responders still show a good radiation effect but with a slight decrease with stage (T1 = 3/3 ; T2 = 23/24 ; T3 = 13/14 ; T4 = 20/24). Minor responders have less probability of control (T1 = 5/6 ; T2 = 5/8 ; T3 = 1/5 ; T4 = 6/14). Similar correlations are observed for nodes. Among major responders to chemotherapy, rates of radiotherapy complete regression are 100 % for N1, 71 % for N2 and 75 % for N3 (AJC classification). On the other side, N2 and N3 chemotherapy minor responders have only 10 % probability of control by radiotherapy alone.

Logistic discrimination analysis points out the prime importance of chemotherapy response for the prediction of radiation effect (chi square = 41. 67), the second selected parameter being node stage (chi square = 22. 98). Fifteen other possible prognostic factors were found redundant or meaningless. The prognostic index (PI) of control by irradiation equals 5.0606 − (1.5221 × chemoresponse) − (0.8416 × Najc) where « chemoresponse » varies from 1 to 3 (major to minor) and « Najc » varies from 0 to 3 (N0 to N3). The probability of radiocurability is given as the quotient exp (PI)/[1 + exp(PI)] ; calculation shows that it ranges from 97 % to 12 % according to the different situations of N stage and levels of chemosensitivity.

Disease early clearance and survival

For a population of 145 advanced cases (51 stage III and 94 stage IV), complete regression after radiotherapy (estimated within 1 month after treatment completion) appears as the prominent prognostic factor of survival in Cox model (chi square = 19.21). The only other significant parameter is Karnofsky index (chi square = 18.62).

Comparing well with the literature, survival after exclusive irradiation amounts, at 2 years, to 65 % (stage III), 47 % (stage IV) and 54 % (all advanced), at 3 years, to 58 % (stage III), 30 % (stage IV) and 42 % (all advanced).

The importance of disease clearance obtained after irradiation is illustrated by a significant different survival observed in advanced cases between complete and incomplete regressors ($p < 0.001$, log rank test) with a median survival time varying from 42 to 12 months.

The survival of 34 stage IV larynx cancers shows a similar pattern : 70 % of complete regressors survive at 3 years with larynx preservation while incomplete regressors are all dead ($p < 0.001$, log rank test). Results for the whole group are 58 % at 2 years and 47 % at 3 years.

Conclusion

In a serie of advanced cases treated by exclusive irradiation, early control of disease appears to be the prominent prognostic factor of survival. This control of primary tumours and nodes by radiotherapy is highly correlated to chemosensitivity. A logistic discrimination model can estimate the radiation effect according to the level of chemotherapy response, a complete response being not a prerequisite of radiocurability. Neo-adjuvant chemotherapy may be of value to select cases that might be cured by exclusive radiotherapy, therefore without undergoing mutilating surgery when the latter is not necessary.

Abstract. Low dose neo-adjuvant chemotherapy combining Bleomycin, Etoposide, Cisplatinum, Fluorouracil and Ifosfamide has been administred to 261 untreated patients with a 70 % rate of response. A 63 Grays irradiation has been subsequently delivered in 181 cases with unchanged tolerance. Logistic discrimination analysis shows that the prominent parameter of tumour control after radiotherapy is the degree of response to chemotherapy (81 % in chemoresponders as opposed to 37 % in non responders). A mathematical model gives the probability of disease clearance by irradiation alone. Neo-adjuvant chemotherapy may help to select cases curable without undergoing unnecessary mutilating surgery.

Neo-Adjuvant chemotherapy with Cisplatin and 5-Fluorouracil, both in continuous 96 hours perfusion, in the multidisciplinary treatment of locally advanced head and neck cancer

E Fonseca, JJ Cruz, A Gómez, P Sánchez, G Martin, P Santos, * A Nieto, ** A Muñoz

The introduction of induction chemotherapy in the treatment of locally advanced head and neck cancer with protocols based on Cisplatin has increased the number of patients in which complete control of the disease can be attained [1].

Among the most efficient protocols is that designed by Al-Sarraf with Cisplatin and 5-Fluorouracil perfusion over 96 hours [2]. The synergism between the two drugs when administered together in continuous perfusion has been confirmed [3]. In the present study we employed a Cisplatin and 5-FU protocol, both substances in continuous perfusion for 96 hours, in an attempt to increase the response rate.

Material and method

From April 1986 to December 1989, 79 patients with locally advanced carcinomas of the head and neck were treated with Cisplatin plus 5-FU as induction chemotherapy.

The mean age of the patients was 57 years. All of them had a Karnofsky index higher than 80 %. Seventy-four of them were males and five female. Histologically, 73 were epidermoid cancers and 5 were undifferentiated. According to the AJC classification, 19 were in stage III and 60 in stage IV. The initial locations of the lesions were as follows : hypopharynx 11 ; nasopharynx 10 ; larynx 31 ; oropharynx 9 ; oral cavity 14 ; paranasal sinuses 2 ; and multifocal 2.

The protocol consisted in the administration of Cisplatin at 25 mg/m²/day in 1,000 cc of physiologic saline serum and 5-FU at 1,000 mg/m²/day in 1,000 cc of glucosaline serum, both in continuous perfusion of 24 hours over 96 hours. The cycle was repeated every 21 days up to a total of 4 cycles.

After the chemotherapy, and according to the results obtained, the patients underwent surgery and/or radiation therapy. After each cycle, the response and degree of the toxicity were evaluated according to the criteria of the WHO.

Results

Of the 79 patients, 72 received 4 cycles of the treatment, 7 of them discontinuing treatment after the third cycle (3 due to progression of the disease and 4 due to toxic effects).

Service of Medical Oncology, * Radiotherapy, and ** ORL University Hospital of Salamanca, Spain

Thirty-nine CR (49 %) were achieved, of which 22 were histological (56 %), and 23 PR (29 %). The total of OR was 62 (78 %). The responses according to the location of the lesions, stage, and T and N can be seen in the Table 1. The CR after the third cycle comprised 30 % and after the fourth, 49 %.

Table 1. Response by characteristics of patients

	n°	CR %	CR + PR %
Location			
Hypopharynx	11	73	82
Nasopharynx	10	60	80
Larynx	31	45	74
Oropharynx	9	50	100
Oral cavity	14	35	70
Paranasal s	2	35	70
Multifocal	2	50	100
Stage			
III	19	63	84
IV	60	45	68
Tumor			
T1	3	66	66
T2	13	70	100
T3	22	45	76
T4	39	43	71
Nodes			
N0	18	55	66
N1	21	63	95
N2	29	41	75
N3	11	36	81
Courses			
1		5	56
2		13	77
3		30	81
4		49	79

With a maximum follow-up period of 44 months, the actuarial global survival is 50 %, remaining stabilized from 24 months. The survival of the patients with CR and PR is 70 % and 51 %, respectively, at 44 months. The patients with NR have a survival of 12 % at 24 months. These differences are statistically significant.

The toxicity in a total of 129 cycles was moderate, with the finding of 1 death due to toxicity after the fourth cycle, owing to sepsis. The most frequent side effects were nauseas and grade 1-2 vomiting, stomatitis and grade 1-2 leucopenia.

Conclusion

The protocol employed is efficient in the multidisciplinary treatment of locally advanced carcinoma of the head and neck. A high percentage of CR is attained with an important number of histological responses. The fourth cycle increases the number of CR. Survival at 44 months is high, those that achieved CR benefiting. Toxicity is low and unimportant.

References

1. Bernal AG, Cruz JJ, Sánchez P et al (1989) Four-day continuous infusion of Cis-platinum and 5-Fluorouracil in head and neck cancer. Cancer 63 : 1927-1930
2. Weaver A, Fleming S, Kish J et al (1982) Cisplatinum and 5-Fluorouracil as induction therapy for advanced head and neck cancer. Am J Surg 144 : 445-448
3. Forastiere AA, Belliveau JF, Goren MP et al (1988) Pharmacokinetic and toxicity evaluation of five day continuous infusion versus intermittent bolus of cis-diaminedichloroplatinum (II) in head and neck cancer patients. Cancer Res 48 : 3869-3874

Organ preservation in the treatment of hypopharyngeal squamous cell carcinoma. Preliminary results of a randomized trial

JL Lefebvre, L Adenis, D Chevalier*, B Castelain, J Ton van, J Stern, JJ Piquet*

Squamous cell carcinoma of the hypopharynx and lateral epilarynx (HLESCC) is a disease that is usualy diagnosed at a very advanced stage and, as a result, carries a very poor prognosis. In 1986 we initiated a prospective randomized trial to determine the effect of induction chemotherapy on local control, overall survival, and organ preservation in responders.

Previously, a chart review of 884 patients with HLESCC treated over a 10 year period at our center showed that only 40 % of patients were resectable at time of diagnosis ; and of these, 90 % must undergo total pharyngolaryngectomy (TPL) with radical neck dissection (RND) and post-operative radiotherapy (RT). Survival rates after this treatment were 84 % at one year, 45 % at 3 years, and 31 % at 5 years.

We tested the classical Cisplatinum-5-FU protocol (three cycles of Cisplatin 100 mg/m^2 on day one and 5-Fluorouracil 1,000 mg/m^2 on days 1 through 5) on 184 previously untreated patients with inoperable head and neck cancer. We obtained a complete response rate in 17 % of cases, and a partial response rate in 38 % of patients. Tumors that responded best to the protocol were HLESCCs : complete response in 21 %, and partial response in 53 % of cases.

Methods

Encouraged by the above mentioned preliminary results, we initiated the « HYPOMAR » trial ; a prospective randomized trial comparing induction chemotherapy to the standard surgical treatment for patients with advanced HLESCC.

Eligibility criteria : Operable but previously untreated patients with HLESCC free of distant metastases and of any other simultaneous cancers. Patients who could be cured by partial surgery or who required more extensive surgery such as circular total pharyngolaryngectomy were excluded.

Randomization was based on a thorough clinical work up and panendoscopy. The surgery arm consisted of TPL with post operative RT. The chemotherapy arm consisted of 3 cycles of Cisplatin/5-FU (as described above) followed by panendoscopy and work up to determine the response rate. Complete and « near complete » (80 % response with complete recovery of laryn-

Centre Oscar Lambret, BP 307, 59020 Lille, France and * Hôpital Claude Huriez, Place de Verdun, 59037 Lille, France

geal mobility) responders received a full course of external beam RT — all other patients were treated by salvage TPL, RND and post-operative RT. One hundred and thirteen patients were randomized, 56 in the surgical arm (AJC stage II : 5, stage III : 30, stage IV : 21) and 57 in the chemotherapy arm (stage II : 2, stage III : 35, stage IV : 20) with a similar distribution of primary sites in both groups.

Results

All patients in the surgical group underwent TPL, RND (with contralateral modified neck dissection in 3 cases), and post operative RT (59 g +/- 4 g) as planned, except for one patient who was found to have an unresectable neck mass during surgery, and one patient who refused surgery after randomization. All margins of resection were free of tumor, and there were no post operative complications or deaths. At the end of the trial, 54 patients could be evaluated in the surgery arm.

Out of the 57 patients randomized into the chemotherapy group, two refused treatment after randomization. Among the remaining 55 patients, 7 patients completed only one cycle of Cisplatin/5-FU, 11 completed two cycles, and 37 (65 %) completed all three cycles. There was a 25 % toxicity rate (14 cases, including 2 deaths) — cardiovascular : 5 (one death), general : 5 (one death during the ensuing RT), hematological : 3, and renal : 1. At the end of the trial, 44 patients could be evaluated. There were 15 complete responses of the primary, and 8 near complete responses (43 % combined). Ten patients had a 50 % response, and 9 patients had less than a 50 % response (one patient had progression of the primary, and one developed distant metastases). Response of the nodal disease was the following : 11 out of 38 patients with palpable neck nodes had a complete response (29 %), 4 had a 50 % response, 7 less than 50 %, 13 no change, and 2 had progression of their neck disease. Overall, 4 patients had progression of their disease (either at the primary, in the neck, or distant metastases) during chemotherapy.

Responders to chemotherapy (23 patients total) were given a full course of RT (61 g +/- 6 g). In addition, 8 patients (6 patients with a poor response to chemotherapy, one with severe toxicity, and one who refused chemotherapy), refused a salvage TPL. These patients were treated by RT. Twenty-three non-responders underwent salvage TPL, RND, and post operative RT. Of the 23 responders to chemotherapy, who as a result were spared a TPL, 13 are alive with no evidence of disease (NED) and a functional larynx, one is alive and NED after salvage TPL. Seven are dead — 1 of local evolution, 1 of neck evolution, 1 of distant metastases, 1 of intercurrent disease, and 3 from unknown causes.

Comparison of the two treatment arms

There were no deaths or complication in the surgery arm. In contrast, among patients randomized in the chemotherapy arm, there were 2 treatment deaths (1 during chemotherapy, and 1 during the ensuing RT).

Although there was no statitical difference in locoregional control between the 2 treatment arms, there was a greater number of distant metastases that developed in patients randomized to the surgery arm (18/56 vs 7/55).

The survival is significantly greater in the chemotherapy group : 67 % at two years, compared to the surgery group : 45 % at two years (p = .05).

Conclusion

We are encouraged by the results of this preliminary randomized trial comparing treatment of advanced HLESCC with chemotherapy to the standard treatment with radical surgery. Patients who show a good response to chemotherapy retain a functional larynx in 56 % of cases. In addition, patients treated with chemotherapy seem to develop distant metastases less frequently, than those treated by surgery and RT alone.

To confirm these findings, we look forward to the results of an international trial funded by the European Organization of Research and Treatment of Cancer (EORTC), head and neck group : « Is laryneal preservation with induction chemotherapy safe in the treatment of hypopharyngeal SCC ? a randomized phase III trial. » EORTC 24891, opened in March 1990.

Regional control after induction chemotherapy for advanced squamous cell carcinoma of the head and neck (SCCHN): a retrospective analysis of 303 patients

P Busse, J Clark, C Norris Jr, A Dreyfuss, C Beard, J Lucarini, J Andersen, D Miller, D Casey, E Frei III

Induction chemotherapy for squamous cell carcinomas of the head and neck has been the subject of a number of clinical trials with ambiguous results. Response data from phase II studies suggest a 20-40 % complete response rate which has lead to an association between chemotherapy and survival and an improvement in survival when compared to historical controls. Eight separate prospective randomized trials have been published to date. Although these have yet to show an improvement in survival, there are critical flaws in each, which limit their interpretation and leave the role of induction chemotherapy an open question [1].

Aside from the issue of overall survival, induction chemotherapy may have an impact on other therapeutic endpoints, i.e., the management of primary and regional disease. Can patients who achieve a complete response avoid surgery ? Does the magnitude of the clinical response to chemotherapy have any predictive value in the ability of patients to be effectively treated with radiation therapy ? This study addresses these questions with respect to the management of regional disease and relates an extensive experience at the Dana-Farber Head and Neck Tumor Clinic.

Materials and methods

Three hundred and three patients with Stage III-IV (American Joint Committee on Cancer) untreated advanced SCCHN were treated at the Dana-Farber Cancer Institute between 10/79 and 3/90. All patients were seen prior to study entry by a multidisciplinary team and were entered into one of four studies of induction combination chemotherapy (Table 1) followed by surgery and/or radiation therapy. All patients were required to have measurable (except one patient with a carcinoma of the middle ear), pathologically confirmed SCCHN, adequate bone marrow reserve, 24 hour creatinine clearance > 50 ml/min, and bilirubin < 2 mg/dl. Patients with multiple primary cancers of the head and neck and those with a prior history of cancer at any site other than skin epithelium were excluded.

During treatment, patients were evaluated monthly. At the end of induction chemotherapy, responses were quantified by clinical and radiographic examinations. Primary site and lymph node responses to chemotherapy were sco-

Dana-Farber Cancer Institute, Joint Center for Radiation Therapy, Harvard Medical School, Boston, MA 02215, USA

P Busse et al

Table 1. Chemotherapy Schedules

Protocol	80-016	83-084		84-119	87-005
Patients	114	104 (randomized phase II trial)		25	60
		52	52		
Regimen	PBM	PBM	PF	PFM	PFL
≠ Cycles	2	2-4	2-4	2-3	2-3
Cycle Length	28 days	28	28	28	28

P : Cisplatin, B : Bleomycin, M : Methotrexate, F : 5-fluorouracil, L : Leucovorin

red separately. A patient's overall response to chemotherapy was determined by the least-responding tumor site — primary or lymph node. Responses, either complete (CR), partial (PR), or none (NR), were defined by standard criteria [2]. Following treatment, patients were evaluated monthly for the first year and every two months thereafter.

Results

A regional response to chemotherapy was recorded in 171/226 (76 %) patients with at least N1 disease ; of these, 91 (40 %) patients were able to achieve a complete response. This correlated with N-stage (26/44 [59 %] with N1, 23/55 [42 %] with N2A, 19/46 [41 %] with N2B, 11/31 [31 %] with N2C, and 12/50 [24 %] with N3 lesions). Regional control of disease in the ipsilateral neck was determined in 281 evaluable patients after either surgery and radiotherapy or radiotherapy alone. At 3 years, the actuarial regional control rates were 83 %, 77 %, 70 %, and 47 % for N0, N1, N2, and N3 disease respectively. The likelihood of maintaining regional control was dependent upon the magnitude of the initial response : actuarial 3 year control ates were 88 % for patients who obtained a CR, 62 % for a PR, and 28 % for non responders. The ability of radiotherapy alone to control regional disease was examined and was found to depend strongly on the magnitude of the response to induction chemotherapy (Figs. 1, 2).

Discussion and conclusion

While the role of induction chemotherapy in improving the overall survival for head and neck cancer patients remains controversial, we feel there is a considerable impact with respect to regional disease control. It appears that a response to chemotherapy, in particular, is a strong biological marker for an improved clinical outcome. Of great interest is the finding that irrespective of the magnitude of regional disease at presentation, a complete response to

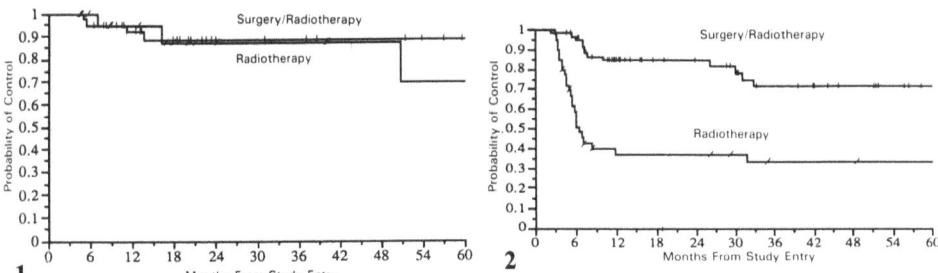

Fig. 1. Regional control of N_{2-3} disease after a complete response

Fig. 2. Ipsilateral regional control of N_{2-3} disease after a partial or non-response chemotherapy followed by radiation therapy achieves a regional control rate of approximately 90 %. This is in contrast to regional control rates of 33 % for patients with N2 and N3 disease, who achieved less than a complete response and were treated with radiation therapy. The anticipated regional control following radiation alone is 60-70 % for N2 and N3 disease [3].

References

1. Clark J, Dreyfuss A (1991) Cisplatin for squamous cell carcinoma of the head and neck. Semin Oncol : (in press)
2. Dreyfuss A, Clark J, Wright J, Norris C, Busse P, Lucarini J, Fallon B, Casey D, Anderson J, Klein R, Rosowsky A, Miller D, Frei III E (1990) Continuous infusion high-dose leucovorin with 5-Fluorouracil and cisplatin for untreated stage IV carcinoma of the head and neck. Ann Intern Med 112 (3) : 167-72
3. Million R, Cassisi N (1984) Management of head and neck cancer ; a multidisciplinary approach. Lipinscott, Philadelphia

Abstract. Between 10/1979 and 3/1990, 303 patients with advanced SCCHN (82 % Stage IV) received 2-4 cycles of Cisplatin-based induction chemotherapy prior to surgery and/or radiation therapy according to 1 of 4 defined treatment schedules. All patients are evaluable for response, local-regional control and survival with a median follow-up of 58 months. A response to induction therapy was recorded in 230 (76 %) patients including 104 (34 %) complete responses. Responses were quantified separately in both the primary site and neck. A regional response to chemotherapy was recorded in 171/226 (76 %) patients with > N1 disease. Achieving a complete regional response was correlated with N-stage (26/44 [59 %] with N1, 23/55 [42 %] with N2A, 19/46 [41 %] with N2B, 11/31 [31 %] with N2C, and 12/50 [24 %] with N3 lesions). Regional control of disease in the ipsilateral neck was determined in 281 evaluable patients, at 3 years, the actuarial regional control rates were 83 %, 77 %, 70 %, and 47 % for N0, N1, N2, and N3 disease respectively. The likelihood of maintaining regional control was dependent upon the magni-

tude of the initial response : actuarial 3 year control rates were 88 % for patients who obtained a CR, 62 % for a PR, and 28 % for non responders. In patients who obtained a CR, radiation therapy was as effective as surgery in controlling regional disease, irrespective of the initial N-stage. These data suggest that neck dissections be reserved for patients with regional disease of any degree that fails to completely respond to chemotherapy. In the setting of completely responding regional disease, neck dissections do not appear to enhance regional control over radiation alone.

Exclusive chemotherapy in head and neck cancer

V Bassot***, P Bonfils**, O Laccourreye*, E Chabardes*, M Menard*, D Brasnu*, D Khayat***, C Jacquillat***, H Laccourreye*, J Trotoux**

Over the past decade, with the important development of neo-adjuvant chemotherapy associating cisplatin and 5 FU (CF), a major change in the indication of chemotherapy in head and neck cancer has taken place. There is still an ongoing discussion regarding the results in term of survical. Despite these controversies, some facts appear to be obvious :
— prognosis is better for patients with complete clinical response (CCR) ;
— rate of CCR is better in small tumors (T1 - T2) than in large tumors (T3 - T4).
It is currently recognized that only patients with a good prognosis are responders to chemotherapy.
Consequently it is reasonable to state that the increasing rate of CCR with progress of chemotherapy efficiency would influence favorably head and neck cancer survival.
The locoregional treatment was therefore modified in CCR patients as follows :
— partial laryngeal surgery could be performed instead of initial radical surgery ;
— radiation therapy administered instead of radical surgery ;
— surgery for residual tumor after induction chemotherapy ;
— attempted prolongation of chemotherapy, in case of well defined conditions.
We report herein the preliminary results of Laennec and Boucicaut groups.

Patients and methods

Prolongation of chemotherapy was indicated in 75 patients with head and neck carcinomas.
When is it logical to pursue chemotherapy as initial treatment ? Well defined criterias are necessary :
— patients without palpable cervical nodes ;
— CRR must be achieved after 2 or 3 chemotherapy courses. In our experience, it is well demonstrated that no complete sterilisation occurred for CCR patients after 4 courses ;

* Department of Otolaryngology, Head and Neck Surgery, Laennec Hospital, 42, rue des Sèvres, 75007 Paris. France. ** Department of Otolaryngology, Head and Neck Surgery, Boucicaut Hospital, 78, rue de la Convention, 75015 Paris. *** Department of Medical Oncology, Salpétrière Hospital, 47, boulevard de l'Hôpital, 75013 Paris, France

— patients must accept the prolongation of chemotherapy for several months as well as a monthly follow-up for a minimum of two years.

Management of chemotherapy treatment

At present time CF is the most common association. We used two different protocols for inpatients and outpatients (Tables 1, 2).

Table 1. Inpatients protocol

CDDP	: 15 mg/m²/24 h (continuous perfusions) × 4 days.
5 FU	: 1 g/m²/24 h (continuous perfusions) × 4 days.

Table 2. Outpatients protocol

CDDP	: 15 mg/m²/24 h (continuous perfusions) × 6 days.
5 FU	: 750 g/m²/24 h (continuous perfusions) × 6 days.

Chemotherapy doses adjustement

Drugs doses must be adjusted for each course depending on biological and clinical side effects. Doses increase is progressive for patients with no side effects. If major side effects occur one must reconsider the therapeutic protocol.

Tumor regression analysis

Regression analysis must be done between each course in order to select CRR patients after 1, 2 or 3 courses and to stop chemotherapy in case of tumor evolution.

When to stop chemotherapy ?

Up to now, there is no argument to definite the optimal number of chemotherapy courses. Once the CRR is obtained, treatment efficacy on microscopic disease cannot be controlled.

Presently, we use to extend chemotherapy to 8 to 10 courses according to biological and clinical tolerance for patients with no clinical residual disease.

What are the risks of prolonged chemotherapy ?

In our experience, the main risks are mostly :

Local recurrence : delay for local recurrence is variable, as well during the treatment time, as after completion of chemotherapy. In our practice most local recurrences occur within the first year after chemotherapy completion. In case of local recurrence, surgical indication is decided in regard to the tumoral extention. In some cases, partial surgery or surgery of residual disease are performed, even if a radical surgery was initially indicated.

Chemotherapy side effects and morbidity : the side effects with the CF protocol are well known. The most important are :

— 5 FU cardiac toxicity : this complication is rare (1 - 3 %) and arise most often after the first or second courses. In some cases, death related to cardiotoxicity may occur (myocardial infarction) (2 %).

— Hematopoietic depression and subsequent infection may occur. But their frequency is rare with the CF protocol if a dose adjustment between each course is respected (2 %).

— Aggravation of associated disease such as arteritis or cardiac vascular disease.

— Renal and neurologic impairment are rare and have to be detected clinically and biologically.

— Metastatic cervical lymph node recurrence : for the last 10 years, neoadjuvant chemotherapy has clearly demonstrated a less effectiveness on cervical metastatic nodes as opposed to the tumoral site. Risk of nodal recurrence lay on a strict cervical control after chemotherapy completion. Surgical treatment of cervical nodes should be performed for CRR patients with clinical metastatic nodes at initial evaluation.

What are the benefits of exclusive chemotherapy ?

One of the most interesting benefit with exclusive chemotherapy is the lack of therapeutic complications, except in the case of definitive cardiac or neurological toxicity.

Local and cervical evaluation is easier after exclusive chemotherapy that after radiotherapy.

Local recurrence and second primary treatments are easier for patients not treated previously either by surgery or radiation therapy.

Results

Study of the department of Otolaryngology, head and neck surgery, Boucicaut Hospital.

Fourty-two patients were treated by prolonged chemotherapy. Classification is showned in Table 3.

Table 3. Patients classification

Oropharynx	10	T1	2	N0	30
Oral cavity	3	T2	14	N1	5
Hypopharynx	13	T3	14	N2	5
Larynx	11	T4	7	N3	2
Simultaneous	5				
Localisations					

Twenty patients were alive and locally controlled after exclusive chemotherapy (range 1-8 years, median : 26 months) (Table 4). Four patients with local recurrence were alive after surgical and radiotherapy treatment (range 1-4 years) (Table 5).

Table 4. Exclusive chemotherapy

Patients disease free : 20
Range : 1-8 years
Median : 26 months

Table 5. Exclusive chemotherapy

Patients disease free after recurrence : 4
Patients disease free after second localisation : 3

Three patients after surgical (2) or radiotherapy (1) treatments for second primary were alive (range 1 — 5 years) (Table 5).
Eight patients died (Table 6).
Two patients were lost for follow-up.
Five patients are still under treatment for metastatic disease (3) or recurrence (2).

Table 6. Exclusive chemotherapy

Causes of death. Nb : 8
4 intercurrent disease
2 local recurrence
1 second primary
1 myocardial infarction

For 53 patients an attempt of chemotherapy prolongation was decided. Classification is shown in Table 7.
Twenty-two patients were disease free (range 1 - 5 years) ; 15 were disease free after local recurrence treatment (Table 9) ; 11 dead patients (Table 8) ; local recurrence treatment failure : 5.

Table 7. Patients classification

Larynx	20	T1	6	N1	9
Hypopharynx	5	T2	8	N2	2
Oropharynx	12	T3	19	N3	4
Oral Cavity	1				
Simultaneous	7	T4	12	N0	29
Head and neck					
Cancer					

Table 8. Causes of death

Nb = 11
1 reccurrence
2 second primary
1 metastatic disease
2 septicemia
1 radiotherapy complications
1 cardiac toxicity (5 FU)

Table 9. Patients disease free after recurrence treatment

Nb = 15   range 2 – 4,5 years
5 surgical resection of residual tumor
5 surgical resection as planned at initial evaluation
1 surgical resection + radiotherapy
4 radiotherapy

Table 10. Recurrence treatment failure

Nb : 5
1 after surgery
1 after surgery + radiotherapy
3 after radiotherapy

Conclusion

For 95 patients an attempted chemotherapy prolongation was tried. Forty-two patients (44.2 %) were free of disease after exclusive chemotherapy (range 1 - 8 years). Twenty-two patients (23 %) were free of disease after recurrence (19) or second primary (3), 15 after surgical treatment, 1 after surgery and radiotherapy, 6 after radiotherapy. In most cases, disease free patients after chemotherapy were initially classified as T1T2 and N0 neck. Over all, disease free patients for the 95 cases are 67 %. For some patients, exclusive chemotherapy seems to be an interesting option. Further studies are needed to define patient selection for exclusive chemotherapy.

Neo-Adjuvant Cisplatin, 5-Fluorouracil and high-dose Leucovorin for advanced head and neck cancer : response, toxicity, survival and comparison with historical controls

J Clark, A Dreyfuss, C Norris Jr, P Busse, C Beard, J Lucarini, J Andersen, D Miller, D Casey, E Frei III

The role of neo-adjuvant chemotherapy for squamous cell carcinoma of the head and neck (SCCHN) remains controversial. While results from randomized trials of neo-adjuvant combination chemotherapy have confirmed the association between response and treatment outcome, an increase in survival has not been reported. Critical review of latter studies, however, reveals flaws which limit the value of their findings [1]. An improvement in the survival of patients who receive neo-adjuvant therapy for advanced SCCHN may not however be confirmed, until the rate of complete response is consistently over 50 %.

The objective of this report is to update published results [2] of a new neo-adjuvant regimen, infusion Cisplatin, 5-Fluorouracil (5-FU) and high-dose Leucovorin (PFL), which has been under phase II evaluation at the Dana-Farber since 1987, and to compare these results to those of an institutional control group.

Materials and methods

Between 7/87 and 3/90, 60 patients with untreated stage III-IV (M0) SCCHN received PFL (excluding T3N0 exophytic lesions of the tonsil or T1N1 tumors), followed by surgery or RT. Criteria for eligibility, staging and response as well as the specifics of PFL administration (Fig. 1) and dose-reduction have been published [2].

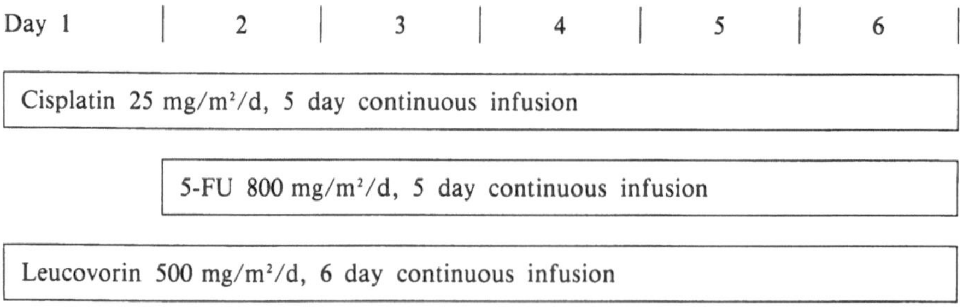

Day 1	2	3	4	5	6

Cisplatin 25 mg/m²/d, 5 day continuous infusion

5-FU 800 mg/m²/d, 5 day continuous infusion

Leucovorin 500 mg/m²/d, 6 day continuous infusion

Fig. 1. Dana-Farber Protocol 87-005 : PFL

Dana-Faber Cancer Inst., Harvard Medical School, Boston MA, USA

PFL was administered for a maximum of 3 cycles prior to surgery and/or RT. PFL was discontinued upon evidence of tumor progression or excessive toxicity, or after 2 cycles if response was less than partial.

Treatment outcomes after PFL were compared to those from three previous studies of Cisplatin-based therapy conducted at the Dana-Farber in 243 similar patients with advanced SCCHN (Table 1). Treatment failure was defined as : a) tumor progression, the end of local-regional treatment or death, whichever came first, for patients not rendered free of disease ; b) relapse for patients rendered free of disease ; and c) death that was treatment associated. Failure-free and overall survival were measured from treatment onset.

Table 1. PFL vs Historical Controls : Responses Rates

Protocol	80-016	83-084	84-119	Total controls	87-005
Chemotherapy [1]	PBM	PBM vs PF	PFM		PFL
Duration	2 m	2-4 m	2-3 m		2-3 m
Patients	114	104	25	243	60
Complete Response	29 %	26 %	40 %	28 %	62 %*
Total Response	86 %	68 %	88 %	75 %	80 %

[1] P = cisplatin, B = bleomycin, M = midcycle moderate-dose methotrexate with leucovorin rescue, F = 5-FU
* PFL was independently associated with a CR in a step-up, step-down multivariate analysis

Results

One hundred and sixty-three cycles of PFL were administered. A response to PFL was noted in 48/60 (80 %), including 37 (62 %) with 95 % C.I., 49 % to 74 % complete responses and 11 (18 %) partial responses prior to surgery or RT. Twelve patients did not respond to PFL including 1 who expired due to sudden death in the absence of associated toxicity on day 16 of the first cycle of therapy. The rate of CR to PFL is significantly higher ($p < 0.0001$) than that observed in the historical control group (Table 1).

Forty-three out of 59 (73 %) patients with evaluable primary site disease developed a CR at the primary. Of these, 38 (88 %) had pathologic evaluation of their primary site after PFL and among them 29/38 (76 %) had no evidence for residual disease upon rebiopsy prior to RT or surgical resection.

The principal toxicity of PFL is oral mucositis which was experienced by 97 % of patients during the first cycle (90 % moderate or severe). Diarrhea and rash were less frequent. These toxicities were controlled with dose-reductions of F and L which were required by 40 % of patients. Clinically important myelosuppression was unusual. A serum creatinine increase > 1.4 mg/dl prompted termination of PFL in one patient. The dose-intensity of PFL remained high for all patients (> 90 %) despite dose-reductions.

At the end of surgery and RT, 51/60 (85 %) patients were disease free in contrast to only 179/243 (74 %) of controls (p = 0.07). With a median follow up of 18 months for PFL patients and > 5 years for controls, overall and failure-free survival are increased after PFL (2 year overall est., 64 % vs 55 %, p = 0.05 ; 2 year failure est., 66 % vs 52 %, p = 0.09, Fig. 2).

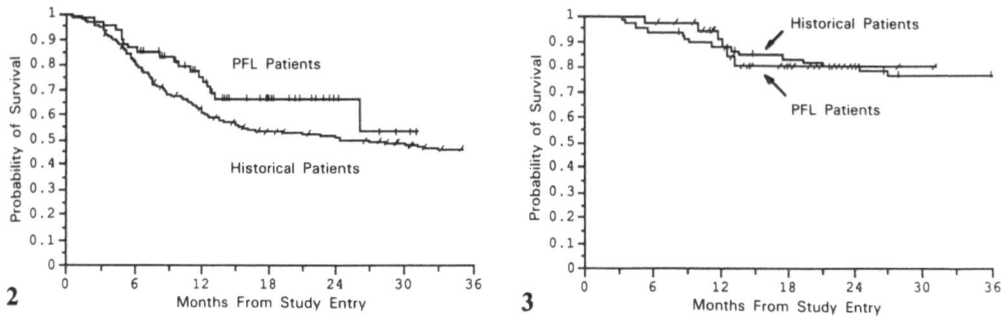

Fig. 2. Failure-free survival : PFL vs controls

Fig. 3. Failure-free survival after a CR to chemotherapy

Discussion and conclusion

These data indicate that PFL is a new and highly active regimen in patients with untreated SCCHN that warrants further study. Although associated with a significant degree of mucositis, PFL was tolerated by the majority of patients without a need for dose reduction. At this time, survival after PFL is increased compared with controls treated with previous Cisplatin-based neo-adjuvant therapy. With continued follow up a significant increase in survival should emerge given the increase in the rate of CR from 28 % to 62 % with PFL and the fact that survival after a CR is comparable between PFL patients and controls.

These data support the contention that highly active regimens of neo-adjuvant therapy impact favorably on the natural history of this disease. The potential for neo-adjuvant chemotherapy to improve the survival of patients with SCCHN remains sound.

Abstract. Cisplatin (P) with 5-Fluorouracil (F) is a synergistic regimen active against squamous cell carcinomas of the head and neck (SCCHN). Leucovorin (L) potentiates 5-FU cytotoxicity. We designed a new induction regimen, PFL (P 25 mg/m²/d, d1-5 ; F 800 mg/m²/d, d2-6 and L 500 mg/m²/d, d1-6) which is administered by continuous infusion every 28 days for 2-3 cycles prior to definitive surgery or radiotherapy (RT). As of 10/90, 60 patients with advanced

(M0) SCCHN (83 % Stage IV) completed 163 cycles of PFL and local-regional therapy. Clinical responses after PFL were recorded in 80 % : CR 62 % (95 % C.I., 49 % to 74 %) and PR 18 %. Forty-three of 59 (73 %) evaluable patients had a clinical CR at the primary site. Pathologic confirmation of a primary site CR was recorded in 29 of 38 (76 %) patients from whom tissue was available. Oral mucositis was common. Diarrhea and rash occurred less frequently. These toxicities were controlled with dose reductions of F and L. Clinically important myelosuppression was unusual. One death occurred during chemotherapy. Comparison of these results to those of 243 comparable patients treated with previous P-based therapies reveals increases in CR rate (62 % vs 28 %, p < 0.001) and increases in the percent of patients disease-free after surgery and RT (85 % vs 179/243, 74 %, p = 0.07). With a median follow up of 18 months for PFL patients, overall and failure-free survival are increased after PFL (2 year overall est., 64 % vs 55 %, p = 0.05 ; 2 year failure est., 66 % vs 52 %, p = 0.09). These data support the contention that highly active regimens of neo-adjuvant therapy impact favorably on the natural history of SCCHN.

References

1. Clark J, Dreyfuss A (1991) Cisplatin for squamous cell carcinoma of the head and neck. Semin Oncol (in press)
2. Dreyfuss A, Clark J, Wright J et al (1990) Continuous infusion high-dose leucovorin with 5-fluorouracil and cisplatin for untreated stage IV carcinoma of the head and neck. Ann Intern Med 112 (3) : 167-72

5-Fluorouracil modulation in head and neck cancer

EE Vokes*, WR Panje**, RR Weichselbaum***

We have attempted to increase the efficacy of available chemotherapy for head and neck cancer through modulation of 5-FU. We took the combination of Cisplatin and 5-Fluorouracil as our base, since it had proven activity and a moderate toxicity profile that might allow for modulation [1, 2]. Our goal was to identify a regimen that would have a higher degree of activity resulting in improved survival.

5-FU can be sequentially phosphorylated and incorporated into RNA as 5-FUTP. This pathway can be modulated by Methotrexate, which increases intracellular UTP-pools. Another pathway is its activation to 5-FdUMP which binds to the enzyme thymidylate synthase (TS), thus inhibiting the conversion of uridine to thymidine. In the presence of reduced folates, a stable ternary complex is formed, greatly increasing inhibition of TS. This pathway might also be modulated by the use of hydroxyurea (HU). HU is a ribonucleotide reductase inhibitor which depletes the cell of dUMP, the substrate competing with 5-FdUMP for binding to TS.

Our first trial focused on the addition of MTX to the combination of 100 mg/m^2/day of Cisplatin and a 5-day continuous infusion of 5-FU at 1,000 mg/m^2 (MPF) [3]. We scheduled MTX to be administered 24 h prior to the administration of Cisplatin and 30 h prior to beginning of the 5-FU infusion. The use of intermediate dose MTX (120 mg/m^2) necessitated leucovorin rescue at 25 mg/m^2 every 6 h for 6 doses given during days 1 and 2 of the 5-FU infusion. Leucovorin was not given with the intent of modulation.

Thirty-eight patients were entered on this trial. Three cycles of neo-adjuvant chemotherapy were followed by response evaluation and standard local therapy [4]. Nine patients had a CR (24 %), 21 a PR (55 %), and 2 patients (5 %) had a minor response for an overall response rate of 79 %. With a median follow-up of 39 months, the estimated median survival was 20 months. The toxicities of neo-adjuvant MPF consisted of mild to moderate myelosuppression and transient renal toxicity. Mucositis, however, was moderate to severe, with 82 % of patients having grade 2 or worse mucositis. As a result, the 5-FU dose had to be decreased to an average of 86 % of the intended dose in the neo-adjuvant setting. In the adjuvant setting, mucositis was further aggravated with a mean 5-FU dose of only 61 %. We subsequently treated 29 patients with 4 cycles of MPF as neo-adjuvant chemotherapy. The CR-rate to 4 cycles of neo-adjuvant MPF was 34 %, and 38 % had a PR (overall response rate 72 %). While this numerical CR-rate was higher than that seen with 3 cycles of neo-adjuvant MPF, the 95 % confidence intervals were overlapping

* Department of Medicine, Section of Hematology/Oncology, ** Department of Surgery and Otolaryngology, Head and Neck Surgery, *** Department of Radiation and Cellular Oncology, The University of Chicago, Chicago, IL, 60637, USA

and the CR-rate was unlikely to approach 50 %. A high incidence of moderate to severe mucositis was again seen. Given these response data and the high incidence of severe mucositis, we decided that modulation of 5-FU with methotrexate in this regimen had resulted in increased toxicity but no substantial increase in activity.

We also investigated the addition of leucovorin to the Cisplatin and 5-FU combination (PFL) [5-7]. Starting in 1985, we initially conducted a dose finding study in patients with recurrent and/or metastatic disease [5]. We identified 800 mg/m²/day of 5-FU as MTD with mucositis being the dose-limiting toxicity ; renal toxicity and myelosuppression were generally mild to moderate. Diarrhea was not a frequent or severe toxicity. Our recommended dose of LV was 50 mg/m² every 4 h. Eighteen patients were evaluable for response ; one had a pathological CR and 9 had a PR for an overall response rate of 56 %. The median response duration was 3 months. Four of 6 patients who had received prior cisplatin and 5-FU as neo-adjuvant chemotherapy responded in this trial.

Our next step was to study this combination in previously untreated patients. Since mucositis had been dose-limiting in previously irradiated patients (raising the possibility of « radiation recall »), we also wanted to study the feasibility of further dose escalation of 5-FU in this group of previously unirradiated patients. This trial involved patients with locally advanced head and neck cancer [6, 7] and aimed at intensifying local and systemic therapy by using both neo-adjuvant chemotherapy and concomitant chemoradiotherapy. Since the latter involved 6 to 8 cycles of chemotherapy administered during radiotherapy, we limited the number of cycles of neo-adjuvant chemotherapy to 2.

While we are waiting for longer follow-up before conducting a final analysis of this trial, we have analyzed response and toxicity following 2 cycles of neo-adjuvant PFL [6]. Of 31 patients treated with PFL, 9 had CR (29 %) and 17 a PR (55 %) for an overall response rate of 74 %. This CR-rate was similar to that previously achieved with 3 to 4 cycles of MPF. It was also similar to the 26 % CR rate reported by Dreyfuss et al following 2 cycles of a similar PFL regimen using continuous infusion Cisplatin and Leucovorin [8]. In their trial, the CR rate increased to 66 % with the addition of a third cycle. The addition of a third cycle had previously also been reported to increase the CR rate with Cisplatin and 5-FU [1].

The toxicities of PFL in previously untreated patients were similar to those observed in previously treated patients. Mucositis was again dose-limiting and necessitated a reduction of 5-FU on cycle 2 to ≤ 80 % in 22 of 29 patients. Thus, administration of 5-FU at 1,000 mg/m²/day with oral LV, as attempted in this trial, was feasible in only a small portion of previously untreated patients.

We consider the PFL regimen to be of high activity in head and neck cancer, based on our own data following 2 cycles of this regimen in the neo-adjuvant setting, and the additional increase in CR rate reported with the addition of a third cycle. We are, therefore, presently continuing its use as a base regimen for neo-adjuvant chemotherapy in head and neck cancer.

In another group of trials, we have studied the interaction of 5-FU, hydroxyurea and concomitant radiotherapy based on their single agent activity, the potential of both drugs to enhance radiotherapy, and the possibility of 5-FU modulation by HU [9-11]. The outcome of these trials is summarized by Haraf et al in this book.

Acknowledgements. We wish to thank Susan Jarman for the preparation of the manuscript and our many co-workers who have contributed to this work.

References

1. Rooney M, Kish J, Jacobs J et al (1985) Improved complete response rate and survival in advanced head and neck cancer after three-course induction therapy with 120-hour 5-FU infusion and cisplatin. Cancer 55 : 1123-1128
2. Vokes EE, Mick R, Lester EP, Panje WR, Weichselbaum RR (1991) Cisplatin and 5-Fluorouracil does not yield longterm benefit in locally advanced head and neck cancer : results from a single institution (in preparation)
3. Vokes EE, Moran WJ, Mick R, Weichselbaum RR, Panje WR (1989) neo-adjuvant and adjuvant methotrexate, cisplatin and fluorouracil in multimodal therapy of head and neck cancer. J Clin Oncol 7 : 838-845
4. Vokes EE, Panje WR, Mick R, Kozloff MF, Moran WJ, Sutton HG, Goldman MD, Tybor AG, and Weichselbaum RR (1990) A randomized study comparing two regimens of neo-adjuvant and adjuvant chemotherapy in multimodal therapy for locally advanced head and neck cancer. Cancer 66 : 206-213
5. Vokes EE, Choi KE, Schilsky RL, Moran WJ, Guarnieri CM, Weichselbaum RR, and Panje WR (1988) Cisplatin, fluorouracil, and high-dose leucovorin for recurrent or metastatic head and neck cancer. J Clin Oncol 6 : 618-626
6. Vokes EE, Schilsky RL, Weichselbaum RR, Panje WR (1990) Induction chemotherapy with cisplatin, fluorouracil, and high-dose leucovorin for locally advanced head and neck cancer : a clinical and pharmacologic analysis. J Clin Oncol 8 : 241-247
7. Vokes EE, Panje WR, Mick R, Haraf DJ, Moran WJ, McEvilly JM, Kozloff M, Weichselbaum (1990) neo-adjuvant chemotherapy surgery and concomitant chemoradiotherapy for locally advanced head and neck cancer. Proc ASCO 9 : 174
8. Dreyfuss AI, Clark JR, Wright JE, Norris CM, Jr, Busse PM, Lucarini JW, Fallon BG, Casey D, Andersen JW, Klein R, Rosowsky A, Miller D, Frei E, III (1990) Continuous infusion high-dose leucovorin with 5-Fluorouracil and cisplatin for untreated stage IV carcinoma of the head and neck. Annals of Internal Medicine 112 : 167-172
9. Vokes EE and Weichselbaum RR (1990) Concomitant chemoradiotherapy : rationale and clinical experience in patients with solid tumors. J Clin Oncol 8 : 911-934
10. Vokes EE, Panje WR, Schilsky RL, Mick R, Moran WJ, Awan AM, Goldman MD, Tybor AG, Weichselbaum RR (1989) Hydroxyurea, fluorouracil, and concomitant radiotherapy in poor-prognosis head and neck cancer : a phase I-II Study. J Clin Oncol 7 : 761-768
11. Haraf DJ, Vokes EE, Panje WR, Weichselbaum RR (1990) Survival and analysis of failure following hydroxyurea, 5-Fluorouracil and concomitant radiation therapy in poor prognosis head and neck cancer. Am J Clin Oncol (in press)

Abstract. 5-FU modulation has succeeded at increasing response and survival rates in patients with metastatic colorectal cancer. We have conducted a series of trials investigating modulation of the Cisplatin and 5-FU regimen with Methotrexate or Leucovorin in patients with head and neck cancer. In addition, we have studied the interaction of Hydroxyurea with 5-FU and concomitant radiotherapy (± Leucovorin). The combination of Cisplatin, 5-FU and Leucovorin (PFL) and 5-FU, Hydroxyurea and concomitant radiotherapy (FHX), in particular, looks promising and deserves further investigation.

Cisplatin, 5-Fluorouracil and high dose oral Leucovorin (PFL) with Methotrexate and Piritrexim as Neo-Adjuvant chemotherapy for head and neck cancer

EE Vokes, DJ Haraf, WR Panje, J-M McEvilly, MF Kozloff,
D Goldman, N Clendeninn, AG Tybor, M Collier, RR Weichselbaum

Studies in head and neck cancer at the University of Chicago have focused on the biochemical modulation of 5-Fluorouracil (5-FU). This has included the addition of high dose oral Leucovorin to the combination of Cisplatin and continuous infusion 5-FU (PFL). After establishing the pattern of toxicities, the recommended doses, and the efficacy of PFL in recurrent and/or metastatic disease [1], we treated patients with locally advanced disease with this PFL regimen and identified a high degree of activity [2, 3]. Piritrexim (PTX) is a MTX-analogue with single agent activity in head and neck cancer [4]. Since it is lipid soluble, it requires no active transportation and, therefore, may be able to overcome transport-related MTX resistance. In this phase II study, we added MTX and PTX to the PFL regimen (PFL-MP) hoping to further increase its activity.

Patients and methods

Patients had stage III or IV [5] squamous cell cancer of the head and neck or nasopharyngeal cancer. Patients were previously untreated and had a performance status of 0 to 2, normal end organ function, and signed informed consent. Chest X-ray and a CT or MRI scan of the head and neck were also obtained. The tumor plan called for 2 cycles of neo-adjuvant PFL-MP, followed by response evaluation and local therapy. This included surgery (for resectable disease) and/or radiotherapy with concomitant 5-FU and hydroxyurea [6, 7].

For PFL-MP, patients received Cisplatin, 100 mg/m^2 over 6 hours, followed by a 120 hour continuous infusion of 5-FU at 800 mg/m^2/day and Leucovorin administered orally at 100 mg every 4 hours from the start of Cisplatin until 24 hours after completion of 5-FU. MTX was administered on day 15 at 50 mg/m^2 and PTX on days 22 to 26 for 10 doses every 12 hours by mouth at 100 mg/m^2 with a cycle duration of 28 days. Response to PFL-MP was assessed clinically. Standard response criteria were used [2].

Departments of Medicine, Section of Hematology/Oncology, of Surgery, Section of Otolaryngology Head and Neck Surgery, of Radiation and Cellular Oncology. The University of Chicago Medical Center, Chicago, IL 60637 1470, USA and Burroughs Wellcome Co., Research Triangle Park, N.C., 27709, USA

All Correspondence to :
Everett E Vokes, MD, Assistant Professor of Medicine and Radiation Oncology, University of Chicago, 5841 S. Maryland Ave., Box 420, Chicago, IL 60637-1470

Results

Twenty-eight patients (19 male, 9 female) were treated. The median age was 57 years ranging from 30 to 77. Eight patients had a performance status of 0 and 10 patients had a performance status of 1 or 2. The sites of origin included the oropharynx or hypopharynx in 18 patients, and the supraglottic larynx in 4 patients ; only 1 patient had nasopharyngeal cancer.

Of 28 patients treated, 4 were unevaluable for response. Eleven patients (39 %) had a clinical CR. Nine patients (32 %) had a PR and 2 patients each had NR or PD.

All patients were evaluated for toxicity. Mucositis was dose-limiting as previously described for PFL, with 11 patients having grade 3 mucositis and 1 patient grade 4 mucositis. Other toxicities, including myelosuppression and renal toxicity, were mild to moderate in degree.

Discussion and conclusion

In an attempt to increase the CR-rate to neo-adjuvant chemotherapy, we have added two antifolate drugs to the PFL regimen. In a small study cohort of 28 patients, we identify a 39 % CR-rate to only 2 cycles of this combination. This suggests that this combination may be highly active in this disease. However, the percentage of patients having NR is unchanged from previous trials (~ 20 %) and this trial does not allow a conclusion that the activity of PFL-MP exceeds that observed with PFL, since 95 % confidence intervals overlap. Since mucositis was frequently severe, the further use of regimens such as PFL or PFL-MP will, ultimately, be justified only if improved survival can be demonstrated with longer follow-up.

Acknowledgements. We wish to thank Susan Jarman for preparation of the manuscript.

References

1. Vokes EE, Choi KE, Schilsky RL, Moran WJ, Guarnieri CM, Weichselbaum RR, and Panje WR (1988) Cisplatin, 5-Fluorouracil and high-dose leucovorin for recurrent or metastatic head and neck cancer. J Clin Oncol 6 : 618-626
2. Vokes EE, Schilsky RL, Weichselbaum RR, Kozloff M, Panje WR (1990) neo-adjuvant cisplatin, fluorouracil and high-dose leucovorin for locally advanced head and neck cancer : a clinical and pharmacologic analysis. J Clin Oncol 8 : 241-247
3. Vokes EE, Panje WR, Mick R, Haraf DJ, Moran WJ, McEvilly JM, Kozloff M, Weichselbaum (1990) neo-adjuvant chemotherapy surgery and concomitant chemoradiotherapy for locally advanced head and neck cancer. Proc Am Soc Clin Oncol 9 : 174
4. Vokes EE, Dimery I, Jacobs DC, Karp D, Collier MA, Eble M, Clendeninn NJ (1990) A phase II study of piritrexim in combination with methotrexate in recurrent head and neck cancer. Cancer (in press)

5. American Joint Committee on Cancer (1988) Manual for Staging of Cancer. 3rd Edition, Lippincott, Philadelphia, pp 25-62
6. Vokes EE, Panje WR, Schilsky RL, Mick R, Moran WJ, Awan AM, Goldman MD, Tybor AG, Weichselbaum RR (1989) Hydroxyurea, 5-Fluorouracil and concomitant radiotherapy in poor prognosis head and neck cancer : a phase I-II study. J Clin Oncol 7 : 761-768
7. Haraf DJ, Vokes EE, Panje WR, Weichselbaum RR (1990) Survival and analysis of failure following hydroxyurea, 5-Fluorouracil and concomitant radiation therapy in poor prognosis head and neck cancer. Am J Clin Oncol (in press)

Abstract. Methotrexate (MTX) and its lipophilic analogue Piritrexim (PTX) have single agent activity in head and neck cancer. We added these 2 antifolate drugs to our previously reported regimen of Cisplatin, 5-FU and high-dose oral Leucovorin (PFL). Patients were treated with 2 cycles of Cisplatin followed by a 5-day continuous infusion of 5-FU and Leucovorin administered. MTX was administered on day 15 and PTX on days 22 to 26, with cycle 2 starting on day 28. Twenty-eight patients were entered on study. Four patients were unevaluable for response, 4 patients had NR, 9 (32 %) had a PR, and 11 patients (39 %) a CR. Mucositis following PFL was dose-limiting. This regimen has shown a high CR-rate following only 2 cycles in the neo-adjuvant setting.

Efficacy of concomitant chemoradiotherapy in poor prognosis head and neck cancer

DJ Haraf, EE Vokes, WR Panje, RR Weichselbaum

Since 1986 we have conducted trials investigating chemoradiotherapy in poor prognosis head and neck cancer. The first study employed 5-Fluorouracil, hydroxyurea and concomitant radiation therapy given on an alternate week schedule in patients with locally advanced or recurrent head and neck cancer. These two drugs were chosen for their potential synergism with each other and to enhance the effectiveness of radiation [1]. A second phase I trial attempted to modulate the original regimen through the addition of Cisplatin. Cisplatin was chosen as the third agent based on high single agent activity in many solid tumors, radiation enhancing properties and synergistic action with 5-FU in vitro [1]. We now present an analysis of the long term results in 65 patients treated on these two trials.

Methods

Between 1986 and 1989 two phase I trials were conducted at the University of Chicago to study concomitant chemoradiotherapy. The initial study (FHX) was designed as a dose escalation study employing 5-FU, HU, and radiation therapy, administered on an alternate week schedule, in patients with poor prognosis head and neck cancer. The study design has been previously reported and will be summarized [2]. Thirty-nine patients treated with FHX were divided into 2 groups for analysis. Group 1 contained patients with recurrent disease who had failed previous curative intent local therapy. Group 2 contained patients with stage IV disease not eligible to receive neo-adjuvant chemotherapy because of poor pulmonary or renal function or metastatic disease. Treatment consisted of continuous infusion of 5-FU at 800 mg/m² on days 1-5 and μ 500 to 3,000 mg/day in divided doses on days 0-5 in a dose escalation study [2]. The study identified 2,000 mg/day as our recommended dose for HU. Radiotherapy was administered in 180-200 cGy fractions by a 4 or 6 mV linear accelerator on days 1-5 approximately. This 5 day course of treatment was followed by a 9 day rest period and constituted 1 cycle. Previously irradiated patients received doses of 40 to 60 Gy to areas of gross disease. Patients without a history of prior radiation received 66 to 75 Gy to areas of gross disease and 45 to 50 Gy to areas of potential microscopic disease.

In the second study (C-FHX) we attempted to modulate the original study through the addition of a third agent (Cisplatin). The study design and toxicity have been reported [3]. Patients received 600 mg/m² of 5-FU by infusion

All correspondence to : Daniel J Haraf, M.D., The University of Chicago Hospitals, Department of Radiation and Cellular Oncology, 5841 South Maryland Ave., Box 442, Chicago, IL 60637 USA

on days 1-5 and 500-1,000 mg HU in divided doses on days 0-5. Cisplatin was added as a continuous infusion at a dose of 10-20 mg/m² on days 0-5. Radio-therapy was identical to the FHX study. Acute hematologic toxicity preven-ting dose escalation of Cisplatin and the treatment plan was altered to admi-nister Cisplatin only on odd numbered cycles (1, 3, 5 and 7). Leucovorin was substituted for Cisplatin on even numbered cycles (2, 4 and 6). The 5-FU dose was decreased to 400 mg/m²/day during the Leucovorin containing cycles. Twenty-six patients who were treated on the C-FHX protocol are divided into group 1 and 2 as in the FHX study for analysis. Standard criteria were used to assess response to therapy.

Results

Overall 39 patients were treated with FHX and 26 patients with head and neck cancer were treated with C-FHX. The median follow-up for both studies is 40 months and 30 months respectively. Patients within each study are separa-ted into 2 groups for analysis. Group 1 patients (20 FHX, 11 C-FHX) had developed recurrent disease after curative doses of radiation, radical surgery or both. Group 2 (19 FHX, 15 C-FHX) patients had not received prior local therapy but presented with advanced disease considered to have a poor pro-gnosis. All 19 patients in FHX group 2 had stage IV disease at the start of treatment and 5 had biopsy proven distant metastases. Of 15 C-FHX patients, 14 had stage IV disease, 1 stage III disease and 2 had distant metastases.

Response rates

The response rate was 91 % (31/34) and 82 % (14/17) for FHX and C-FHX respectively. Five patients in FHX group 1 were unevaluable for response. Four patients had no measurable disease after attempted resection and one who deve-loped chest pain during chemotherapy received radiotherapy alone are exclu-ded. Of the 15 evaluable FHX group 1 patients, six (40 %) had a complete response (CR) and eight (53 %) had a partial response (PR). Five C-FHX group 1 patients were evaluable. Exclusions include : 4 patients without mea-surable disease after attempted resection, 1 patient who died of aspiration pneu-monia during the second cycle of therapy, and 1 patient who developed pro-gressive facial edema and refused treatment or response evaluation after three cycles. Of the 5 evaluable patients in C-FHX group 1 there were two CRs and one PR. One patient was a nonresponder and another progressed at the mar-gin of the radiation portal.

   Two patients in FHX group 2 were excluded from response analysis. Both had received two treatment cycles at the maximally tolerated dose of HU (3,000 mg daily) then refused further therapy. There were 12 complete responses (71 %) and five partial responses (29 %) in the 17 evaluable patients. Three patients in C-FHX group 2 had no measurable lesion after resection of the primary lesion as part of the planned therapeutic approach prior to the start of protocol and were excluded from response analysis. Of the remaining 12 patients, 9 (75 %) had a CR and 2 (17 %) had PRs. Only 1 C-FHX group 2 patient was a non-responder.

Survival

Three deaths during treatment occured with FHX (two aspiration pneumonia and one respiratory insufficiency). One patient was lost to follow-up after 6 months. Two patients in group 1, and 3 group 2 patients, expired after the completion of treatment of non-malignant causes. One group 1 patient and 5 group 2 patients are alive from 35 to 50 months after the start of therapy. The remaining 15 group 1 patients and 9 group 2 patients died of progressive head and neck cancer. The median survivals for FHX groups 1 and 2 were 8 months and 14 months respectively.

One death in each group occured during treatment with C-FHX (one pulmonary embolism and one aspiration pneumonia). One group 2 patient was lost to follow-up at 14 months after a complete response. In group 2, one patient expired from a second malignancy of the distal esophagus while an additional 3 patients died of non-malignant causes. Two group 1 patients and 7 group 2 patients remain alive from 23 to 32 months after the start of therapy. The remaining 8 group 1 and 2 group 2 patients died of progressive head and neck cancer.

Analysis of failure

Four patients in FHX group 1 died without disease progression. Nine patients (45 %) developed isolated local failure, 5 patients (25 %) developed local and distant failure and 1 patient developed isolated distant failure. One FHX group 1 patient is alive and well 35 months following treatment. Four FHX group 2 patients died without evidence of failure and 1 patient was lost to follow-up 6 months after achieving a complete response. Three (16 %) FHX group 2 patients developed isolated local failure. Two of these failures were in patients who received the maximally tolerated dose of HU and refused any further therapy after the initial cycle. Isolated distant failure was recorded in 6 patients. Five patients remain alive and well 36 to 50 months following treatment.

Nine of the eleven patients in C-FHX group 1 progressed after treatment. Isolated local failure occurred in 3 patients (27 %) while 4 patients (36 %) failed in both local and distant sites. One patient, progressed at the margin of the radiation treatment portal, underwent surgical salvage and is currently alive and well 32 months following treatment but is counted as having local and distant failure. One patient is alive 32 months after treatment without evidence of failure. Two C-FHX group 2 patients progressed in distant sites and no local failures have been recorded. One patient was lost to follow-up after 14 months and 7 are alive and well after treatment. Five patients have died of non-malignant causes.

Discussion and conclusion

The results presented here provide evidence that concomitant chemoradiotherapy with 5-FU and HU with or without Cisplatin administered on a split course schedule is a tolerable, acceptable and effective regimen in the treatment of head and neck cancer. The activity of the regimens described was impressive considering the advanced stage and high incidence of prior therapy in these patients. Group 1 patients remain a difficult group to treat with an exceptionally poor prognosis. Recurrences following aggressive local therapy often results in symptoms requiring palliation. Frequently these patients receive chemotherapy alone with disappointing results. The reported response rate of 56 % (6 % CR) after Cisplatin, 5-FU and Leucovorin in recurrent head and neck cancer with no long term survivors [4] is inferior to the 85 % response rate (40 % CR) seen in group 1 patients after chemoradiotherapy. In addition, 1 patient in FHX group 1 has remained free of disease after treatment and 2 patients are alive and well after C-FHX (one after surgical salvage).

The results in group 2 have been impressive in both studies. The overall response rate for group 2 patients was 97 % (72 % CR). The local failure rate after FHX was 16 % (3/19) including 2 patients treated at the MTD of Hydroxyurea who refused further therapy after the initial cycle. This is similar to the 100 % local control observed in C-FHX group 2. The better local control seen in group 2 is most likely related to the radiotherapy administered. Group 1 patients tend to receive fewer cycles of treatment and lower doses of radiation to smaller volumes because of concerns for normal tissues than group 2. Overall group 1 patients receive a median of 5 000 cGy in 5 cycles which is in contrast to the median of 7 000 cGy in 7 cycles given to group 2 patients.

Acknowledgements. We wish to thank the Geraldi Norton Memorial Corporation, The Center for Radiation Therapy and The Chicago Tumor Institute for their support.

References

1. Vokes EE, Weichselbaum RR (1990) Concomitant chemoradiotherapy : rationale and clinical experience in patients with solid tumors. J Clin Onc 8 : 911-934
2. Vokes EE, Panje WR, Schilsky RL et al (1989) Hydroxyurea, fluorouracil and concomitant radiotherapy in poor prognosis head and neck cancer : a phase I-II study. J Clin Onc 7 : 761-768
3. Moormeier JA, Vokes EE, Haraf DJ et al Cisplatin (CDDP), 5-Fluorouracil (FU), and hydroxyurea (HU) with concomitant radiotherapy (RT) for advanced solid tumors. Third International Conference on the Interaction of Radiation Therapy and Systemic Therapy, Monterey, CA
4. Vokes EE, Choi KE, Schilsky RL et al (1988) Cisplatin, fluorouracil and high-dose leucovorin for recurrent or metastatic head and neck cancer. J Clin Onc 6 : 618-626

Abstract. *Since 1986 we have studied chemoradiotherapy treatment of poor prognosis head and neck cancer in 2 phase I trials. The median follow-up is 40 months and 30 months respectively. The initial trial employed Hydroxyurea (HU), 5-Fluorouracil (5-FU) and concomitant radiotherapy on an alternate week schedule. Thirty-nine patients were treated on this study. Treatment was well tolerated and an overall response rate of 97 % was observed. Subgroup analysis revealed local control rate of 84 % (16/19) in previously untreated patients and 30 % (6/20) in those who had failed prior therapy. The second trial attempted to add infusional Cisplatin to the regimen in an effort to improve local and distant control. Twenty-six patients with head and neck cancer were enrolled on this phase I study. The overall response rate was 82 %. Local control was 100 % (15/15) in previously untreated patients and 36 % (4/11) in those who had failed prior local therapy. We conclude that concomitant chemoradiotherapy is effective in poor prognosis head and neck cancer.*

Radiotherapy (RT) with concomitant Cisplatin (CDDP) in the management of locally advanced or recurrent head and neck cancer (LARHNC)

G Gasparini, S Dal Fior, G Recher, G Panizzoni, V Cristoferi, A Testolin, R Squaquara, F Pozza

There are several advantages in combining RT and chemotherapy, particularly with CDDP, in LARHNC. In fact, CDDP given concurrently with RT leads to a potentiation of cell killing, based on an inhibition of the recovery of the radiation-induced damage and which is more evident in inherently sensitive cells to CDDP alone [1]. Furthermore, the simultaneous administration of RT and chemotherapy minimizes the duration of the induction treatment and maximizes the dose intensity [2]. On this rationale we began the present Phase III study.

Materials and methods

Between 1987 and 1990, 48 consecutive patients were evaluable. Eligibility criteria were : diagnosis of squamous cell carcinoma, untreated stage III-IV or loco-regional rd, PS > 50, normal renal function, adequate bone marrow function and patients informed consent. Patients received CDDP 80 mg/m^2 i.v. on days 1,21, ± 42 with parenteral hydratation and antiemetics. RT by supervoltage equipment with Co 60 or 4 MeV linear accelerator was started on day 1 at 2 Gy daily fractions for 5 days a week for 6-8 weeks, until total doses of 60-70 Gy. A « boost » of 10 Gy was given in patients with primary of diameter > 4 cm or in those with persistent primary or nodes after 30 Gy. Response and toxicity were defined according to the WHO criteria [3]. A X^2, testing homogeinity, was employed to evaluate differences in response rate. Differences in time events were evaluated by the Mantel-Haenszel test and the time events were plotted using the Kaplan-Meier estimates.

Results

The main characteristics of the patients were : median age : 58.5 yrs (39-75) ; median PS : 90 (60-100) ; 46 male and 2 female ; 52 % had stage IV ; 37.5 % stage III and 10.5 % rd (recurrent disease) ; 52 % had primary in oropharynx, 19 % in hypopharynx ; 19 % in oral cavity and 10 % in larynx. No treatment related death was observed. 40 % of cases had grade III and only 6 % (1 patient) had grade IV stomatitis ; 16 % had grade III nausea and vomiting ;

St. Bortolo Hospital, Vicenza, Italy

16 % had grade III leukopenia. Transient acute renal toxicity was observed in 31 % of patients. Response to treatment in the 43 stage III-IV patients was : complete response (CR) in 27 (63 %) ; partial response (PR) in 15 (35 %) and stable disease in 1. The median duration of response was 10 months (2-34) in CR and 8 months (2-15) in PR. After a median follow up of 18 months (6 to 34), 22 patients are still alive, 15 free of disease. The estimated 1 and 2 year OS probability was 59 % and 38 %. A higher 2 year OS was observed in CR vs PR patients (p = 0.037) and in those receiving 3 vs 2 cycles of CDDP (p = 0.085). Among the 5 patients with rd, only 1 achieved CR and 2 had PR. Median time to progression was 4 months. In the group of 50 patients treated with RT alone (historical controls) the main characteristics were comparable with those of that treated with RT-CDDP. Response rate was : CR in 28 %, PR in 56 % and progression in 16 %. The median survival was 8 months, with 31 % and 12.5 % patients alive respectively at 1 and 2 years ; 25 % cases died for distant metastases.

Discussion and conclusion

Our results suggest that the synchronous combination of intermittent high-dose CDDP with conventional RT is an effective and tolerable regimen. We obtained a CR rate of 63 % in inoperable stage III-IV patients, better than that obtained in the historical group treated with RT alone (28 %). Comparable results have been reported in other Phase I-II trials using different schedules of chemotherapy plus RT with CR varying from 59 % to 82 % [4, 5]. With the combined approach we obtained a probability of OS of 59 % and 37 % at 1 and 2 years and a DFS at 2 years of 36 % compared to a median survival of only 8 months and to a 1 year OS of 33 % in the 50 stage III-IV patients treated with RT alone in years 1985-87. The frequency of distant failure appears lower in the CDDP-RT group (12.5 %) than in the historical control (25 %). In the palliative group of patients with rd, RT-CDDP obtained a transient local control (CR + PR) in 3 out of 5 patients. Overall, acute toxicity of this combined treatment was acceptable and patients' compliance to treatment was high, permitting the completion of the planned schedule in 90 % of patients. In conclusion, the present Phase II trial suggests benefit from CDDP given simultaneously with RT. To clearly define real survival advantages of CDDP-RT in LARHNC, a randomized comparison with RT alone is needed.

References

1. Coughlin CT and Richmond RC (1989) Biologic and clinical development of cisplatin combined to radiation : concepts, utility, projection for new trials and the emergence of carboplatin. Sem Oncol 16 (suppl 6) : 31-43
2. Clark JR and Frey III E (1989) Chemotherapy for head and neck cancer : progress and controversy in the management of patients with Mo disease. Sem Oncol 16 (suppl 6) : 44-57

3. Miller AB, Hoogstraten B and Staquet J (1981) Reporting results of cancer treatment. Cancer 47 : 207-214
4. Al-Sarraf M, Pajak TF, Marcial VA et al (1987) Concurrent radiotherapy and chemotherapy with cisplatin in inoperable squamous cell carcinoma of the head and the neck. An RTOG study. Cancer 59 : 259-265
5. Taylor SG, Murthy AK, Caldarelli DD et al (1989) Combined simultaneous cisplatin/fluorouracil chemotherapy and split course radiation in head and neck cancer. J Clin Oncol 7 : 846-856

Abstract. We planned a Phase II study of concurrent RT, for a total dose of 60-70 Gy with CDDP 80 mg/m² for 2 or 3 doses to improve the locoregional control of patients with LARHNC. Forty-eight patients were evaluable : 18 had stage III, 25 stage IV and 5 recurrent disease (rd). Complete response rate (CR) was 63 % (27/43) in cases with stage III-IV and only 20 % (1/5) in those with rd. In patients with stage III-IV the overall probability of 1 and 2 year OS was 59 % and 38 %, respectively. Disease-free survival at 1 and 2 year was 46 % and 38 %, respectively. Gastrointestinal and hematologic toxicity were the most common side effects. Comparing data of this present trial with that of 50 patients treated with RT alone in the years 1985-87 (historical control), we observed that the CR rate, OS and DFS were better in the patients treated with RT-CDDP. In conclusion, RT with concurrent CDDP is an effective and safe treatment in LARHNC and needs to be evaluated in a Phase III randomized trial vs RT alone.

Primary chemotherapy and surgery in advanced oral cavity squamous cell carcinomas : retrospective analysis

L Licitra, C Grandi, V Bonfante, MI Grosso, M Guzzo, R Molinari, G Bonadonna

Chemotherapy is usually employed for head and neck squamous cell carcinomas only in the advanced disease setting. The best regimen has not yet been defined, due to the lack of controlled trials and to differences in reported results within the uncontrolled published series [1-4]. One reason for such differences may lie in a different patient selection, and tumor site may be one of the factors contributing to the selection bias. For this reason, we decided to perform a retrospective case series analysis on the patients with squamous cell carcinoma arising from one site, the oral cavity, receiving chemotherapy at our institution over the last ten years. In order to obtain a homogenously treated series, we selected only those patients who received primary chemotherapy and subsequent surgery.

Patients and methods

Eligible patients had previously untreated advanced squamous cell carcinoma and received primary chemotherapy and subsequent surgery at our institution from 1980 to 1989. Therefore they had an advanced disease, i.e. a disease which either was difficult to surgically excise or required very demaging interventions. It follows that patients with stages III and IV were included, as well as some patients with less advanced disease, i.e. stage II.

Thirty-nine patients were included in this case series analysis (M/F : 30/9 ; median age 56 yrs). Six patients had stage II (T2N0), 22 patients had stage III (T2N1, 3 ; T3N0, 11 ; T3N1, 8) and 11 had stage IV (T2N2, 2 ; T3N2, 2 ; T4N0-2, 7). Nine patients had mandibular bone involvement. All patients received primary chemotherapy for at least 2 cycles. Twenty-eight patients received Cisplatin + Fluorouracil (Table 1), and 11 patients received a non Cisplatin-including regimen (Vincristine + Bleomycin + Methotrexate or Vinblastine + Bleomycin) [5]. Locoregional treatment was radical surgery alone in 20 patients and surgery followed by radiotherapy in 19. Radiotherapy was used whenever surgical margins were histologically positive and/or peri-lymphnodal invasion was documented.

Results

Overall response rate to primary chemotherapy was 64 % (CI, 48 % to 77 %). Only 1 (pathologically proven) complete remission was recorded (3 %).

Division of Medical Oncology and Division of Head and Neck Surgical Oncology, Istituto Nazionale Tumori, Milano, Italy

Table 1. Treatment regimens

FU	1,000 mg/m²	day 1 2 3 4 5	(continuous infusion)
CDDP	100 mg/m²	day 1	(30 min infusion)
			every 3 weeks
VCR	1 mg	day 1	(i.v. bolus)
BLM	15 mg	day 1 2	(i.m.)
MTX	30 mg	day 3	(p.o.)
			weekly

At a median follow-up of 20 months, 10 patients are alive and disease-free, 5 were lost to follow-up, one is alive with disease, 21 died with active disease, 2 died for other causes. Twenty patients had a loco-regional recurrence (14 to the primary site, one both to the primary site and lymphnodes, 5 to lymphnodes only) and 3 patients died with distant metastases. The actuarial overall survival is 28 % at 5 years.

Discussion and conclusion

This case series analysis shows a low complete remission rate in squamous cell carcinomas arising from the oral cavity. The overall response rate was similar to that recorded in other published series. Chemotherapy can contribute to the feasibility of surgery in some cases, and the response rate may be higher for smaller tumors than for those included in this series. The site of origin of the tumor, however, can be a critical factor in determining the complete response rate. Therefore, the role of primary chemotherapy in oral cavity squamous cell carcinomas remains to be fully assessed by randomized studies. One of such studies, enrolling only patients with oral cavity tumors, is ongoing at our institution.

References

1. Weaver A, Flemming S, Kish J et al (1982) Cisplatin and 5-Fluorouracil as induction therapy for advanced head and neck cancer. Am J Surg 144 : 445
2. Al-Sarraf M (1988) Head and neck cancer : chemotherapy concepts. Sem Oncol 15 : 70-85
3. Jacobs C (1989) Adjuvant chemotherapy for head and neck cancer. J Clin Oncol 7 : 823-824
4. Olasz L, Szabo I, Horvath A (1988) A combined treatment for advanced oral cavity cancers. Cancer 62 : 1267-1274
5. Molinari R, Mattavelli F, Cantù G et al (1980) Results of low-dose combination chemotherapy with vincristine, bleomycin and methotrexate (V-B-M) based on cell kinetics in the palliative treatment of head and neck squamous cell carcinoma. Eur J Cancer 16 : 469-472

Neo-Adjuvant intra-arterial chemotherapy by Cisplatin and 5-FU for squamous cell carcinoma of the oral cavity

MH Gaspard, J Santini, O Dassonville, A Thyss, F Demard, M Schneider

The association of Cisplatin with continous 5-FU infusion has led to an improved response rate in previously untreated head and neck cancer [1, 2]. However, this combination protocol is accompanied by a significant incidence of systemic toxicity that is often acceptable but sometimes severe, depending on dose or on specific site. Moreover, our experience with this chemotherapy protocol indicated that the best results were obtained for tumors of the oropharynx and hypopharynx and that oral cavity lesions were the most refractory [3]. These limitations in treatment tolerance and response suggest that the intra-arterial route may be an interesting alternative to the intravenous route for the delivery of this combination. This approach is further justified by pharmacological characteristics of both Cisplatin and 5-FU. Cisplatin is highly bound to plasma proteins so that when given intravenously, only a limited part of the active drug (free drug action) is accessible to target tissues. Thus, it is not surprising that higher platinum levels were found in tumor biopsies after infra-arterial administration, as compared with the intravenous route in head and neck cancer patients [4]. On the other hand, 5-FU systemic clearance is particularly high and, thus, represents a drug of choice for intra-arterial chemotherapy [5].

Our objective in this work was to evaluate the effects of this combination when administered by an intra-arterial route to patients with squamous cell carcinoma of the oral cavity.

Methods

Criteria for admissibility

Patients with histologically confirmed squamous cell carcinomas of the oral cavity (tongue, floor of mouth buccal mucosa) were involved in this study. None had been treated previously. They had a TNM stage II or above, with MO disease, including only metastatic lymphnodes of the upper neck. Patients were in good general condition and had normal renal function. The fixed upper age limit was 75 years. Patients with previously documented vascular cerebral attack were excluded.

Centre Antoine Lacassagne, Nice, France

Chemotherapy

The scheduled first protocol consisted in 24 hours continuous infusion of 60 mg of Cisplatin followed by a 120 hours continous infusion of 5-FU 150 mg per day. Due to the locoregional toxicity (stomatitis and, or cutanenous toxicity) observed in the 7 first entered patients, the daily dose of 5-FU was reduced to 120 mg. The protocole called for 3 consecutive courses and a 7 day free interval was set between each course.

Infusion technique

Intra-arterial catheter insertion was done by a retrograde catheterisation of the superficial temporal artery. The correct site of perfusion was confirmed by fluorescin dye for all patients. For half of the patients, 99 technetium was delivered via the catheter ; this was followed by radionuclide scanning of the head and neck. This allowed not only the determination on the infused area, but also permitted the detection of unwanted CNS infusion. In addition, an implanted specific chamber of intra-arterial drug delivery from Cordis lab was placed : catheter was tunneled through the subcutaneous tissue of the neck and upper chest wall, and connected to the chamber implanted in the subclavicular area.

Before treatment, lesions were biopsied during a panendoscopy. Two weeks after the completion of chemotherapy the lesions were reexamined, measured and assessed for the degree of regression.

Pharmacokinetics study

Systemic 5-FU blood levels were measured twice daily and for 8 patients, the locoregional 5-FU extraction was evaluated according to the Collins formula comparing intra arterial and intravenous AUC.

Patients characteristics

Twenty-six patients have been treated between january 86 and may 89, 24 males and 2 females, mean age 59 (range 30 to 66) with 7 stage II, 10 stage III and 9 stage IV.

Results (Table 1)

Table 1. Intra-arterial chemotherapy ; overall results ; clinical response

---

25 patients evaluable for response to IAC
1 patient died of intercurrent non specific complication
Response rate [CR + PR] 23/35 [92 %]

CR 13/25 [52 %]
PR 10/25 [40 %]
NR 2/25 [8 %]

Twenty-five patients were evaluable for response. One patient died of inter-current non specific complication. The total response rate was 92 % (23/25). There were respectively 52 % of complete response (13/25), 40 % of partial response (10/25) and 8 % of no response (5/25).

Histological response (Table 2)

Table 2. Histological responses in 23 patients who underwent surgery after iac

No detectable disease = 8/23
Microscopic disease [< 5 mm] = 3/23
Macroscopic disease = 12/23

Twenty-three patients undergone surgery after IAC. The histological examina-tion of the resected specimen demonstrated respectively 8/23 cases free of can-cer, 3/23 cases with macroscopic residual material.

For the 3 patients with palpable nodes of the upper neck, the response on nodes was partial for 2 and absent for 1. This was confirmed by histology.

Toxicity

The one and only toxicity was locoregional with 7/26 patients (27 %) having grade III-IV stomatis and regional cutaneous toxicity.

It must be kept on mind that 5 of those patients were treated with the initial chemotherapy protocol with 150 mg 5-FU.

Pharmacokinetics data

Within an important interpatient variability, drug concentrations are gradually increased from the beginning to the end of their treatment period ; this indi-cating a progressive saturation of the local captation of the drug.

An estimation of the local extraction of 5-FU has been performed for 8 patients. There was a high interpatient variability of the extraction ratio ran-ging from 0 to 80 %. For a given patient, the ratio was also variable from 1 course to the other and the amplitude of the extraction ratio was not rela-ted to the response.

Follow-up (Table 3)

Twenty-one patients were available for follow-up with a mean duration of 26 months. The 5 missing patients were 1 death during chemotherapy, 2 deaths during the immediate post-operative course and 2 patients lost of follow-up. Fourteen patients are alive and disease free within a 12 36 months period. Seven

MH Gaspard et al

Table 3.

Intra-arterial chemotherapy follow-up

21/26 Patients

1 death during induction chemotherapy
2 post-operative deaths
2 lost for follow-up

14/21 Alive and disease free [12-36 months]

7/21 Deaths

Local reccurence = 2
Metastases = 1
2nd primary = 2
Cancer unrelated = 2

Among 8 histologically complete responders

6/8 Alive disease free [18-36 months]
2/8 deaths [1 post-op, cancer unrelated]

---

died : 2 of them from loco-regional recurrence, 1 from distant metastases, 2 from a second primary and the last 2 from a non carcinogenic etiology.

More interestingly among the 8 complete responders confirmed by histology, 6 are alive and disease free after 18 to 36 months of survey. The 2 deaths were not due to the evolutive neoplastic disease. One was in the immediate post-operative course and the other due to a myocardial infarction.

This study demonstrates that the combination chemotherapy Cisplatin 5-FU given by an intra-arterial route in squamous cell carcinoma of the oral cavity allows the obtention of a very interesting tumoral response rate = 92 %, with 52 % of clinical complete response and 8 out of 13 patients with clinically complete response, who show histological evidence of the complete eradication of lesions, a longer DFS and whole survival.

The toxicity was slight and only locoregional with 120 mg 5-FU.

Conclusion

Squamous cell carcinomas of the oral cavity are theorically ideal candidates for intra arterial chemotherapy. They are agressive cancers and often easily amenable to vascular access and the implanted specific access system allows an easy repeatibility of intra-arterial chemotherapy from course to course.

The consequent dose reduction in both 5-FU and Cisplatin in comparison with systemic IV protocols represents a strong argument in favor of intra-arterial route. This relative dose reduction would also permit a better benefit of further chemotherapy in this group of patients who are predisposed to a second primary. In total, this pilot study suggests a reconsideration of intra-arterial chemotherapy in squamous cell carcinoma of the head and neck according to the specific modalities herein described.

References

1. Al-Sarraf M, Amer MH, Vaishampayan G, Loh J and Weaver A (1979) A multidisplinary therapeutic approach for advanced previously untreated epidermoid cancer of the head and neck. Preliminary report. Int J Radiat Oncol Biol Phys 5 : 1421
2. Thyss A, Schneider M, Santini J, Caldani C, Vallicioni J, Chauvel P, Demard F (1986) Induction chemotherapy with cisplatinum and 5-Fluorouracil for squamous cell carcinoma of the head and neck. Br J Cancer 54 : 755
3. Demard F, Schneider M, Thyss A, Chauvel P, Vallicioni J, Santini J, Caldani C (1988) Cisplatinum and continous 5-FU infusion for the treatment of head and neck cancer. In : Jacquillat C (ed) Neo-Adjuvant Chemotherapy, Paris, pp 321-325
4. Gouyette A, Apchin, Foka M, Richard JM (1986) Pharmacokinetics of intra-arterial and intravenous cisplatin in head and neck cancer patients. Europ J Cancer Clin Oncol 22 : 257
5. Collins JM (1984) Pharmacologic rationale for regional drug delivery. J Clin Oncol 2 : 498

Abstract. Twenty-six previously untreated patients with squamous cell carcinoma of the oral cavity were treated by an intra arterial protocol : Cisplatin 60 mg D1 and 5-FU 150 mg/D, D2 to D6 by continous infusion. This protocol called for 3 consecutive courses. Due to local toxicity observed in the 7 first patients, the 5-FU daily dose was reduced from 150 to 120 mg/D. The total response rate [PR + CR] was 92 % [23/25] including 52 % of CR [13/25].

After surgical resection in 23 cases, there was an histological sterilization in 8/23 cases. Owing to the high complete response rate observed in this study, intra-arterial chemotherapy should be reconsidered for therapeutic management of squamous cell carcinoma of the oral cavity.

Treatment of locally advanced head and neck cancer with Neo-Adjuvant Cisplatin (CDDP) and 5-Fluorouracil (5-FU) chemotherapy (CT)

C Balana, J Minguell, B Massuti, A Arrivi, B Sanchez

The efficacy of neo-adjuvant CT with CDDP-5-FU is widely recognized [1-4]. The role of local treatment and its impact on results and overall survival (OS) must still be defined. Response to initial Cisplatin combination has been considered an indicator of response to radiation therapy (XRT) [5].

Material and methods

After October 1987 patients with diagnosis of head and neck cancer are revised by a Tumor Committee. Patients with tumors T3 or T4, N1-3 MO or not resectable by its location, are treated with induction CT previous to local treatment. Chemotherapy schedule consists of CDDP 100 mg/m² on day 1 and 5-FU 1,000 mg/m²/24 h for a 120 h infusion. Antiemetic treatment is standard for all patients. Before each course, complete blood count, renal function and assessment of toxicity are done. The course is delayed if WBC are less than 2,000/mm³ or platelets are < 100,000/mm³. After 3 courses patients are revised by Tumor Committee and are evaluated for response. Local treatment : radical surgery or XRT are selected individually. Surgery includes all initial tumors. Radiation therapy portals include cervical and supraclavicular bilateral lymphatic areas. WHO criteria are used to evaluate toxicity and response. Statistics are processed with the SPSSPC + package, and OS and remission duration by the Kaplan-Meier method.

Results

Characteristics of 50 treated patients are outlined in Table 1. Total number of courses : 142. Two patients received only 1 course : they were included in the toxicity analysis but they were not evaluated for response (Table 2). Forty-eight patients are evaluable for response to CT (Table 3). Median OS by response to CT was 19.2 for partial response (PR) and not reached at 23 min for complete response (CR) (p = 0.15) (Fig. 1). After CT, 40 patients had XRT, 3 had surgery and 3 patients surgery plus XRT. Thirty-six patients are evaluable for response to XRT. XRT increased response in 12 patients (33.4 %) ; 2 patients with no response (NR) to CT reached a PR with XRT and 10 patients with PR to CT reached a CR to XRT. Furthermore, XRT maintained all previous CT CR. Only 3 patients with previous response to CT

Hospital General Alicante C/Maestro Alonos 109, 03010 Alicante, Spain

Table. 1. Patients characteristics

Characteristic	Number	%	Characteristic		Number	%
Stage II	3	6	Performance st	0	2	4
III	10	20		1	19	28
IV	37	74		2	16	32
Site of disease				3	2	6
Oropharynx	10	20	Histological type			
Oral cavity	8	16	Squamous		41	82
Larynx	14	28	Undiferentiated		7	14
Nasopharynx	9	18	Transitional		1	2
Pharynx	7	14	Other		1	2
Salivary gl	1	2	Histological grade	1	8	16
Lymph node	1	2		2	4	8
				3	14	28
Sex 47M/3F			Unknown		24	48

Table 2. Toxicity (142 courses)

Type-degree		%	Courses	Type-degree		%	Courses
Leucopenia	1		4	Mucositis	1		15
Anemia	1		11		2		9
	2		4		3		3
Thromboc	1		1	Neurological	1		6
Emesis	1		20		2		2
	2		42	Renal	1		5
	3		12				
Diarrhea	1	4	3	Cardiac failure	1		
	2	4	3	Ototoxicity	1		

Table 3. Chemotherapy responses (%) (n = 48) and median overall survival (months)

Type	N	T	Total response	Overall survival	p
NR	14.3	12.8	16.7		
PR	60.0	48.9	60.4	19.2 months	
CR	25.7	38.3	22.9	not reached 23 m	0.15

Table 4. Results after systemic and local treatment (n = 42) : responses (%) and median overall survival (months)

Type	N	T	Total response	Overall survival	p
NR	3.3	7.3	7.1		
PR	26.7	17.1	26.2	14.3 months	
CR	60.0	68.3	57.1	not reached 23 m	0.0000

showed progressive disease with XRT. After CT and local treatment patients
were evaluated as beeing in NR 7.1 %, PR 26.2 % and CR 57.1 % (total response rate 83.3 %) (Table 4). Complete responses were reached with CT in
11 cases, with CT and XRT in 10 cases and CT, XRT and surgery in 1 case.
OS at the end of treatment showed significant differences depending on the
type of response obtained. Duration of response was 8.7 min for PR and 19.4
min for CR (p = 0.0057 Cox-Mantel). OS was : NR 7 min, PR 14.3 min and
CR not reached at 23 min (67 % at 23 min) (p = 0.0000) (Fig. 2). Patients
with the best OS were those who reached complete response after systemic and
local treatment. Thirteen patients needed local treatment to reach CR and benefit from better survival.

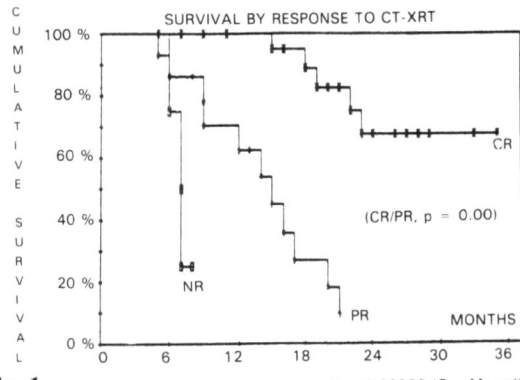

Fig. 1.   P = 0.00000 (Cox-Mantel)

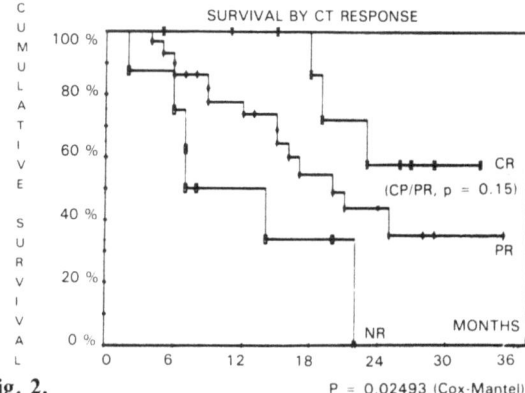

Fig. 2.   P = 0.02493 (Cox-Mantel)

Discussion and conclusion

The responses we report to CDDP-5-FU CT are similar to the results reported
by other authors with the same schedule [1-4]. Patients who reach a CR have

a better survival. Local treatment XRT or surgery can increase the response primarily obtained by CT, turning PR's in CR's, thus increasing the survival probability of these patients. OS must be estimated according to the patients state at the end of treatment in order to include the increase of responses provided by local treatment and measure its effect over results. Advantages of the neo-adjuvant approach must be demonstrated not only over standard treatment but also over chemotherapy alone.

References

1. Kish J, Drelichman A, Jacobs J et al (1982) Clinical trial of cisplatin and 5-FU infusion as initial treatment for advanced squamous cell carcinoma of the head and neck. Cancer Treat Rep 66 : 471-474
2. Decker DA, Drelichman A, Jacobs J et al (1983) Adjuvant chemotherapy with cis-diamminodichloroplatinum II and 120-hour infusion 5-fluorouracil in stage III-IV squamous cell carcinoma of the head and neck. Cancer 51 : 1353-1355
3. Demard F, Schneider M, Thyss A et al (1988) Cisplatinum and continous infusion 5-fluorouracil for treatment of head and neck cancers. In : Jacquiilat Cl, Weil M, Khayat D (eds) neo-adjuvant chemotherapy. Colloque Inserm/John Libbey Eurotext Ltd, Paris, vol. 169, p 231
4. Cappelaere P, Lefèbvre JL, Buisset E (1988) Induction cisplatin-5-FU chemotherapy as initial treatment for advanced head and neck squamous cell carcinoma. In : Jacquillat Cl, Weil M, Khayat D (eds) Neo-Adjuvant Chemotherapy. Colloque Inserm/John Libbey Eurotext Ltd, Paris, vol. 169, p 339
5. Ensley JF, Jaccobs JR, Weaver A (1984) Correlation between response to cisplatinum-combination chemotherapy and subsequent radiotherapy in previously untreated patients with advanced squamous cell cancers of the head and neck. Cancer 54 : 811-814

Abstract. After 1987, 50 locally advanced head and neck cancer patients (P) have been treated with CDDP-5-FU-CT previous to local treatment. A 83.3 % total response rate with 57.1 % complete response (CR) rate have been noted after CT and local treatment. Overall survival (OS) is significantly better for P in CR if systemic and local treatment are considered but not if survival is only estimated according to CT response.

T3T4 operable cancers of oral cavity and oropharynx. Randomised trial for surgery and radiotherapy

D Nizri*, H Szpirglas, JP Lacoste, A Thomas, S Godeau, L Benslama

In a previous trial performed from 1981 to 1987 in the oncology and medical stomatology department and the radiation department of the Salpétrière Hospital in Paris (with a grant of INSERM), we studied 114 patients with T3T4 unoperable cancers of the oral cavity and oropharynx. Neo-adjuvant chemotherapy and 3 different modalities of radiotherapy (time and doses) were randomised. We concluded that a good response to chemotherapy was predictive of better efficiency of radiotherapy and we don't find any difference between the 3 tested modalities of radiotherapy especially for complete response.

Two facts must be pointed out :

— trials for oral cavity and oropharynx cancers presented in september 1987 at the second head and neck oncology meeting in Arlington USA had shown a 27 % overall survival at 3 years ;

— three years after the end of the « INSERM » study, there is only one patient living, out of the 58 patients in the radiotherapy group, and one also out of the 56 patients in the chemotherapy group.

Our conviction was that the advanced T3T4 cancers of the oral cavity and oropharynx involved very different patients and we decided to considere separetely the operable and the non operable ones.

Our further purpose was to study the place for radiotherapy in operable patients and, considering the INSERM trial results, we reserved this study, because of ethical reasons, only to patients responding to neo-adjuvant chemotherapy.

Methods

In 1987 a trial was activated in which entered 164 patients with epidermoid T3T4 cancers, of oral cavity and oropharynx, operable and unoperable, all treated first with neo-adjuvant chemotherapy, trial already described (see in Dr H. Szpirglas' article, a randomised trial for surgical or radiotherapeutic treatment after neo-adjuvant chemotherapy in oral and oropharyngeal cancers).

Out of the 109 operable patients, 50 responded to chemotherapy and were randomised beetween surgery and radiotherapy.

These 50 patients were : 40 males ; 10 females ; 57 middle age. They were equally dispatched for following treatment according to age and localisations :

* Radiotherapy department. Oncology and medical stomatology department CHU. Pitié Salpétrière, Paris, France

Table 1.

Age	20/29	30/39	40/49	50/59	60/69	70/80
Surgery	0	0	2	11	6	1
Radiotherapy	0	0	2	15	5	2
Localisations	Mob. Tongue	Floor of M.	Post Tongue	Orop.	Gum	Misc
Surgery	5	7	1	0	5	2
Radiotherapy	4	6	4	3	7	1

Average tumor sizes were 45/26 mm for T3 and 53/35 mm for T4.

The nodes involvement was the same in the two groups.

Results

Out of 50 operable patients responders to neo-adjuvant chemotherapy, 25 had to be and were all irradiated, 25 were to be operated and only 20 could be. Five patients could not be operated because of intercurrent diseases (phlebitis, delirium tremens, heart failure, refusal, delayed treatment).

Out of 20 operated patients, 15 achieved complete remission and 4 reached remission after additional radiotherapy for involved resection limits or positive nodes.

Out of 25 irradiated patients, 18 achieved complete remission and one achieved remission after salvage surgery.

Patients in complete remission were randomised for an adjuvant treatment (2 additional courses with 5FU/CDDP).

Both groups, surgery and radiotherapy, showed no immediate benefit with adjuvant chemotherapy ; rates of local, nodal and metastatic failures or second localisations are equal, and sometimes higher for treated patients.

If we compare the actuarial survival curves of operated and irradiated patients, there is a slight and no significant difference ; better for the operated patients, but 5 of them (25 %) were treated with additional radiotherapy.

If we compare the survival in patients who achieved remission after surgery alone or radiotherapy alone, there is no difference at all.

Conclusion

In conclusion, survival rate is equal for patients, responders to neo-adjuvant chemotherapy, after surgery or after radiotherapy.

Unfortunatlly, up to now, adjuvant chemotherapy for these same patients did not show any usefulness.

Abstract. A randomized trial for surgical or radiotherapeutic treatment has been activated in patients bearing T3T4 tumors of oral cavity and oropharynx considered as operable. All were responders over 50 % to a neo-adjuvant chemo-

therapy with 5-FU Cisplatin three courses. Out of 25 patients in the surgical group, only 20 were operated and 15 reach remission (60 %). Eight had soon relapsed with or without adjuvant chemotherapy (3 additional courses). In the radiotherapy group 18/25 reach remission, 8 also relapsed, among wich 5 had received adjuvant chemotherapy. The immediate result and at short term is the same in operated and irradiated patients. Knowing that some operated patients received an additional radiotherapy because of incomplete resection or spread out cells from node capsula, we can conclude that in patients responders to chemotherapy, chances to survive are equal whathever the locoregional treatment had been and that adjuvant chemotherapy with 3 more courses was of no benefit.

Neo-Adjuvant chemotherapy on T2 cancers in oropharyngeal and oral-cavity

JP Lacoste, H Szpirglas, D Nizri*, A Thomas, S Godeau, L Benslama

Simultaneously, we realised a randomized trial neo-adjuvant chemotherapy concerning tumors T3T4 and compared two groups of tumors T2 (study non randomized) one receiving a neo-adjuvant chemotherapy in association with (CDDP, 100 mg/m^2 and 5-FU, 1,000 mg/day, continuously during 5 days) ; the other receiving surgical treatement from the start.

The first group of patients receiving the neo-adjuvant chemotherapy included 50 patients from 1987 to 1990.

The average was 54 years of age (38 men and 12 women).

The situation of cancer was :

— oral cavity, 41 ;

— oropharyngeal, 9.

Most of the patients received 3 cycles of chemotherapy.

With 64 responders, including 30 with complete response : 22 % of responses under 50 % ; 8 % of non responders ; 4 % increase of response.

The planned treatment was surgery.

Four responders would not undergo an operation.

Radiotherapy, curietherapy, loose sight-of : 28 were operated. Five non responders patients were not operated (30 % : followed-up elsewhere, loose sight-of, died during radiotherapy or waiting for treatment) and 12 % was operated-on.

Patients with complete remission after surgery have been randomised to see if they have more adjuvant treatment or not.

For the responders to the chemotherapy (24 patients) the randomisation took place between adjuvant chemotherapy (5-FU - CDDP).

For the non responders put in remission (9 patients) and without treatment (15 patients), the randomisation was done between radiotherapy and non treatment.

At the same time, a control group (38 patients, carriers of carcinoma graded T2) had to receive the surgical treatment at first.

Thirty-three were able to undergo an operation.

We obtained :

— 70 %, complete remission on the first attempt ;

— 18 % after a complementary treatment by radiotherapy ;

— 6 % start a new evolution ;

— 6 % were lost sight of.

* Département d'Oncologie et de Stomatologie Médicale, Département de radiothérapie. CHU Pitié-Salpêtrière, Paris, France

Conclusion

Patients responders to chemotherapy obtained a better score after surgery with 87.7 % of complete response.

The neo-adjuvant chemotherapy helps to improve the results (surgery alone 69.6 % of complete remission).

Complementary treatments do not necessarily improve the results of remission.

Even for small tumors the response to chemotherapy is predictive from the appearance of remission, that is confirmed by survival curves.

Abstract. A non randomized study on T2 and oropharyngeal compared a group of 50 patients receiving a neo-adjuvant chemotherapy (5-FU Cisplatin) before surgery since 1987 to 1990 to another group (38 patients) receiving a surgical treatment alone during the same time. We obtained in the first group, 64 % of major responses, to chemotherapy and 87 % reached remission after surgical treatment. The second group (38 patients) showed 70 % of complete remission after surgery alone. After analysis, that response appears for operated patients is increased by chemotherapy.

Perioperative chemotherapy in hypopharyngeal squamous cell carcinomas (SCC)

G Mamelle, C Domenge, F Eschwege, AM Leridant, B Luboinski

This study was designed to reduce the rate of distant metastasis and lessen the rate of locoregional recurrences of hypopharyngeal SCC by adding to the initial chemotherapy a post-operative chemotherapy, before radiotherapy, to prevent a possible tumour dissemination during the operation.

Methods

Eligibility

Were eligible : SCC of the pyriform sinus or of the epilarynx, with indication of total laryngectomy, with partial hypopharyngectomy and without prior treatment ; distant metastasis, multiple primaries, general contraindications for chemotherapy or surgery.

Treatment protocol

Patients received 3 consecutive courses of initial infusion (D1, D21, D42) with CDDP (100 mg/m^2) at D1, in 1 h continuous infusion after hyperhydratation, and 5-FU (1 g/m^2/day) at D1, 2, 3, 4, 5 in continuous infusion.

Surgery was performed on day 60. Then, patients received 2 post-operative courses of the same chemotherapy at day 10 and 31 after surgery. Post-operative radiotherapy was initiated at day 50.

No protocol modification was forecasted except for those patients where surgery was threatened by tumour evolution or for those who have major toxicity.

The response was appreciated by clinical examination before each course and by CT-scan and endoscopic examination before surgery.

Patient inclusion

Sixty of the 198 hypopharyngeal cancers screened between 1986 and 1989 were included. Other patients were excluded for multiple primaries (30), distant metastasis (6), prior treatment (35), surgical inoperability (6), partial functional surgical indication (20), medical contraindication (26), patient refusal (11) and inclusion error (4).

Département de Chirurgie Cervico-Faciale, Institut Gustave Roussy, Rue Camille Desmoulins, 94805 Villejuif, France

TN repartition show an important rate of T3 T4 (58/60) with 27/60 staged N2 N3. The mean age is 54 years, with 57/60 men.

The sites are the pyriform sinus (45), epilarynx (13) and postcricoid area (2). General status is OMS 0 for 55 patients and OMS 1 for the 5 last.

During this prospective study, *initial chemotherapy* was completely performed in 46 cases. It was interrupted for hematologic toxicity after 1 course in 4 cases and 2 courses in 5 cases. In 3 cases, chemotherapy was protracted. One patient died after the first course of myocardial infarction. One patient received 5 initial cycles due to temporary refusal of surgery.

In 49 cases the tumoral and nodal response to chemotheray was assessed by CT-scan and endoscopy, in 8 cases only by clinical examination. In one case no evaluation was done, one patient died after the first cycle and one was lost of follow-up after 2 cycles. Concerning the tumour response, 36 objective responses were observed (57 %) of which 11 were complete responses. 40 patients were evaluable for nodes (of which 20 N0), 17 had objective responses of which 6 were complete.

In 21/30 patients who where studied by CT-scan and endoscopy, the radioclinical compliance was good. Residual tumors was found on CT-scan whereas clinical response was complete.

Surgery was performed without modification in 47 cases (2 partial pharyngectomy, 3 total pharyngo-laryngectomy and 42 total laryngectomy with partial pharyngectomy).

Forty-eight patients who demonstrated a response close to 90 % received a radiotherapy (violation of protocol), 2 others with progressive disease were treated by an association of chemo-radiotherapy and the 2 last refused surgery.

The pathological examination of the specimen after surgery demonstrated residual tumors on 45 cases out of the 47 operated on.

In 22/46 (54 %) the nodal involvement was N + R +. There is a discrepancy between the 11 cases with objective responses and the pathologic examination which found 7 cases N + R + of which 4 had vascular embols.

35 out of the 47 patients operated on received the *post-operative chemotherapy*. The compliance was good (2 cycles) for 28 cases, 7 received only one cycle (2 hematologic toxicity, 1 fistula, 1 possible mediastinal node).

The post-operative chemotherapy was not performed in 12 cases : 2 for general contraindication (delirium tremens and cerebral infarction), 2 for toxicity during the pre-operative courses, 1 for bone metastase, 3 for delaying of healing, 3 for progressive disease during the preoperative courses and 2 who ended their treatment outside our hospital.

Only 6 hematologic toxicity were noted : 3 leucopenia grade 3 and 3 grade 2.

Post-operative radiotherapy was initiated in a mean delay of 47 days after surgery. The delay was more than 60 days in 5 cases (1 septicemia, 3 delayed healing, 1 surgery for bone metastase before radiotherapy).

The doses delivered were 50 gy on the tumor bed and the nodes with a boost of 15 gy on the areas of capsular rupture and/or for positive margins.

Radiotherapy was well tolerated and only 4 mucitis and 4 skin burns were observed. Radiotherapy was stopped during one week for only one patient.

Results

Twenty-eight patients (46.6 %) were in perfect compliance with the protocol of treatment. In 39 cases (65 %) the different phases of the protocol were respected.

With a median follow-up of 34 months, the 39 patients demonstrated : 5 local recurrences of which 3 were associated with distant metastases, 3 second primaries (2 of them controlled), 1 acute myeloblastic leukemia.

Nine patients died : 5 by tumor evolution, 3 by intercurrent disease and 1 of iatrogenic cause.

Results, compared with historical series (199 patients) with the same mean delay of follow up (30 months), show the same rate of metastasis (18 % against 20 %), a worse rate of loco-regional recurrences (12 % against 6 %), a better nodal control (no recurrence against 4 %). The 2 years survival rate is the same 78 % against 77 %.

It is interesting to note that among the patients who did not follow the protocol of treatment, 8 with tumour regression > 90 % were treated with exclusive radiotherapy. Three of them died (2 metastases, 1 local and nodal recurrence). One patient was salvaged by surgery for local recurrence. The last is lost of follow-up at 10 months, with a tracheostomia. Three patients are alive NED and without tracheostomia with a follow-up of 21, 38 and 40 months. Two others patients who presented a progressive disease during the preoperative chemotherapy were treated by an association of chemo-radiotherapy. They are alive NED with a follow-up of 11 and 41 months.

Conclusion

Only 1 patient out of 3 is eligible for this study. However it is too soon to conclude. Perioperative chemotherapy does not seem to improve the follow up of these patients. Initial chemotherapy is at present studied in a randomised EORTC trial with the aim to preserve the larynx.

Abstract. The aim of this prospective study was designed to reduce the rate of locoregional recurrences and distant metastasis of hypopharyngeal squamous cell carcinomas (SCC). SCC of the pyriform sinus or the epilarynx with indication of pharyngolaryngectomy without prior treatment, distant metastasis, multiple primaries, general contraindications for chemotherapy or surgery were eligible.

Patients received 3 consecutive courses of initial chemotherapy (CDDP 100 mg/m² D1, 5-FU 1 g/m² D1, 2, 3, 4, 5) before surgery, then 2 post-operative courses of the same chemotherapy at day 10 and 31 after surgery. Post-operative radiotherapy was initiated at day 50. Sixty of the 198 hypopharyngeal cancers screened between 1986 and 1989 were included. Tumour response to the initial chemotherapy was NR : 23, PR : 25, CR : 11. One patient died after the first course. Two patients with tumour progression received a combined radio chemotherapy and are free of disease at 11 and 41 months. Two patients refused surgery. Eight patients with tumour regression > 90 % were treated with exclusive radiotherapy. Three of them died, one other had a pharyngolaryngectomy for local recurrence and one had a tracheostomia for dyspnea. Forty-seven patients underwent surgery. Pathologic data showed only 2 specimens free of tumour and 2 others with keratin debris. For those 39 patients in which protocol treatment was respected 2LR, 3LR and DM, 5DM, 3 second primaries and one acute myeloblastic leukemia were observed. Nine patients died, 5 from tumour evolution, 3 from intercurrent disease and one of iatrogenic cause. Results compared with historical series (199 patients) with the same mean delay of follow up (30 months) show the same rate of metastasis (18 % against 20 %), a worse rate of loco regional recurrences (12 % against 6 %), a better nodal control (no recurrence against 4 %). The 2 years survival rate is the same 78 % against 77 %.

Urology

Chemotherapy for invasive bladder cancer : rationale and results

HI Scher

The development of effective combination chemotherapy regimens, and the observation that patients who succumb to bladder cancer following local treatment modalities such as surgery or radiation therapy and doing so from metastatic disease, led to the integration of chemotherapy in the treatment of locally invasive nonmetastatic (T2-4, N0M0) bladder tumors. When used in either the neo-adjuvant or adjuvant setting, the aim is to treat micrometastases, to exploit the higher sensitivity of small volume-high growth fraction tumors, and the higher cure fraction seen in patients with nodal v.s. metastatic disease [1]. The approaches are contrasted in Table 1.

Table 1. Comparison of neo-adjuvant and adjuvant therapy

	Neo-Adjuvant	Adjuvant
A. Factors favoring neo-adjuvant therapy :		
1. Chemosensitivity determined case by case *in vivo* :		
A. Response assessment *in vivo*	+	−
B. Prognostic information of response vs. non-response	+	−
C. Organ preservation possible	+	−
2. « Downstaging » of the primary tumor can :		
A. Decrease the extent and need for additional therapy	+	−
B. Convert an « unresectable » to a « resectable » lesion	+	−
C. Drug delivery not compromised by previous surgery or radiation therapy	+	−
3. Prognostic importance of response in the primary	+	−
4. Endpoint of treatment more precise	+	−
5. Potential for accelerated growth after surgery	I	
6. Better patient tolerance	+	+ / −
B. Factors favoring adjuvant therapy :		
1. Case selection :		
A. Staging error of « T » vs. « P »	−	+
B. Need based on pathologic as opposed to clinical criteria	−	+
C. Exposure of patients « cured » by local therapy to chemotherapy	−	+
2. Timing of definitive local therapy :		
A. Jeopardize curative therapy by prolonged treatment with inactive drugs	−	+
B. Refusal of potentially curative therapy	−	+

Modified after Scher H : Chemotherapy for Invasive Bladder Cancer : neo-adjuvant vs. Adjuvant. Sem Onc 17 : 555-564, 1990

Genitourinary Oncology Service, Department of Medicine, Memorial Sloan-Kettering Cancer Center, 1275 York Ave. NY, NY 10021 and Department of Medicine, Cornell University Medical College, NY, NY. Supported by CA-05826

Advantages of the neo-adjuvant approach are that an *in vivo* assessment of chemosensitivity is possible. This permits maximal treatment for responding patients, while sparing non-responders continued treatment with ineffective agents. « Downstaging » may decrease the extent of local therapy required, allowing the possibility of organ preservation. Response in the primary provides prognostic information, although a direct cause and effect cannot be implied [2]. A major limitation is that clinical criteria, which are inaccurate, form the basis for treatment decisions.

Patients treated in the adjuvant setting are selected by pathologic criteria, reducing the proportion of patients treated with chemotherapy who may not require it. Response, however, cannot be evaluated, increasing the duration of exposure to ineffective agents. Organ preservation is not possible. The major drawback of both approaches is that the « best » chemotherapy regimens produce long term survival in only 20-30 % of patients with nodal (N+) and 10-15 % of those with metastatic (M+) tumors.

A number of non-randomized phase II trials using neo-adjuvant chemotherapy have been reported. Despite variations in methodology, the trials show that chemotherapy alone can produce complete responses in the bladder, that response proportions vary inversely with depth of invasion, and that non-transitional cell histologies and carcinoma in situ are less responsive than pure transitional cell tumors. However, as the pathologic complete response proportion ($_p$CR) is < 30 % in most series, and because our ability to document which bladders are indeed free of disease is modest, chemotherapy alone cannot replace local treatment for the majority of patients. While standard therapy remains radical surgery, other groups have investigated concurrent chemotherapy and radiation therapy with encouraging results in selected cases [3, 4].

Concurrent with improvements in chemotherapy have been advances in surgery. These include a reduction in operative mortality, and refined case selection due to improvements in pre-operative staging. Further, the survival of patients with microscopic positive lymph nodes, felt to be incurable, is not « zero » as previously believed [5]. The development of continent urinary reservoirs and alternative forms of urinary diversion has reduced interest in the use of chemotherapy, with the aim toward bladder preservation. These approaches, however, are not appropriate for all patients, and when used alone, will not alter the natural history of the disease.

Despite encouraging reports, neo-adjuvant chemotherapy has not been shown to improve the survival of patients with invasive bladder cancer. To do so will require carefully designed, executed and completed randomized trials. Considering the « best » available therapy, a minimum of 300 patients with adequate follow-up will be needed to achieve statistical significance. For these reasons, neo-adjuvant chemotherapy cannot be considered « standard » therapy. When used outside of the protocol setting, case selection, including the ability to deliver adequate doses of chemotherapy, and the aim of treatment — bladder preservation, treatment of micrometastases or both — should be carefully defined at the start of treatment.

Invasive bladder tumors represent a spectrum of diseases. Critical to improved management will be refining our ability to predict metastatic potential, allowing better selection of patients for whom treatment is essential. Advances in identifying which tumors will be sensitive or resistant to a combination, and reversing drug resistance will also improve outcome. Ultimately, more effective systemic therapy will be required before a significant impact on survival can be anticipated. Only then, will the uniform treatment recommendation for all patients become an obsolete approach.

References

1. Scher HI (1990) Chemotherapy for invasive bladder cancer : neo-adjuvant vs. adjuvant. Sem Onc 17 : 555-565
2. Splinter TAW, Scher HI, EORTC-GU group, et al (1990) The prognostic value of the pT-category after combination chemotherapy for patients with invasive bladder cancer who underwent cystectomy. In : Splinter T, Scher HI (eds) Neo-Adjuvant Chemotherapy of Invasive Bladder Cancer. Alan R. Liss, Inc. New York, pp 219-224
3. Shipley WU, Kaufman DS, Heney NM (1990) Radiation therapy in bladder cancer : can its integration with chemotherapy and transurethral surgery make cystectomy unnecessary ? Oncology 4 : 25-32
4. Broderick GA, Stone AR, de Vere White R (1990) neo-bladders : clinical management and considerations for patients receiving chemotherapy. Sem Onc 17 : 598-605
5. Skinner DG, Daniels JR, Russell CA, et al (1990) Adjuvant chemotherapy following cystectomy benefits patients with deeply invasive bladder cancer. Sem Urol 8 : 279-284

Concomitant radiotherapy and Cisplatin in transitional cell bladder cancer

G Fellin, L Luciani, O Caffo, M Amichetti, A Bolner, L Busana, C Graiff, S Maluta, G Pani, G Ambrosini

External beam radiotherapy (RT) is an effective treatment modality for selected patients with invasive bladder cancer. Patients who achieve a complete clinical response (cCR) after full dose RT enjoy a 45-69 % probability of surviving 5 years.

Furthermore, the majority of patients cured of their bladder cancer by RT retained normal bladder function [1, 2, 4, 6]. Recently, encouraging results have been reported using concomitant RT and chemotherapy in patients with transitional cell bladder cancer [3, 5, 7]. Therefore, a protocol of RT with simultaneous Cisplatin (CDDP) administration was started at S Chiara Hospital in Trento in 1987. The aim was to improve local tumor control. The preliminary results are presented here.

Methods and materials

From December 1987 to April 1989, 24 consecutive patients with transitional cell bladder cancer and eligible for radical RT, underwent concomitant full dose RT and CDDP chemotherapy. There were 18 males and 6 females with a median age of 69,3 years (range 51-80).

Pre-treatment evaluation included history and physical examination, complete blood count, blood urea nitrogen, serum creatinine, liver function, audiogram, computed tomography of abdomen and pelvis, excretory urogram, bone scan, chest X-rays, cystoscopy with transurethral tumor resection (TUR) and random biopsies, evaluation under anesthesia.

Clinical stage (UICC 78-82) was : T1 in 2 patients, T2 in 2, T3 in 17 and T4 in 3 ; N0 ; M0. Five patients had some degree of ureteral obstruction. Complete TUR was possible in 4 cases, but microscopic residual was present in all.

All patients were treated on a 10 MeV linear accelerator to the pelvis by four fields box technique and received a dose of 40 Gy using five 2 Gy fractions weekly for 4 weeks. This was followed by a boost to the primary tumor for a total dose of 66 Gy in 6.5 weeks. Simultaneous CDDP was administered in bolus injection at a dose of 20 mg/m^2 every week. The response was evaluated by means of cystoscopy and repeated TUR, 3-4 months after the end of treatment. Patients in cCR underwent cystoscopy with biopsies and urine cytology at 6 months intervals. Median follow-up was 31 months (range 19-38). Survival analysis was performed by Kaplan-Meier method. Early toxicity was graduated by Miller scale.

Depts of oncology-radiotherapy and urology, S Chiara hospital, Trento, Italy

Results

There were 5 cases of grade 2 and 1 of grade 3 vomiting, 5 cases of grade 1 and 1 of grade 2 leukopenia and 1 case of grade 1 renal toxicity.

A cCR was observed in 11 patients (46 %). One of these developed subsequently distant metastases and another one developed distant, metastases and local failure simultaneously. Persistence of disease in the bladder was observed in 10 patients (superficial cancer in 2 and no change in 8). Systemic progression occurred in 3 cases. Of 10 patients with local persistence, 6 underwent salvage cystectomy. Three of these died of disease. The 3 years overall survival was 54.3 % and disease free survival retaining a functioning bladder was 37.5 %. Of 9 patients who obtained and maintained cCR after RT and CDDP, 2 had T2 and 7 had T3 disease. Only 1 of 5 patients with hydronephrosis and 1 of 4 patients with macroscopically complete TUR achieved and maintained cCR.

Late complications developed in 4 patients : mild in 3 (hematuria, cystitis, urethral stenosis) and severe in 1 (delayed healing after cystectomy).

Discussion and conclusion

Full dose RT and salvage cystectomy has been standard treatment for invasive bladder cancer at S Chiara Hospital in Trento since 1960. In a historical series the cCR rate obtained by full dose RT alone was 58 % and definitive local control 44 %. Twenty-three percent of patients were free of disease and retained a functioning bladder 3-18 years after RT. The 3 and 5 years overall survival was 49 % and 36 % respectively [2]. Therefore, this simultaneous combination of RT and CDDP does not appear to have given better results.

Furthermore, higher rates of cCR have been obtained by other authors using different schedules of simultaneous radio-chemotherapy and particularly using higher single doses of CDDP [3, 5, 7]. A possible explanation may be the loss of an adjunctive anti-tumor effect using CDDP at low, not therapeutic doses.

References

1. Blandy JP, England HR, Evans JW, Hopestone HF, Mair GMM, Mantell BS, Oliver RTD, Paris AMI, Risdon RA (1980) T3 bladder cancer — the case for salvage cystectomy. Br J Urol 52 : 506-510
2. Fellin G, Valdagni C (1989) Ruolo della radioterapia nel carcinoma della vescica profondamente infiltrante. In : I tumori genito-urinari. Casa Editrice Ambrosiana, Milano, p 51
3. Jakse G, Frommhold H, Nedden DZ (1985) Combined radiation and chemotherapy for locally advanced transitional cell carcinoma of the urinary bladder. Cancer 55 : 1659-1664
4. Quilty PM, Duncan W (1986) Primary radical radiotherapy for T3 transitional cell cancer of the bladder : an analysis of survival and control. Int J Radiat Oncol Biol Phys 12 : 853-860

5. Sauer R, Dunst J, Altendorf-Hofmann A, Fischer H, Bornhof C, Schrott KM (1990)
   Radiotherapy with and without cisplatin in bladder cancer. Int J Radiat Oncol Biol
   Phys 19 : 687-691
6. Shipley WU, Rose MA (1985) Bladder cancer. The selection of patients for treatment by full-dose irradiation. Cancer 55 : 2278-2284
7. Shipley WU, Prout GR, Einstein AB, Coombs LJ, Wajsman Z, Soloway MS,
   Englander L, Barton BA, Haferman MD (1987) Treatment of invasive bladder cancer by cisplatin and radiation in patients unsuited for surgery. J Am Med Assoc
   258 : 931-935

Neo-Adjuvant chemotherapy for invasive transitional cell carcinoma (TCC) of the urinary bladder

A Figer*, B Nussbaum*, E Mukamel**, E Fenig*, E Kunicevsky***, C Servadio**, H Lurie*, A Sulkes*

The treatment of invasive urinary bladder cancer remains a challenging problem.

In spite of progress achieved over the last 30-40 years with treatment modalities such as surgery and radiation therapy, no substantial impact on survival has been made.

Five-year survival of 40-60 % in patients presenting with stages T2 (B1) and T3a (B2) disease are reported by most authors using either radical surgery [1, 2], a combination of preoperative radiation and radical surgery [2-5] or radiation therapy and salvage cystectomy [6-8]. Most of the patients with recurrence succumb with widespread metastases within 24 months, as the recurrence is truly local in only 10 % of these cases [9, 10]. In recent years various combination chemotherapy programs have been developed for metastatic TCC of the bladder [11-14] ; such chemotherapy regimens were shown to be effective not only for metastatic but also for primary bladder tumors, leading to the design of trials of preoperative neo-adjuvant chemotherapy and radical cystectomy. We initiated such a study in our institution in 1986.

Methods

Patients and tumor characteristics

Twenty consecutive patients, 16 males and 4 females, mean age 63 years (43-76), with operable urinary bladder tumors were seen at our institution between 1986 and 1990. Seventeen patients had pure TCC, two had TCC and squamous cell carcinoma (SCC) and one TCC and adenocarcinoma.

Seventeen patients had T2 — T3a (B) tumors and in 3 patients extravesical growth stage T3b (C) was found both by CT and ultrasound prior to treatment. Eleven patients had grade (G) III tumors and in 9 patients the tumor was G IV.

Treatment design

All patients had cystoscopy with transurethral resection of bladder tumor (TURBT), chest X-ray, CT scan of chest and abdomen, abdominal sonogram (US), bone scan (BS), blood count and blood biochemistry for accurate clinical staging. Prior to the onset of chemotherapy, all patients also underwent

Departments of *Oconlogy, **Urology and ***Pathology, Beilinson Medical Center, Petah Tiqva, 49100, and Tel Aviv University Sackler School of Medicine, Tel Aviv, Israel

a MUGA scan, audiometry and creatinine clearance test. Chemotherapy consisted of two courses of M-VAC (MTX, VLB, ADR, Cisplatin) as first described at the Sloan Kettering Hospital in 1985. Three weeks after the first chemotherapy administration the patients were re-evaluated again. In the absence of metastatic disease, patients were referred to surgery, consisting of radical cystectomy with ileal conduit or cystectomy and urinary bladder replacement.

Results

Toxicity

All patients suffered nausea and vomiting and all had alopecia. Eight patients had grade $\geqslant 3$ bone marrow toxicity, 10 had grade 2 or 3 stomatitis and 2 patients developed symptomatic ototoxicity. No persistent nephrotoxicity was observed.

Treatment results

All patients underwent surgery. In 5 patients no residual tumor was found in the surgical specimen. They are all alive and disease-free at 3, 22, 24, 30 and 36 months post-surgery. Three patients had down-staging and/or down-grading of the tumor and are also alive and disease-free 10, 12 and 19 months post-surgery. In 7 patients the staging and grading remained unchanged. Six of them are alive and disease-free 4, 8, 9, 12 13 and 16 months after surgery, and one patient is alive with metastatic disease occurring 20 months after surgery. Five patients showed progressive disease in the surgical specimen and at the time of analysis were all dead of metastatic disease. The 3 patients whose specimen revealed histopathologic features other than pure TCC were all among this last group.

Adjuvant chemotherapy for operable invasive TCC of the urinary bladder has so far failed to show significant improvement in survival in controlled randomized trials.

In our trial we could demonstrate evidence of antiserum activity with 2 cycles of systemic preoperative M-VAC, as 8 out of 20 patients responded locally in the primary tumor.

The routine use of adjuvant chemotherapy in primary invasive operable TCC of the bladder has yet to be established because of the problem of the accuracy of clinical versus pathological staging and the lack of well controlled, large, randomized studies of preoperative and/or postoperative chemotherapy and surgery versus surgery alone.

Conclusion

In agreement with the latest updates on the status of adjuvant treatment of TCC of the urinary bladder in patients with operable invasive bladder cancer, further prospective randomized studies are needed, using chemotherapy as an adjuvant to local therapy versus local therapy alone, in order to determine whether the addition of currently available systemic therapy improves results over local therapy alone.

References

1. Skinner DG, Lieskovsky G (1984) Contemporary cystectomy with pelvic node dissection compared to preoperative radiation therapy plus cystectomy in the management of invasive bladder cancer. J Urol 131 : 1069-1072
2. Sagalowsky AI, Rœhrborn CG, Peters PC (1989) Long term patient survival after cystectomy for regional metastatic bladder cancer. J Urol 141 : 263A (abstr 373)
3. Bloom HJG, Hendry WF, Wallace DM, et al (1982) Treatment of T3 bladder cancer : Controlled trial of pre-operative radiotherapy and radical cystectomy versus radical radiotherapy : second report and review (for the Clinical Trials Group, Institute of Urology). Br J Urol 54 : 136-151
4. Parsons JT, Million RR (1988) Planned preoperative irradiation in the management of clinical stage B2-C (T3) bladder carcinoma. Int J Radiat Oncol Biol Phys 14 : 797-810
5. Van der Werf-Messing BHP, Friedell GH, Menon RS, et al (1982) Carcinoma of the urinary bladder T3NXM0 treated by preoperative irradiation followed by simple cystectomy. Int J Radiat Oncol Biol Phys 8 : 1849-1855
6. Swanson DA, von Eschenbach AC, Bracken RB, et al (1981) Salvage cystectomy for bladder carcinoma. Cancer 47 : 2275-2279
7. Smith JA Jr, Whitmore WF Jr (1981) Salvage cystectomy for bladder cancer after failure of definitive irradiation. J Urol 125 : 643-645
8. Freiha FS, Faysal MH (1983) Salvage cystectomy. Urology 22 : 496-498
9. Scher H (1990) Chemotherapy for invasive bladder cancer : neo-adjuvant vs adjuvant. Sem Oncol 17 : 555-565
10. Daniels JR, Skinner DG, Russell CA, Lieskovsky G, et al (1990) The role of adjuvant chemotherapy following cystectomy for invasive bladder cancer. A prospective comparative trial. In : Salmon SE (ed) Adjuvant therapy of cancer. Vol. VI. WB Saunders, Tucson, Arizona, p 475
11. Sternberg C, Yagoda A, Scher H, et al (1985) Preliminary results of methotrexate, vinblastine, adriamycin and cisplatin (M-VAC) in advanced urothelial tumors. J Urol 133 : 403-407
12. Loehrer PJ, Elson P, Kuebler JP, et al (1990) Advanced bladder cancer : a prospective intergroup trial comparing single agent cisplatin (CDDP) versus M-VAC combination therapy (INT 0078). Proc Am Soc Clin Oncol 9 : 132 (Abstr)
13. Logothetis CJ, Dexeus FH, Finn L, et al (1990) A prospective randomized trial comparing MVAC and CISCA chemotherapy for patients with metastatic urothelial tumors. J Clin Oncol 8 : 1050-1055
14. Lo RK, Freiha FS, Torti FM (1989) CMV for metastatic urothelial tumors. In : Johnson DE, Logothetis CJ, von Eschenbach AC (eds) Systemic therapy for genitourinary cancers. Year Book Medical, Chicago, IL, pp 59-63

Neo-Adjuvant chemotherapy : Epirubicin in invasive bladder cancer ; four-year follow-up

N Gad-El-Mawla, MA Mansour, S Eissa, NM Ali, N Habbobi, I Magrath

In order to improve the disease-free survival in resectable bladder cancer patients, at the National Cancer Institute (NCI), Cairo, a neo-adjuvant study was conducted starting September 1986. Preliminary results of this study were reported [4]. The importance of bladder cancer in Egypt is due to its prevalence ; 32 % of all cancers are treated at the NCI, Cairo [1]. This tumour has certain characteristics ; the histopathology is mainly squamous cell carcinoma ; 75 %, the transitional 20 % and others 5 % [1]. The tumour is mostly local, distant metastases are only 3 % [2]. The majority of the cases ; 75 % are resectable T2T3 tumours, 24 % are non-resectable, and 1 % are superficial tumours (UICC staging system). The adopted surgery is radical cystectomy and urinary diversion. This yields at the NCI, Cairo, a 36 % five-year disease-free survival [2]. Ninety percent of relapses are local recurrences [2]. Various attempts to improve these results with radiotherapy, either pre-operatively, post-operatively, or both, were tried but without a significant improvement [3].

The present report shows the results achieved, at a follow-up of 34-50 months, median 36 months, of the first trial of neo-adjuvant chemotherapy in this malignancy [4]. Epirubicin was chosen for neo-adjuvant therapy as it yielded 60 % responses in a phase II study in advanced bladder cancer patients [5].

Material and methods

From September 1986 to November 1988, a consecutive series of patients with presumably resectable T2T3 bilharzial bladder cancer, were randomly assigned to be treated by a standard surgical approach, or by surgery and neo-adjuvant Epirubicin.

Group I : patients received 2 courses of Epirubicin at a dose of 120 mg/m² i.v. push every 21 days. At day 22 they were subjected to radical cystectomy with urinary diversion. Resected specimens were sent for histo-pathological examination, which included grading of tissue necrosis due to chemotherapeutic effects. After wound healing, patients received 4 more courses of Epirubicin at the same dose every 21 days, as adjuvant therapy.

Group II : patients were subjected to radical cystectomy. Follow-up was carried out for all patients monthly during the first year, and every 3 months during the second year.

National cancer institute, Cairo ; National cancer institute, Bethesda, Md, USA ; Farmitalia Carlo Erba, Milano, Italia
Mailing address : Prof. Dr Nazli Gad-El-Mawla, M.D., Prof. of medical Oncology, National cancer institute, Fom-El-Khalig, Cairo, Egypt

Results

Between September 1986 and November 1988, 71 patients were entered into the study. Thirty-four patients were assigned to group I, and 37 to group II (Table 1). In group I, 33 patients underwent radical cystectomy and 1 patient electrofulguration. Chemotherapeutic effects in resected specimens are shown in (Table 2). Resected lymph nodes were negative in 28 cases and positive in 5. At a follow-up of 34-50, median 36 months, 2 patients died in the first post-operative week, and 6 patients relapsed with local pelvic recurrences at 4, 6, 7, 8, 13 and 14 months. Five of these patients subsequently died of the disease, and one is currently receiving chemotherapy. During the follow-up, 26 remained free of disease, one died from uremia, and 25 are still alive and disease-free (Table 3). Chemotherapy toxicity was tolerable (Table 4).

Table 1. Patients characteristics

	Group I	Group II
Number	34	37
Males	25	25
Females	9	12
Age range	30-63 y	30-65 y
mean	48-35 y	51-78 y
Squamous cell ca	21	25
Transitional cell ca	12	8
Other histology	1	4
T2/T3 tumour	2/32	3/34

Table 2. Chemotherapy effects in resected specimens

Pathology	Grade 0		Grade I		Grade II		Grade III	
	N	%	N	%	N	%	N	%
Squamous C C	1	4.76	11	52.38	6	28.57	3	14.29
Transitional C C	5	41.67	5	41.67	0	0	2	16.66
Undifferentiated C C			1	100				

C C : Carcinoma

Table 3. Follow-up 34 - 50 months, median 36

	Group I	Group II
No. of patients	34	37
CCR	25	14
Relapse	6	12
Early death	2	3
Died at home	1	3
LFU	0	5

CCR : Continuous complete remission
LFU : Lost to follow-up

Table 4. Toxicities

	Grade I (%)	Grade II (%)	Grade III (%)
Nausea/vomiting	59	8	0
Anemia	23	3	0
Alopecia	21	62	15
Asthenia and Fatigue	47	23	0
Cardiac	3	0	0

Thirty-seven patients were assigned to group II, and all were subjected to surgery, radical in 36 and electrofulguration in one. Resected lymph nodes were negative for tumour in 26 cases and positive in 10 cases. Post-operative complications were similar in both groups. At the same period of follow-up, 3 patients died in the first post-operative week, 12 patients developed recurrent tumour, 63 % within the first 6 months, and 82 % within the first year. Eight patients were lost to follow-up, and 14 are still alive and free of disease (Table 3).

At a median follow-up of 36 months (range 34-50 months) 25 patients from group I, and 14 patients from group II are still alive and disease-free, for a disease-free survival rate of 73.5 % versus 37.9 % (Fig. 1).

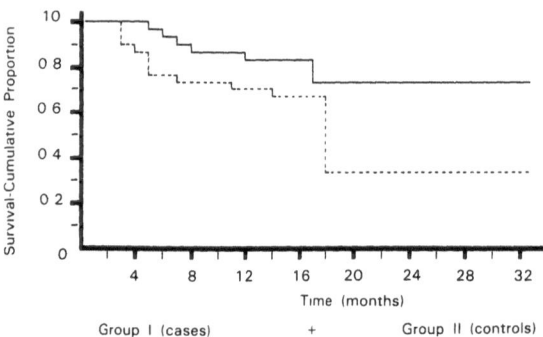

Fig. 1. Disease free rate (Kaplan-Meier)

Discussion and conclusion

In view of our observation that a number of chemotherapeutic agents are active in patients with recurrent or inoperable cancer of the bilharzial bladder [6], we decided to explore the effectiveness of adjuvant chemotherapy, in addition to radical surgery, as a mean of reducing the relapse rate. We chose to use Epirubicin — one of the most active agents in our phase II studies. Doses of 40 mg/m^2 weekly, and 80 mg/m^2 every 3 weeks had achieved response rates of 50 and 60 % respectively, in 2 groups of patients with advanced bladder cancer [5]. Prior to initiating the present study, we concluded an additional phase I-II study, in which we escalated the dose of Epirubicin in successive groups of patients in order to find the maximally tolerable dose in Egyptian patients with bladder cancer. A dose of 120 mg/m² was well tolerated [5], and so was chosen for the present study. The results of the present trial showed a marked reduction in the relapse rate of patients treated with Epirubicin. A total of 6 of the 32 evaluable patients relapsed, 4 in the first year, and 2 in the second. The median time for relapse was 9 months. In contrast, 12 of the 26 evaluable patients in the control group relapsed. Since 8 patients were lost to follow-up in this group, the actual number of relapses could have been greater. An additional finding of interest was that more of the patients who received pre-operative therapy had negative nodes at the time of surgery (5/33), than did those in the control group (10/36).

These results point out that neo-adjuvant chemotherapy, and specifically Epirubicin, will provide a clear advantage in disease-free survival in this common Egyptian cancer. This stimulated us to start a new randomized study with reduction in the extent of surgery allowing continent urinary diversion with the preservation of potency in males. Male patients with T3 bladder cancer are subjected to this modified radical cystectomy, followed by post-operative adjuvant chemotherapy with Epirubicin in group I, and follow-up with no chemotherapy in group II. This study started September 1990.

References

1. Elsebai I (1978) Cancer of the bilharzial bladder. Urologic Research 6 : 233-236
2. Elsebai I (1983) End results of cancer in the bilharzial bladder. Prognosis, Recurrences, and Rehabilitation. In : Elsebai I (ed) Bladder Cancer, vol. II. CRC press, pp 163-197
3. Ghoneim MA, Awwad HK (1983) 2000 rad pre-operative radiotherapy and cystectomy for the treatment of carcinoma of the bilharzial bladder. In : Elsebai I (ed) Bladder Cancer, vol. II. CRC press, p 127-133
4. Gad El Mawla N, Mansour MA, Eissa S, Ali NM, Elattar I, Hamza MR, Khaled H, Habbobi N, Magrath I, Elsebai I (1991) A randomized pilot study of high-dose epirubicin as neo-adjuvant chemotherapy in the treatment of cancer of the bilharzial bladder. Annals of Oncology (Accepted for publication)
5. Gad El Mawla N, Mansour MA, Eissa S, Ali NM, Habbobi N, Magrath I (1988) Eprirubicin in bilharzial bladder cancer : a phase II and neo-adjuvant trials. Proceedings of ASCO 17 : 123
6. Gad El Mawla, Hamza MR, Zikri Z, Elserafi M, El Khodary A, Khaled H, Abdel Wareth A (1989) Chemotherapy in invasive carcinoma of the bladder. A review of phase II trials in Egypt. Acta Oncol 28 : 73-75

Preliminary results of a protocol of pre-operative radiation therapy with concomitant chemotherapy for invasive bladder cancer

M Housset, Y Chretien, C Maulard, P Brunel, AT Lachand, JP Hallez, B Dufour, F Baillet

The classical treatment of T3 Bladder Cancer is surgery. The place of irradiation remains limited, for example in the frame of associated radio-surgery protocol. The incidence of pathological down-staging following 40-50 Gy pre-operative irradiation has been noted in more than 60 % of patients, and the incidence of histologically positive lymph nodes is half of the expected incidence (20 %). But only 30 to 40 % of the patients, with clinical T3 bladder cancer have no tumor in cystectomy specimen after pre-operative irradiation. Furthermore, in the NSABP trial, the survival of patients who were down-staged to pT0 enjoyed a significant survival advantage over patients whose tumors were not down-staged [1].

Several experiments have clearly shown a potentialisation of the effects of radiotherapy, by concomitant chemotherapy. This potentialisation of irradiation is linked to an enhancement of initial DNA target damage and interferenc with DNA damage repair. These experiments have been confirmed through clinical studies notably with 5-FU and CDDP. Based on the above observations, we started at the Necker Hospital in Paris, early 1988, on patients with T3 bladder cancer, a pre-operative protocol associating the two therapies. Our objective was to increase the complete histological response rate and to observe if, in patients with complete response, a conservative treatment excluding surgery was possible. All patients were available for evaluation.

Methods

Patients characritics : 29 T3 bladder cancer patients and 1 T2, with a pelvic adenopathy identified by CT scanner were selected. There were 26 males and 4 females, with a mean age of 66 years (3-82 years). All patients at the time of treatment had their disease confined to the pelvis, as determined by chest X-ray, bone scan, CT scan. Abnormal IVP, with hydronephrosis, were shown in 44 % of the patients. All 30 patients had an initial TUR, with macroscopically satisfactory results (removal of all visible tumor) in 47 % of the patients.

The pre-operative concomitant radio-chemotherapy protocol : all patients were treated, on a 5 MeV linear accelerator, to the whole pelvis by a four fields box technique. The total irradiation dose is 24 Gy over 17 days with 6 Gy on days 1, 3, 15 and 17, with a daily bi-fractionation. In our experiment, this would be equivalent to 40-45 Gy in classical fractionation. Furthermore, 5-FU

Centre de Traitement des Tumeurs, Hopital Necker, 149, rue de Sèvres 75015, Paris, France

(400 mg/m²/d) and CDDP (15 mg/m²/d) were administered from day 1 to day 3 and from day 15 to day 17, by short infusion of 4 to 6 hours.

A second new complete examination, with cytology and with a deep resection of any abnormalities as well as the initial site of the tumor was performed 5 to 6 weeks after the irradiation. Two weeks after this second examination a systematic cystectomy was initially planned in all patients, but we will see that we were able to avoid surgery in a selected number of these patients.

Results

The endoscopic control at 6 weeks shows 23 over the 30 patients (76 %) with complete response. Therefore, 7 patients exhibited an incomplete response. Depending on the quality of the initial resection, the residual tumor rate varies from 7 % for complete macroscopical resection to 37 %.

Cystectomy was performed in all patients with residual tumor. Surgery confirmed in all cases the presence of tumor and, in 4/7 patients, histologically positive associated lymph nodes. In the 23 patients with complete response, 12 did not undergo the planned cystectomy and bladder conservation treatment was attempted. These 12 patients received an additionnal smaller boost field of 12 Gy with concomittant chemotherapy. So far, no patient had a local recurrence. The remaining 11 patients, despite complete response, underwent the planned surgery. None had a residual tumor or positive histologically lymph node, suggesting the ability of this treatment to control both local and regional node disease. Furthermore, it seems that we have a good correlation between the results of the resection at 6 weeks, and the results of surgery. This correlation is obviously a must if, in the future, conservative non surgical treatment is to be performed in a larger population of patients.

Discussion

Our rate of complete response after the 6 weeks resection is twice as high as the rate achieved through classical pre-operative radiotherapy. This is in line with other results from the literature where all types of pre-operative concomittant radio-chemotherapy protocols gave a complete response rates equal or superior to 60 % [2-5].

Does the increase in complete response correlates with an increase in survival rate? Conclusions concerning long term survival cannot be drawn at this moment because of limited follow-up. Nevertheless, for the complete response patients, we observe an increase in short term survival with a 83 % survival rate at 2 years, whereas for residual tumor patients the survival rate is 23 %. This can be explained by a frequency of metastasis far superior in the residual tumor patients (5/7 for residual tumor patients and 3/23 for complete response patients).

Does this pre-operative concomitant radio-chemotherapy increases the rate of post-operative complications for patients undergoing surgery? Not in our experiment compared with our historical records. Five patients could even have an enterocystoplast replacement. By the way, no patient treated by conservative treatment exhibited radiotherapeutic complication.

Is there enough historical experience to prescribe or start prescribing conservative treatment in complete response patients after concomittant radiochemotherapy protocol ? Our results as well as others in the literature allow us to ask the question. However, this concept should be evaluated in randomized studies and long term results should be obtained. It should be noted, that the local recurrence rate in completely responding inoperable patients treated by full dose irradiation with concomittant chemotherapy is between 5 % and 29 % [6-10].

Conclusion

In potentially operable patients, the local efficacy of our neo-adjuvant therapeutical protocol is twice as high as the one obtained by conventionnal preoperative irradiation. The complete response patients, 76 % of our population, exhibited a superior short term survival rate, with a non mutilating treatment in 50 % of the patients. In potentially inoperable patient this type of therapeutic protocol should be systematically discussed, if not to increase the survival rate, at least to increase the quality of this survival.

References

 1. Slack NH, Bross IDJ, Proust GR Jr (1977) Five-year follow-up results of a collaborative study of therapies for carcinoma of the bladder. J Surg Oncol 9 : 393-405
 2. Coppin C, Brown E, the GU Tumor Group (1986) Concurrent cisplatin with radiation for locally advanced bladder cancer : a pilot study suggesting improved survival. Proceedings of ASCO, A 382
 3. Tester W, Porter A, Asbell S et al (1989) Combined modality program with possible organ preservation for invasive bladder cancer : preliminary results of RTOG Protocol 85-12. Proceedings of ASCO, A 548
 4. Venturi M, Merlano M, Michelotti A et al (1989) neo-adjuvant or definitive alternating chemotherapy and radiotherapy for infiltrating bladder cancer. Am J Clin Oncol 12 : 63-67
 5. Marks LB, Kaufman S, Prout GR jr, Heney NM, Griffin PP, Shipley WU (1988) Invasive bladder carcinoma : preliminary report of selective bladder conservation by transurethral surgery, upfront MCV chemotherapy and pelvic irradiation plus cisplatin. Int J Radiation Oncol Biol Phys 15 : 877-883
 6. Wajsman Z, Klimberg I, Parsons J et al (1989) Bladder sparing treatment for muscle invasive transitionnal cell carcinoma : systemic chemotherapy followed by radiation therapy with adjunctive cisplatin. Proceedings ASCO, A 513
 7. Shipley W, Einstein A, Coombs L et al (1987) Cisplatin and full dose irradiation for patients with invasive bladder carcinoma : a multi institutional group experience. Proceedings of the American Radium Society, A 1
 8. Jakse G, Frommhold H, Dieter zur Nedden (1985) Combined radiation and chemotherapy for locally advanced transitionnal cell carcinoma of the urinary bladder. Cancer 55 : 1659-1664
 9. Sauer R, Schrott KM, Dunst J et al (1987) Preliminary results of treatment of invasive bladder carcinoma with radiotherapy and cisplatin. Int J Radiation Oncol Biol Phys 15 : 871-875
10. Eapen L, Stewart D, Danjoux P et al (1989) Intraarterial cisplatin and concurrent radiation for locally advanced bladder cancer. J Clin Oncol 7 : 230-235

Induction chemotherapy with Methotrexate, Vinblastine, Epiadriamycin and Carboplatin (M-VEP) in transitional cell urothelial cancer

G Aravantinos, DV Skarlos, H Linardou, C Christodoulou, C Deliveliotis, A Kostakopoulos, T Vardoulakis, K Dimopoulos

Radical cystectomy remains the standard treatment for patients with transitional cell urothelial carcinoma (TUCC) of the bladder with muscle invasion and/or N 0-2. However, 70-80 % of these patients eventually die of disseminated disease. Systemic treatment might eradicate co-existing metastases [1]. Cisplatin, Methotrexate, Fluorouracil, Vinblastine, Mitomycin and Carboplatin have been used as single agents in metastatic disease, with 20-35 % overall response (OR) being reported. Combinations including Cisplatin yield a relatively high OR (45-70 %) and complete response (CR) rate. A 75 % OR with 35 % CR was reported with the M-VAC (Methotrexate, Vinblastine, Adriamycin, Cisplatin) regimen [2, 3].

Neo-adjuvant induction chemotherapy aims at eradicating micrometastases, debulking the tumor to facilitate surgery or radiation and avoiding amputational procedures. Its disadvantages are its high cost and a delay of the next therapeutic procedure. A 70 % OR with 50 % CR was reported in 2 trials with M-VAC induction [3, 4]. However, the regimen used is associated with severe toxicity. In an attempt to improve patient compliance, we used the M-VEP combination therapy, a modification of M-VAC. The aim of this ongoing study is to obtain an indication on the activity and toxicity of this regimen.

Patients and methods

Twenty-five patients with TUCC were entered between April 1988 and October 1990. Patient characteristics are shown in Table 1. Three patients had been previously irradiated and 6 had received intravesical instillation.

Table 1. Patients characteristics

Sex		male 24	female 1
Age		48-77	median 65
P.S. (WHO) grade			
	0 : 17		
	1 : 7		
	2 : 1		
Stage	T2 (NO) 6		
	T3a 5		
	T3b 7		
	T2-4 (N2) 1		

3 rd Medical Oncology Dept, Agii Anargiri cancer hospital, Kifissia, Athens and Dept of Urology, University of Athens, Greece

Evaluation before treatment and after completion of chemotherapy included physical examination, bimanual examination, chest x-ray, hematology, blood chemistry, computerized tomography of the abdomen and pelvis, isotope bone scan, intravenous urography, cystoscopy with biopsies and, when indicated, transurethral resection. Tumor response was determined according to WHO criteria ; only patients achieving a CR or partial response (PR) were considered as responders.

Four to six cycles of M-VEP were given, consisting of Methotrexate, 25 mg/m^2 i.v., and Vinblastine 2.5 mg/m^2 i.v. on days 1, 15 and 22, Epirubicin, 25 mg/m^2 i.v. and Carboplatin, 250 mg/m^2 i.v.on day 1, and Leucovorin rescue with 15 mg q.i.d. orally to a total dose of 120 mg, 24 h after methotrexate. Treatment was administered on an outpatient basis. Epirubicin was omitted from treatment in one case with cardiopathy.

Results and discussion

Of the 25 patients entered, 24 are evaluable for response ; one has not yet completed treatment. Treatment was interrupted after 2-3 courses in 3 patients. This good compliance could be due to the patients' good performance status and to the tolerable toxicity of the treatment regimen.

A total of 101 treatment courses were administered. Toxicity is indicated in Table 2. Myelosuppression caused a total of 26 weeks treatment delay in 11 patients. One episode of infection necessitated hospitalization for 7 days. Vinblastine was omitted due to neurologic toxicity after the first and 4th course, respectively.

Table 2. Toxicity (percent)

	Grade (WHO)		
	1	2	3
Leucopenia	20	12	8
Thrombocytopenia	8		
Nausea/Vomiting	12	16	4
Neurologic	12	8	
Alopecia	8		
Infection		4	

Complete response was achieved in 6 patients (25 %, approx. confidence limits 10-47 %) and partial response in 10. The overall response rate (66.6 %, confidence limits 44-84 %) was similar to that reported with the M-VAC regimen ; it should be noted, however, that the patient selection is not superposable (inclusion of only N0 disease in the Mayo Clinic study) and that the CR in the Memorial study was estimated postcystectomy, not after the completion of induction chemotherapy [2, 4].

Three patients with CR relapsed after 7.7 and 12 months ; they remain disease-free after a salvage cystectomy. Up to January 1, 1990, disease-free survival after chemotherapy is 13-24 + months (median 20) and time to progression for all responding patients 4 + to 33 + months (median 11). Nineteen patients are still alive ; 5 patients died of tumor progression and 1 from myocardial infarction.

In conclusion, induction chemotherapy with M-VEP in patients with TUCC (stages T2-4a N0-2 M0) is effective, relatively well tolerated and can be administered on an outpatient basis.

References

1. Yagoda A (1988) neo-adjuvant chemotherapy in bladder cancer. Supplement to Urology 31 (2) : 9-12
2. Yagoda A (1988) Chemotherapy of urothelial tract cancer : memorial Sloan-Kettering Cancer Center experience. In : De Vita V Jr, Hellman S, Rosenberg S (eds) Important advances in oncology. Lippincott, Philadelphia, p 143
3. Sternberg CN, Yagoda A, Scher HI et al (1988) M-VAC (methotrexate, vinblastine, doxorubicin and cisplatin) for advanced transitional cell carcinoma of the urothelium). J Urol 139 : 461-469
4. Zincke H, Sen SE, Hahn RG, Keating JP (1988) neo-adjuvant chemotherapy for locally advanced transitional cell carcinoma of the bladder : do local findings suggest a potential for salvage of the bladder ? Mayo Clin Proc 63 : 16-22

Neo-Adjuvant chemotherapy aiming at bladder preservation

CCL Paz-Ares, P Lianes, M Diaz-Puente, J Passas, A Rodriguez, C Gravalos, I Sevilla, H Cortés-Funes

Following reports of significant antitumor activity against metastatic and primary sites of TCC with new chemotherapy (CT) regimens (CMV, M-VAC), we started, in March 1987, a prospective study with neo-adjuvant CMV (Cisplatin, Methotrexate, Vinblastine), hoping to act over micrometastatic disease, cause of death in 50 % of patients with standard treatments, and subsequently increase overall survival. Secondly, we tried to avoid some cystectomies.

Material and methods

Patients with histologically proven urothelial cancer of the bladder of clinical category T2, T3 or T4 (N0 M0) were admitted into the study. Other criteria of eligibility included age < 75 years, performance status < 2, creatinine clearance > 50 ml/min, normal blood counts, bilirubin < 1.5 mg %, no prior irradiation or systemic chemotherapy. Clinical staging included a cystoscopy with transurethral resection of the tumor (TURB) and multiple biopsies (selected at random), bimanual palpation of the pelvis under anesthesia, urinary cytology, chest x-ray, CT scan of the abdomen and pelvis. Transrectal sonography, radionucleide scan were optionally performed or when clinically indicated. The same work-up was made after 3 and 6 CT cycles and quaterly in non-cystectomised patients.

The followed treatment response criteria were : CR ; complete disappearance of all evidence of disease (including no T_{is}) for > 1 month, PR ; > 50 % decrease in tumor size of downstaging of > 1 category, PROG ; > 25 % increase in tumor size, and NR ; other categories.

Initially, all patients received 3 cycles of Cisplatin (C) 100 mg/m^2 day 1, Methothrexate (M) 30 mg/m^2 days 1 and 8, Vinblastine 4 mg/m^2 days 1 and 8 every 3 weeks (dose modifications were done according to Harker). Thereafter, a re-evaluation was made and patients, judged to have a complete clinical remission (cCR), received 3 additional CMV courses. At this point, patients who mantained CR were closely followed-up, but those who showed clinical progression suffered cystectomy. Non-cCR at first reevaluation were also cystectomised (Fig. 1).

Between March 1987 and March 1990, 43 patients were recruited and all but 4 are evaluable (2 protocol violations and 2 short follow-up). There were 37 males and 2 females, with a median age of 62 years (range 33-75). Performance status was 0 or 1 (ECOG) in 37. Macroscopical complete TURB of the tumor was done in 21 patients before chemotherapy. One third had prior

Hospital « 12 de Octubre ». Servicio de Oncología Médica E-28041 Madrid, Spain

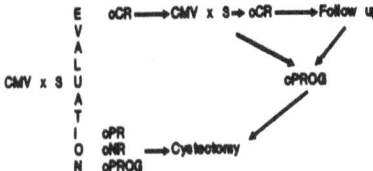

Fig. 1. Therapeutic scheme

	cCR	cPR	cNR/prog	
NED	17 (B+ 16)	3 (B+ 1)	2	22
Alive with Disease	2	2		4
Dead with Tumor	4	1	8	13
	23	6	10	

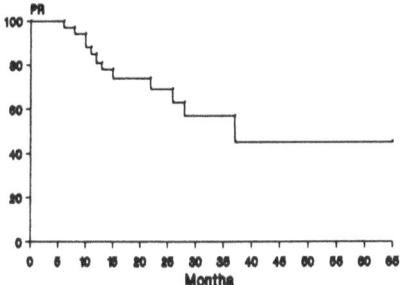

Fig. 2. Current status vs initial response

Fig. 3. Overall survival

superficial bladder carcinoma treated with TURB and/or intravesical therapy. Histological review showed 37 transitional Ca and 2 anaplastic Ca : (5 had synchronous in situ Ca). Grade was G3 in 30 (76 %) patients and G2 in 9 (24 %) patients. The initial clinical stage was T1 in 5 patients (13 %), T2 or T3 in 18 patients (46 %), T3b in 13 patients (33 %) and T4 in 3 patients (8 %).

Results

Following administration of the first 3 CMV cycles, 29 patients (74 %) responded (26 cCR and 6 cPR) and 10 (26 %) were non responders (8 cCR and 2 cProg).

Presently, with a median follow-up of 16 months (4-43), 26 of the total group are alive (67 %) and 16 of them preserve their bladder (41 %). Current status according to initial response to chemotherapy is illustrated in Figure 2. It should be remarked that 8 out of the 10 NR-patients died, in a median time after initial treatment of 12 months (7-22).

Estimated overall survival after 4 years of the 39 patients is 45 % (Fig. 3), being 62 % for CR and 0 % for NR ($P < 0.001$). There were no differences in response rate or survival depending on the grade of resection of the tumor before chemotherapy, clinical stage or histological grade. Cystectomy was performed in 18 cases. All the pathological specimens showed viable tumor. Comparing preoperative clinical stage versus pathological stage, we found 13 patients were correctly staged, 2 overstaged and 2 understaged.

Toxicity

The toxicity analysis of the 183 administered cycles revealed nausea and vomiting (g. III-IV) in 80 % and haematological depression (g. III-IV), renal disfunction (g. I), neuropathy (g. I) and mucositis in 8 %, 7 %, 8 % and 20 % of the patients. No toxic deaths were seen.

Conclusions

CMV chemotherapy induces high clinical response rates.

The obtention of cCR predicts « good prognosis » for survival and bladder preservation.

NR patients could be considered for second line treatment and/or bladder preservation.

Local radiotherapy may help to maintain local control.

Randomized studies (some in course) are needed to know the effect of − 2 chemotherapy on survival and bladder preservation.

References

1. Harker WG, Meyers FJ, Freiha FS et al (1985) Cisplatin, Methotrexate and Vinblastine (CMV) : an effective chemotherapy regimen for metastatic transitional cell carcinoma of the urinary tract. J Clin Oncol 3 : 1463-1470
2. Meyers FJ, Palmer JM, Freiha FS et al (1985) The fate of the bladder in patients with metastatic bladder cancer treated with Cisplatin, Methotrexate and Vinblastine : a Northern California Oncology Group Study. J Urol 134 : 1118-1121
3. Scher HI (1989) Chemotherapy for invasive bladder tumors. In : Splinter TAW, Scher HI (ed) neo-adjuvant chemotherapy in invasive bladder cancer. Progress in clinical and biological research, Volume 353. Wiley-Liss, New York, p 1

Immunotherapy in metastatic renal cell cancer. The Lyon's experience on 100 patients

S Negrier* ** A Mercatello**, M Bret**, P Thiesse*, R Oskam***,
CR Franks***, JF Moskovtchenko**, T Philip*

It is now accepted that cytokine therapy i.e. Interferon α (IFNα) and Interleukin 2 (IL2) are active in metastatic kidney cancer [1, 2, 3]. Significant questions remain, however, about the optimal application of these therapies as well as their real impact in this disease. Since october 1987, we have developed in Lyon an important evaluated immunotherapy program and more than 100 patients with metastatic renal cell cancer have been included in different successive protocols. Between october 1987 until august 1990, 135 patients were referred to our institution. Thirty-five (26 %) were excluded according to the protocol criteria and 100 were eligible. Three different groups of patients have to be considered.

Group 1

Twenty-six patients received a continuous infusion of IL2 according to the West schedule [2] and were included in the European Eurocetus trials. In this group of 25 evaluable patients, 5 partial responses were achieved (response rate : 20 %). In addition, 15 patients in progression or in relapse after this therapy received a rescue protocol with Interferon α and Vinblastine. In 12 evaluable patients, 9 were in progression despite both cytokine therapy, whereas 3 patients with prior objective responses to IL2 achieved, with this protocol, an important partial response in 2 cases, and a long lasting stabilisation of the lesions in one.

These results evidence that the same patients are sensitive to both cytokines. Toxicity was not negligible in this group, but acceptable since no toxic death and only 2 grade 4 (WHO) toxicities were registered.

Group 2

Thirty-two patients received a combination of bolus I.V. doses of IL2 and IFN together with LAK cells. In 28 evaluable patients, 2 complete and 5 partial responses were observed (one is now in complete remission after surgery). The response rate is of 25 %. Toxicity was more significant than in the previous group with 4 grade 4 (WHO) toxic events including one toxic death. Seven patients who were progressive after this protocol together with 10 patients previously treated with IFN, received a rescue protocol, combining IL2 and TNF (Tumor Necrosis Factor). The results were disappointing with only one partial and short response.

---

* Centre Léon Bérard. ** Hôpital E. Herriot Lyon France. *** Eurocetus Amsterdam, The Netherlands

These results show that the combination of IL2 and IFNα do not significantly improve the response rate. Of note, the non significant gain (25 % vs 20 %) observed between the results of groups 1 and 2, could be related to the increased doses of cytokines as well as the combination. The results of the combined therapy IL2 and TNF were disappointing and TNF is not more considered in our protocols.

Group 3

This group corresponds to the ongoing protocols and 3 different studies are undergone.

— Continuous infusion in patients above 65 years of age. At this point of time, 17 patients were treated without any life-theatening toxicity. In 16 evaluable patients, 1 partial and 2 complete responses were observed. The response rate in the oldest patients is comparable to that obtained in the other groups.

— Low doses of subcutaneous IL2 and IFNα according to the schedule described by Atzpodien et al [4]. This new ambulatory schedule was done in collaboration with Fondation Bergonié in Bordeaux. The preliminary response rate is of 3/13 (23 %) with 1 complete response ans 2 partial responses. No grade 4 toxic event was yet registered but general toxicity was present in almost all the patients (fever, fatigue, anorexia, weight loss).

— IL2 alone in patients with previously treated brain metastases. This is a pilot study that will be realized as a multicentric french trial. Three patients have already been treated in Lyon without any specific complication.

Although IL2 and IFN are approved and registred by Health Authority in France, the biological and clinical evaluation of these therapies have to be actively pursued. However, our results have evidenced some points of concern i.e. the same patients are able to respond to both IFN and IL2 and consequently the combination of those cytokines do not improve the response rate. In addition, the oldest patients are potential responders as well as younger patients and age cannot be a selection criteria.

References

1. Rosenberg SA, Lotze MT, Muul ML et al (1989) A progress report on the treatment of 157 patients with advanced cancer using lymphokine-activated killer cells and interleukin-2 or high-dose interleukin-2 alone. New Engl J Med 316 : 889-897
2. West WH, Tauer KW, Yanelli JR, Marshall GD, Orr DW, Thurman GB, Oldham RK (1987) Constant infusion recombinant Interleukin-2 in adoptive immunotherapy of advanced cancer. New Engl J Med 316 : 898-905
3. Negrier S, Philip T, Stoter G, Fossa SD, Janssen S, Iacone A, Cleton FS, Eremin O, Israel L, Jasmin C, Rugarli C, Masse HVD, Thatcher N, Symann M, Bartsch HH, Bergmann L, Bijman JT, Palmer PA, Franks CR (1990) Interleukin-2 (IL2) with or without LAK cells in metastatic renal cell carcinoma : a report of a European multicentre study. Eur J Cancer Clin Oncol 25 : 21-28
4. Atzpodien J, Korfer A, Franks CR, Poliwoda M, Kirchner H (1990) Home therapy with recombinant interleukin-2 and interferon α-2b in advanced malignancies. Lancet 335 : 1509-1512

Breast

Induction chemotherapy prior to definitive treatment improves outcome in stage III carcinoma of the breast

GF Schwartz*, SL Carter, J Panico

The uniformly dismal outcome of patients with locally advanced carcinoma of the breast has been recognized since Haagensen and Stout described criteria of operability fifty years ago. In an attempt to reverse these almost inevitably unfavorable results, in 1979 we began to treat women with locally advanced breast cancer, AJC Stage III, by induction (neo-adjuvant) chemotherapy before any surgical treatment other than initial (incisional) biopsy to confirm the diagnosis and determine hormone receptor status (as well as flow cytometry when it became available) [1]. All women presenting initially with Stage III breast cancer were considered candidates for this study. Patients, entered between 1979 and 1988, were reclassified per the AJC 3rd edition guidelines [2], so that only patients currently classified as Stage III, regardless of classification at time of entry, are included. Serial measurements of tumor are involved ; lymph nodes were used to assess response ; responders were defined as patients whose tumors decreased in diameter by at least 25 %, or whose lymph nodes decreased by 50 %. Three cycles of therapy determined this decision, and responders were continued on this regimen until a plateau was reached. Definitive surgery was then performed, tailored to the response, with a larger number of patients being treated by irradiation following local excision and axillary dissection through the years of the study.

Between mid-1979 and June 30, 1990, 137 women with Stage III cancer of the breast (AJC 3rd edition, 1988, definition), between the ages of 22 and 83, were entered into this study group. If the older classification of Stage III had been used, the group would have included 154 patients ; thus, 17 women were deleted from the group constituting this report, regardless of their outcome, since they no longer fit the current Stage III definition. These 137 women have been followed from 1 month to 11 years from the time of definitive treatment or determination that they were not responders. Patients currently « on treatment » have not been included. For responders, the mean number of cycles of chemotherapy before definitive treatment was six. Follow-up after definitive treatment ranged from 1 month to 11 years, with mean follow-up of 3.5 years. Of the entire group, 71 % responded, and 76 % of these women have remained disease-free. Non-response was almost inevitably followed by recurrence and death.

Induction chemotherapy produces significant tumor regression in a majority of patients with Stage III breast cancer, permitting definitive local therapy

The department of surgery, Jefferson Medical College, and the Breast Health Institute, Philadelphia, PA 19107 USA
* GF Schwartz, Professor of Surgery, Jefferson Medical College, 1015 Chestnut Street, Suite 510, Philadelphia, PA 19107 USA

with greater success than heretofore expected. A more optimistic attitude has replaced our previously dismal outlook for this group of patients.

References

1. American Joint Committee on Cancer (1988) Manual for Staging of Cancer, Third Edition, JB Lippincott Company, Philadelphia, pp 145-150
2. Schwartz GF, Cantor RI and Biermann WA (1987) neo-adjuvant chemotherapy before definitive treatment for Stage III carcinoma of the breast. Archive of Surgery, 122 : 1430-1434

Multimodality treatment of stage II, III and IV breast cancer with biochemical modulation of 5-FU/Leucovorin and estrogen recruitment

S Swain, S Honig, L Walton, C Berg*, T Spitzer

This study was designed to evaluate the efficacy of an intensive induction regimen in patients with locally advanced breast cancer (LABC) as defined by the UICC 1987 staging [1] which includes Stage IIIA and IIIB disease, clinical T3N0, pathologic Stage II with ≥ 4 + nodes, and Stage IV disease (T3N0 is now considered Stage II). This induction regimen included the use of a high-dose Leucovorin to biochemically modulate 5-Fluorouracil. This has been shown to have a response rate of 24 % in heavily pretreated patients with metastatic breast cancer [2]. A previous study in the Medicine Branch, at NCI, treated patients with a combination of Cyclophosphamide, Doxorubicin, Methotrexate, 5-Fluorouracil, and hormonal synchronization with Tamoxifen and Premarin (CAMFTP) to best response [3]. This yielded high overall response rates of 95 %, but median disease-free survival was 34 months and was approximately equivalent in both Stage IIIA and IIIB disease. The extent of response (i.e. CR or PR, or CR with negative biopsy) did not predict response duration. Therefore we designed this study using a more intensive regimen to give patients nine cycles of induction chemotherapy (96 % of patients on a previous NCI study had best response by nine cycles) followed by local therapy. Patients received approximately two cycles of chemotherapy during their local therapy.

The long doubling time of human breast cancer cells may be one reason why these tumors are unresponsive to chemotherapeutic agents, especially cell cycle specific agents. Ethinyl estradiol was incorporated into the current regimen in an attempt to recruit cells into the S-phase of the cell cycle. Estrogens have been shown to cause an increase in parameters of cell proliferation, such as thymidine incorporation, in hormone-dependent human breast cancer cell lines [4]. A previous study done at the National Cancer Institute on LABC in which serial biopsies were taken suggested an increase in the thymidine labeling index with estrogen priming. Conte et al have also evaluated a cytokinetically-oriented regimen using DES followed by chemotherapy [5]. He found that the proliferative activity of tumor biopsy samples showed a significant increase in thymidine labelling in 8 of 16 patients, and a primer-dependent -DNA polymerase labelling index in 13 of 16 tumors. These observations suggest that estrogen may increase cell proliferation, therefore increasing the likelihood that more tumor cells will be killed by the chemotherapy.

Accelerated hyperfractionated radiation therapy (twice daily treatments at slightly lower than standard dose per fraction) has the theoretical advantages of improving the therapeutic ratio by minimizing tumor growth during treat-

Division of Medical Oncology*, Division of Radiation Oncology, Vincent T. Lombardi Cancer Research Center, Georgetown University Medical Center, Washington, D.C. 20007, USA

ment and causing less late-occurring normal tissue damage. In one study of BID radiation, the local-regional recurrence rate of inflammatory breast cancer decreased from 46 % to 26 % [6]. The patients at highest risk of recurrence, Stage IIIB inflammatory and IIIB non-inflammatory, were treated with accelerated fractionation.

Left-sided chest wall or intact breast irradiation has been associated with cardiac toxicity in patients in the Medicine Branch, NCI LABC and other series [7]. Treatment planning by computed tomography scans excludes the left ventricle from the tangential treatment volume in most patients and was performed in this study. If that was not feasible, a volumetric analysis of the ventricle in the port was performed. This could then be correlated with toxicity. To decrease the treatment volume and decrease mediastinal and cardiac irradiation, the internal mammary nodes were not treated in patients with left-sided disease. Right-sided breast lesions were treated with tangents that included the internal mammary nodes. This allowed the value of internal mammary node irradiation to be assessed.

The use of combination alkylating agents with bone marrow rescue in high-dose therapy trials has been based on the demonstration of anti-tumor synergy against multiple solid tumor and leukemic cell lines using combined agents [8, 9]. Included in this data is a demonstrated in vitro synergy between Cyclophosphamide and Cisplatin against the L1210 leukemia cell line [8]. Clinical experience has, moreover, demonstrated impressive anti-tumor efficacy in a variety of solid tumors using Cyclophosphamide and Cisplatin combination alkylating regimens [10-12]. Initial studies by Peters et al, which evaluated the toxicities of various alkylating agents in a Phase I fashion, showed the maximally tolerated dose of Cyclophosphamide, Cisplatin, and BCNU to be 525 mg/m^2, 165 mg/m^2, and 600 mg/m^2, respectively. Impressive anti-tumor responses were observed with this regimen as well, including a recent report of a 73 % response rate including 54 % complete responses (with 14 % of the patients in unmaintained remission beyond 16 months at the time of the reporting) in premenopausal patients with previously untreated metastatic breast cancer. However, toxicities remained formidable with a reported mortality incidence of 20 % in one series [11].

In an attempt to maintain anti-tumor efficacy but reduce toxic complications, the present trial utilized high-dose Cyclophosphamide in combination with high-dose Carboplatin at the end of induction therapy. Cyclophosphamide is an alkylating agent with significant anti-tumor activity in a wide variety of solid neoplasms. Moreover, most high-dose combination alkylating agent regimens have utilized Cyclophosphamide at maximally or near maximally-tolerated doses [10, 11]. Carboplatin is a Cisplatin analogue with a broad scope of anti-tumor activity [13, 14]. Advantage over the parent compound is that it is significantly less nephrotoxic and neurotoxic than Cisplatin, and doses can be escalated to considerably higher levels than can be achieved with Cisplatin.

Methods

Patient selection

Between May 1989 and November 1990, 36 patients with Stage II, III or IV breast cancer were entered onto a protocol which used a multimodality approach. The study was open to 1) patients with Stage III or clinical Stage T3N0 with histologically documented breast carcinoma and evaluable disease in the breast, 2) patients with pathologic Stage II disease with an axillary lymph node dissection which revealed 4 or more positive lymph nodes, 3) patients with Stage III disease with mastectomy, and 4) patients with evaluable or measurable metastatic breast cancer. Patients could not have had previous cytotoxic therapy, or a history of previous malignancy except for cured non-melanoma skin cancer and cervical cancer in situ. They had a performance status of ECOG 3 or better, a WBC of 4,000/mm^3, platelets of 100,000/mm^3, and normal hepatic and renal function unless due to tumor involvement in Stage IV patients. Patients gave informed consent.

By November 1990, 36 patients had been entered onto the study. Four patients had Stage IIIA disease, 8 Stage IIIB (6 inflammatory and 2 non-inflammatory), 6 Stage IV, 3 Stage II with 4 or more positive nodes, and 3 Stage III with previous mastectomy. The median age was 50 years. The menopausal status included 16 premenopausal women, 17 postmenopausal women, and 3 perimenopausal women. Twenty-two patients were estrogen receptor positive, and 14 were estrogen receptor negative.

Chemotherapy

For systemic chemotherapy, all 36 patients received the following regimen as induction therapy: Ethinyl Estradiol 50 mcg. po on days 1-8, Leucovorin 500 mg/m^2 IV on days 4-8, 5-Fluorouracil 375 mg/m^2 IV on days 4-8 one hour after the termination of Leucovorin, Cyclophosphamide 500 mg/m^2 IV on day 5, and Doxorubicin 40 mg/m^e IV on day 5. This was repeated every 28 days. Patients were to receive 9 cycles of induction therapy. After 9 cycles, if the patient was Stage III or clinical T3N0, the breast was re-biopsied with an open biopsy. If the patient had achieved a complete clinical response and the biopsy was negative, local radiation and 2 additional cycles of chemotherapy were given. If the biopsy was positive or there was no change in evaluable disease, the patient underwent a mastectomy followed by radiation therapy and 2 additional cycles of chemotherapy. If the patient had no evaluable disease at the completion of radiation therapy and the 2 additional cycles of chemotherapy, they were given the option of receiving high-dose chemotherapy with autologous bone marrow rescue.

Patients with Stage II disease already had mastectomy or lumpectomy with axillary dissection upon referral. Patients who received radiation after lumpectomy started chemotherapy within 4 weeks of surgery and received chemotherapy along with radiation therapy. Those treated with mastectomy (including

Stage III patients who already had a mastectomy) had chest wall and regional nodal irradiation after 9 cycles of chemotherapy. All Stage IV patients received 9 cycles of chemotherapy, after which they were assessed for response. If they had a CR or a convertible PR, they were offered the high-dose therapy with ABMT protocol. If they had stable disease or a non-convertible PR, they received chemotherapy until progression.

All ER-positive patients who were NED received Tamoxifen 20 mg po q day for 5 years after the completion of the chemotherapy.

Thirteen patients completed the above multimodality approach and were eligible for autologous bone marrow transplant. Six patients chose to receive high-dose chemotherapy, and 7 refused. Fourteen patients were not eligible for high-dose therapy because of age or stage of disease, and 9 patients are still receiving induction therapy.

The treatment schedule for high-dose chemotherapy and autologous bone marrow rescue began with a bone marrow harvest. Cyclophosphamide was administered at a dose of 1.6 g/m² dissolved in 250 ml of D5W over 2 on days -5, -4 and -3. Carboplatin was administered at a dose of 400 mg/m² dissolved in D5NS to a final concentration of 10 mg/ml over 2 hours on days -5, -4, and -3, immediately following the Cyclophosphamide. In order to prevent hemorrhage cystitis [15, 16], MESNA (sodium 2-mercaptoethane sulfonate) was administered at dose of 20 mg/kg, 15 min prior to, and 3, 6, and 9 hours following Cyclophosphamide. Hydration began with 150 ml/h, 12 hours before Cyclophosphamide, and ended 12 hours after the last dose. On days -2 and -1 the patient rested, and on day 0 the autologous bone marrow was reinfused. Bone marrow was not purged. Four patients were also treated with granulocyte-macrophage colony stimulating factor.

Radiation therapy

All radiation therapy was delivered using high-energy photons from a linear accelerator or a ⁶⁰Co unit. Electron treatment of an appropriate energy was permitted to optimize treatment. Computerized treatment planning was used in all patients to maximize dose homogeneity and spare normal tissues. Radiation treatment started 2 weeks after surgery or as soon as possible after the repeat biopsy, preferably on day 1 of chemotherapy cycle 10. Doxorubicin was deleted during chemotherapy cycle 11 during radiation. Patients with Stage II or IIIA disease, or patients requiring chest wall irradiation were treated with conventional fractionation. The entire breast was treated to 5,040 cGy and, if a boost was needed, it was given to 6,040 cGy. For patients with inflammatory or IIIB non-inflammatory disease, radiation was given twice daily (Monday through Friday) and continuously, unless breaks were required for standard local toxicity (desquamation). Dose per fraction was 160 cGy to the 100 % isodose. The dose of radiation was at least 5,120 cGy to areas of low but potential risk, and 6,080 to areas of involvement, depending on the original sites of disease. For patients with inflammatory disease and those needing chest wall treatment, a bolus was used daily to 3,200 cGy to bring the skin reaction to deep erythema at the completion of treatment.

Statistical considerations

A major objective of this study was to characterize the response rates of patients with Stage II (clinical T3N0), Stage III locally advanced breast cancer, and Stage IV breast cancer to the CALF-E regimen. Data from the previous study has suggested that CR rates may be approximately 45 % in patients with these stages of disease. If we accrue 50 patients in any of the 3 categories of disease, then if between 18 and 28 complete responses are noted in any stage, they will demonstrate a clinical complete response rate for that stage which is consistent with 45 % (with 95 % confidence and power).

Results

Eighteen patients had evaluable disease and could be followed for clinical response to induction chemotherapy. Six of these patients (33 %) achieved a clinical complete response, 10 patients (56 %) a partial response, and 2 patients (11 %) had progressive disease. Four of the patients who had clinical complete responses in the breast required a mastectomy because of a positive biopsy. The median number of cycles to best response was 3.5 cycles.

Toxicities

Thirty-six patients were evaluable for toxicity and, as of November 1990, had received 297 cycles of chemotherapy. Twenty-seven patients (75 %) required a dose reduction due to neutropenia in 7 (19 %), mucositis in 4 (11 %), diarrhea 3 (8 %), neutropenia and mucositis combined in 10 (28 %), and 3 (8 %) for other causes. Most of these patients had 5-FU reduced by 25 % as their only dose reduction. There were no toxic deaths. Hematologic toxicities included WBC Grade I (3.0-3.9) 0 %, Grade II (2.0-2.9) 25 %, Grade 3 (1.0-1.9) 50 %, and Grade 4 (.0) 25 %; and platelets Grade I (75K-normal) 14 %, Grade II (50-74.9 K) 8 %, Grade 3 (25-49.9 K) 6 %, and Grade 4 (<25 K) 6 %. Seven patients (19 %) had neutropenic sepsis.

Gastrointestinal toxicities included nausea Grade III (8 %) and Grade IV (0 %), vomiting Grade III (6 %) and Grade IV (0 %), diarrhea Grade III (17 %) and Grade IV (0 %), and stomatitis Grade III (33 %) and Grade IV (8 %).

Two patients (6 %) had deep venous thromboses. Three patients had infections and 3 had clots at the site of their venous access devices.

One patient required hospitalization and transfusions for severe vaginal bleeding related to estrogen treatment. The estrogen was initially given for 28 days, and she received a full dose. After this incident, all patients received estrogen for 8 days as described in Methods. Ten patients experienced vaginal bleeding, 5 had vaginal discharge, and 3 had heavier menses.

Two patients (6 %) developed cardiac toxicity. The Doxorubicin doses they had received were 360 mg/m^2 and 370 mg/m^2. One patient developed the cardiac toxicity after receiving the high-dose therapy with Cyclophosphamide.

Four patients have completed high-dose therapy and autologous bone marrow rescue. The median length of hospital stay was 37 days. There were no deaths. Two patients are currently in the hospital receiving treatment.

Discussion and conclusion

Locally advanced, non-metastatic breast cancer is associated with poor local control and dismal survival. The results of Haagenson and Stout [17,18] emphasize the poor outlook for this group of breast cancer patients. They have reported that radical mastectomy failed to cure even a single patient in their series of 120 patients followed up to 8 years. They regard these lesions as « categorically inoperable » and suggest that they be treated by other measures. Improved radiotherapy techniques have allowed the delivery of higher doses of radiation to these patients' tumors with acceptable rates of local complications, thus increasing the chance of achieving and maintaining local control.

Patients with an earlier clinical stage of breast cancer but with greater than 3 positive lymph nodes are also in a known poor prognostic category. The results of the NSABP [19] and Milan [20] studies reveal. a 17 % and 15 % relapse-free survival, respectively, in all patients with greater than 3 positive nodes not treated with adjuvant chemotherapy. Multiple trials examining the efficacy of high-dose chemotherapy and autologous bone marrow transplantation for breast cancer, either as adjuvant therapy in women with a high number of lymph nodes at high risk of relapse, or in patients who have achieved a complete remission of metastatic disease with conventional chemotherapy, are currently in progress. Early results are promising, but follow-up is too short to evaluate the effect on overall survival.

The current multimodality protocol was developed to fill a gap in available therapy. It provides an intensive induction chemotherapy regimen, radiation therapy to maximize local control, and a high-dose chemotherapy regimen at the end to eliminate micrometastases. The objective response rate to conventional doses of chemotherapy was high (89 %), indicating therapeutic efficacy ; however, in previous studies the response rates have also been high, with little change in overall survival. The intent of the current protocol was to increase overall survival by providing maximal anti-tumor activity compared to conventional chemotherapy. The results so far have been encouraging, but it is too early to make definitive statements regarding survival advantages from this regimen.

References

1. TNM classification of malignant tumours (1987) Hermanek P, Sobin LH (eds), Springer-Verlag, Berlin, pp 93-99
2. Swain SM, Lippman ME, Egan EF, Drake JC, Steinberg SM, Allegra CJ (1989)

Fluorouracil and high-dose leucovorin in previously treated patients with metastatic breast cancer. J Clin Oncol 7 (7) : 890-899

3. Swain SM, Sorace RA, Bagley CS, Danfort DN, Bader J, Wesley MN, Steinberg SM, Lippman ME (1987) neo-adjuvant chemotherapy in the combined modality approach of locally advanced nonmetastatic breast cancer. Cancer Research 47 : 3889-3894

4. Lippman ME, Bolan G, Huff K (1976) The effects of estrogens and anti-estrogens on hormone-responsive human breast cancer in long-term tissue culture. Cancer Research 36 : 4595-4601

5. Conte PF, Alama A, Bertelli G (1987) Chemotherapy with estrogenic recruitment and surgery in locally advanced breast cancer : clinical and cytokinetic results. Int J Cancer 40 : 490-494

6. Barker JL, Montagne ED, Peters LJ (1980) Clinical experience with irradiation of inflammatory carcinoma of the breast with and without elective chemotherapy. Cancer 45 : 625

7. Loprinzi CL, Carbone PP, Tormey DC et al (1984) Aggressive combined modality therapy for advanced local-regional breast carcinoma. J Clin Oncol 2 : 157-163

8. Dykes DJ, Griswold DP Jr, Peters WP, Frei E III (1985) Response of B-16 melanoma to high dose chemotherapy. Proc Am Assoc Can Res 26 : 833

9. Schabel FM Jr, Skipper HE, Trader MW et al (1984) Establishment of cross resistant profiles for new agents. Cancer Treat Rep 68 : 453-459

10. Eder JP, Antman K, Peters W et al (1986) High dose combination alkylating agent chemotherapy with autologous bone marrow support for metastatic breast cancer. J Clin Oncol 4 : 1592-1597

11. Peters WP, Eder JP, Henner WD et al (1986) High-dose combination alkylating agents with autologous bone marrow support : a phase I trial. J Clin Oncol 4 : 646-654

12. Edem JP, Antman K, Elias A et al (1988) Cyclophosphamide and thiotepa with autologous bone marrow transplantation in patients with solid tumors. J Nat Cancer Inst 80 : 1221-1226

13. Evans BD, Raja KS, Calvert AM et al (1983) Phase II study of JM8, a new platinum analog in advanced ovarian carcinoma. Cancer Treat Rep 67 : 957-1000

14. Canetta R, Bragman K, Smaldone L et al (1988) Carboplatin : current status and future prospects. Cancer Treat Rev 15 (suppl B) : 17-32

15. Blacklock H, Ball L, Knights S et al (1983) Experience with mesna in patients receiving allogeneic bone marrow transplants for poor prognostic leukemia. Cancer Treat Rev 10 (suppl A) : 45-52

16. Hows JW, Mehta A, Ward L (1984) Comparison of mesna with forced diuresis to prevent cyclophosphamide induced hemorrhagic cystitis in marrow transplantation : A prospective randomized study. Br J Cancer 50 : 753-756

17. Haagensen CD (1971) Diseases of the breast, Ed 2. W.B. Saunders Co., Philadelphia, pp 629

18. Haagensen CD, Stout AP (1943) Carcinoma of the breast II. Criteria of operability. Ann Surg 118 : 859-879, 1032-1051

19. Wolmark N, Fischer B (1985) Adjuvant chemotherapy in stage II breast cancer : a brief overview of the NSABP clinical trials. World J Surg 9 : 699-706

20. Bonadonna G, Rossi A, Valagussa P (1985) Adjuvant CMF chemotherapy in operable breast cancer. Ten years later. World J Surg 9 : 707-713

Ten years of breast preserving management in infiltrative breast cancer : results in 412 patients treated by Neo-Adjuvant chemotherapy and radiation therapy with or without hormonotherapy

Cl Jacquillat, M Weil, G Auclerc, Ch Borel, Cl Soubrane, F Baillet, D Khayat

The studies that Claude Jacquillat undertook in 1980 in infiltrative breast cancers were inspired by two concepts : breast cancer should be considered in most women as a two components disease, a visible locoregional disease and an invisible systemic disease which constitutes its main danger and its therapeutic priority ; since it is not an exclusive locoregional disease, breast preservation must be focused on.

These concepts were based on solid backgrounds. The data of Niessen-Meyer [1] and Fisher [2] were the first to demonstrate that short perioperative chemotherapy could modify the natural history of breast cancer. Since 1972 several adjuvant studies have been performed, most of them in node-positive patients. Their overview by Peto et al [3] demonstrates that medical treatment could produce moderate but highly significant improvement in 5-year survival. Overall reductions in the odds of death during the first 5 years were 16 % SD 3 for Tamoxifen versus no Tamoxifen (p = 0.00001), and 11 % SD 4 for chemotherapy versus no chemotherapy (p = 0.003). In Tamoxifen trials, there was a clear reduction in mortality only among women aged 50 or older, for whom allocation of Tamoxifen reduced the annual odds of death during the first 5 years by about one-fifth. In chemotherapy trials, there was a clear reduction only among women aged under 50, for whom allocation of polychemotherapy reduced the annual odds of death during the first 5 years by about one-quarter. The improvements in recurrence-free survival produced by Tamoxifen and by cytotoxic therapy were, however, statistically definite both for older and for younger women.

More recently, the prognosis of node-negative patients has been reexamined. It has been found that adjuvant Tamoxifen and adjuvant chemotherapy significantly improve disease-free survival (DFS) and overall survival (OS) [4-7].

However, the adjuvant setting is not the optimal strategy, and this consideration prompted Claude Jacquillat to propose neo-adjuvant or primary chemotherapy in breast cancer management [8-11]. The main advantage of neo-adjuvant chemotherapy, given before any locoregional treatment, is to preserve the major indicator of effectiveness, the complete remission rate [11]. In addition, neo-adjuvant chemotherapy has the potential to downstage tumors by decreasing the size and extent of the tumor mass, thereby allowing the proposal of breast-conserving treatment, whatever the initial tumor size. Earlier drug

Service d'Oncologie Médicale, Hôpital de la Salpétrière, 47, boulevard de l'Hôpital, 75013 Paris, France

administration also may have the advantage of a lesser likelihood of drug-resistant lines being present.

The local treatment chosen in these studies is radiotherapy. It has already been demonstrated that the 10-year survival achieved by irradiation alone is similar to that obtained by standard surgical procedures [12]. It has also been shown that the combination of external and endocurietherapy with Iridium 192 allows a much higher rate of breast conservation for T2 and T3 patients who have had no previous tumorectomy [13].

Material and methods

Four hundred and twelve evaluable patients entered 2 successive protocols 03SR80 between 1980 and 1986 and 02SR86 since 1986. The median follow-up is thus 75 months (ranges 1-126) for the first protocol and 26 months (ranges 3-49) for the more recent protocol. Two hundred fifty patients who have been reported previously have now been observed for a longer time period [14].

The aims of the first protocol were as follows : to extend breast-sparing management to all patients with breast cancer, whatever the initial size of the cancer ; to study the correlation between the tumor volume decrease (tumor regression) that was induced by chemotherapy before the start of radiation therapy and the outcome (local recurrence or metastasis) ; to prolong DFS. In addition, the aim of protocol 02SR86 was to induce more clinical regression before radiotherapy by trying a rescue protocol using alternative more intensive combinations in slow responders.

Thus, no surgery was planned (no tumor excision, nodes dissection or mastectomy) except in the eventuality of local failure after the completion of radiation therapy.

Diagnosis relied in most patients on cytology by fine needle aspiration and in some patients on histology by drill-biopsy.

FNA allows to stratify the patients to 3 cytopronostic grades index (CPI) and there is a close correlation between the Scarf Bloom and Richardson grades (SBR) and CPI. In addition since 1985, FNA allows to quantify ER and PR and since 1990 it allows to study cathepsin D.

Hormone receptors thus could be studied in 99 patients from 02SR80 and cathepsine D level could be determined in the 20 most recent patients.

There are major similarities and minor differences between both protocols :

a) *drugs combination* including Velbe, Thiotepa, Methotrexate, Fluoro-5-Uracil, Adriamycin and Prednisone (VTMFAP) is the same,

b) *the treatment general schema* is the same, namely induction chemotherapy followed by teleradiotherapy and boost by bradytherapy then consolidation, the duration of which is adjusted to the prognostic parameters ; but there are minor differences concerning patients stratification, drugs schedules, the duration of consolidation, the availability of a rescue treatment in the most recent protocol.

— In protocol 03SR80 stratification was based on tumor size and clinical lymphnode status that defined group 1 (tumors $\leqslant 3$ cm No) Group 2 (tumors $> 3 \leqslant 27$ cm and/or N1), group 3 (tumors > 7 cm and/or N2), group 4 (T4 whatever the N status).

— In protocol 02SR86, tumor differenciation expressed by CPI or SBR was combined to tumor size and lymphnode status to define 3 groups : group 1 (T1 N0 CPI or SBRI), group 2 (T2 or T3 and/or N1 and/or CPI II or SBRII), group 3 (T4 and/or N2 and/or CPI III or SBRIII).

— In protocol 03SR80 (Fig. 1) the number of induction doses varied as well as their schedule according to the therapeutic groups.

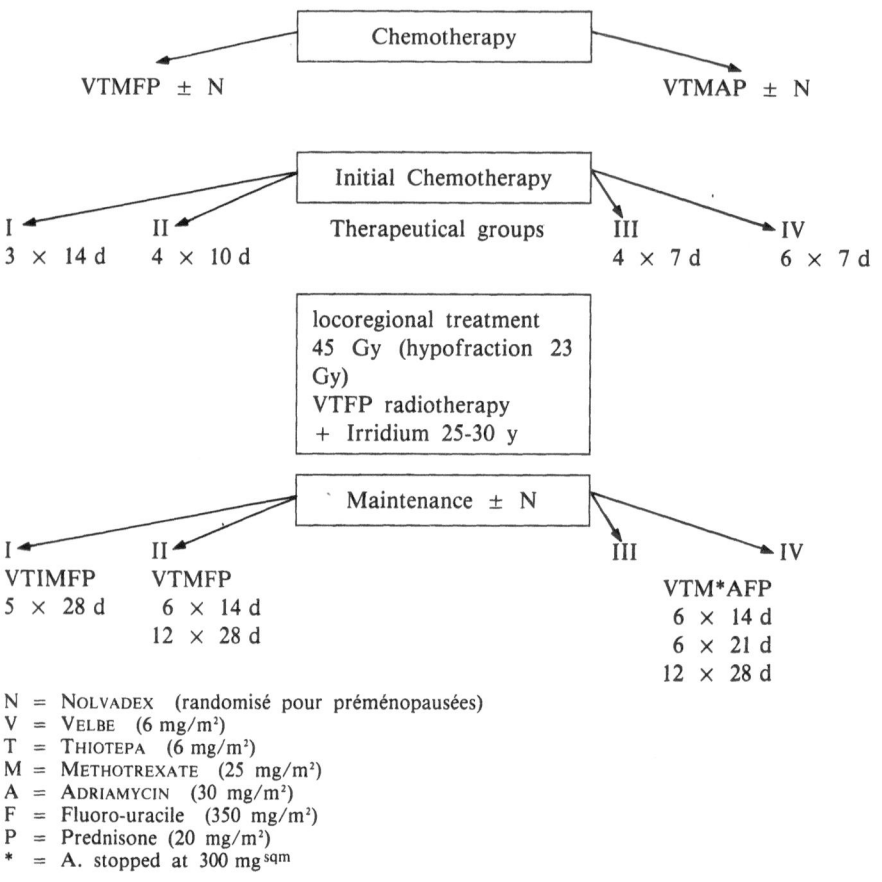

N = Nolvadex (randomisé pour préménopausées)
V = Velbe (6 mg/m²)
T = Thiotepa (6 mg/m²)
M = Methotrexate (25 mg/m²)
A = Adriamycin (30 mg/m²)
F = Fluoro-uracile (350 mg/m²)
P = Prednisone (20 mg/m²)
* = A. stopped at 300 mg sqm

Fig. 1. Protocol 03 R 80 (19)

Tamoxifen was planned for all post-menopausal women and its administration was randomized in premenopausal patients.

Cobaltotherapy was delivered according to the classic schedule or in four sessions in group 1 and 2.

In group 3 and 4 this hypofractioned schedule was applied to all patients and chemotherapy was interspersed between the two courses of teleradiotherapy and between teleradiotherapy and brachytherapy. Maintenance was planned for 5, 16 or 20 months according to the therapeutic groups.

— In protocol 02 SR 86 (Fig. 2, p. 131) the projected treatment schedule was the same for all patients and 8 doses were planned before radiotherapy started on day 100. Adriamycin was given to all patients except those belonging to group 1 (T1 SBRI) ; but because of the prognosis significance of tumor regression that we had observed previously [14, 15] tumor shrinkage evaluation was performed after 3 doses and the rescue protocol was undertaken in those patients whose tumor regression was less than 50 %. The rescue protocol which combined Cisplatin, Etoposide, continuous 5-FU and alternatively Mitomycin or Adriamycin is detailed elsewhere in this book (Khayat D, Borel Ch, Weil M et al) The modalities of radiotherapy have been described in previous publications and is detailed in another section of this manual (Baillet F, Jacquillat Cl, Housset M et al). The patients characteristics are shown on Table 1. The distribution of TNM status is shown on Table 2, and indicates that over half of our patients had locally advanced breast cancer.

Table 1. Patients characteristics

Number of patients (%)

	03SR 80	02 SR 60
No of patients total	250	162
Age		
20-39	31	22
40-59	141	97
60-79	78	43
Clinical T :		
T1	23 (9)	26 (16)
T2	112 (45)	57 (35)
T3	57 (23)	58 (36)
T4	58 (23)	21 (13)
Clinical N :		
N0	140 (56)	107 (66)
N1	100 (40)	48 (38)
N2	10 (4)	7 (4)
SBR or CPI		
I	40 (16)	32 (20)
II	109 (44)	68 (42)
III	40 (16)	43 (27)
IV	61 (24)	19 (11)
Unspecified		
Hormone receptors		99
ER + and/or PR +		80 (80)
PeV		
1	25 (11)	19 (12)
2	29 (12)	10 (6)
3	7 (3)	9 (6)

Table 2. TNM stage (AJC, 1988)

	03 SR 80	02 SR 86
I	19 (8)	25 (15)
IIa	68 (35)	54 (33)
IIb	51 (20)	40 (25)
IIIa	36 (14)	22 (14)
IIIb	58 (23)	21 (13)
Total	250	162

Results

During primary chemotherapy the successive clinical measurement of the tumor volume at the time of each drug infusion showed the rapid shrinkage of the tumor. As shown on Table 3 there were 91 % responders in the first protocol whom 30 % had complete clinical regression and 94 % in the second protocol whom 40 % were complete responders.

Table 3. Clinical tumor regressions (CTR) after induction chemotherapy

	TR < 50 %	TR > 50 %	CCR
03 SR 80	22 (9)	154 (61)	74 (30)
02 SR 86	20 (12)	79 (49)	63 (39)
	PEFAM	9	2
Total	9 (6)	88 (54)	65 (40)

The rescue protocol that was applied to 20 patients induced 2 complete remission and 9 partial remission. After radiotherapy all patients of the first protocol were in complete clinical remission whereas a mastectomy was indicated in 4 patients of the second protocol who had a persistant tumor after the completion of radiotherapy.

Figures 3 and 4 show the DFS according to stages in 03SR80 and in 02SR86. The 5 year DFS in 03SR80 are 92 % for stage I, 81 % for stage IIA, 65 % for stage IIB, 44 % for stage IIIA and 52 % for stage IIIB. In 02SR86 the data are still premature but there are already obvious differences according to stage. The 2 year DFS is thus 100 % for stage I, 95 % for stage IIA, 90 % for stage IIb, 64 % for stage IIIA and 54 % for stage IIIB.

The univariate predictors for 5 years DFS in protocol 03SR80 and for 2 years DFS in protocol 02SR86 are figured on Table 4.

T and N are the best prediction parameters in both protocols and inflammatory symptoms (PeV2 or PeV3) are more important for early relapses which

TREATMENT SCHEDULES

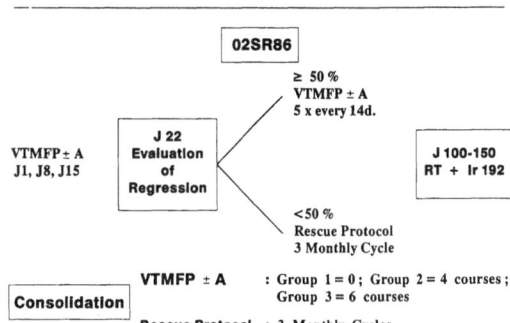

Fig. 2.

Table 4. Univariate predictor of DFS

	03 SR 80		02 SR 86	
	5 years DFS	p value	2 years DFS (%)	p value
T				
T1	93 %		100	
T2	74 %	0.0004	95	0.0001
T3	56 %		79	
T4	52 %		54	
N				
N0	76 %		91	
N1	55 %	0.0008	23	0.0001
N2	40 %		17	
CPI				
I	88 %		94	
II	63 %	0.0146	94	0.01
III	60 %		72	
Pev				
PeV0	71 %	0.0034	94	0.0001
PeV +	51 %		56	
Tumor regression				
< 50 %	46 %	0.0169	66	0.02
> 50 %	69 %		87	

is not surprising. Tumor regression is a significant factor in both protocols. The multifactorial analysis according to the Cox model applied to the more mature protocol confirms its independant significance and underlines the value of tumor differenciation (Table 5).

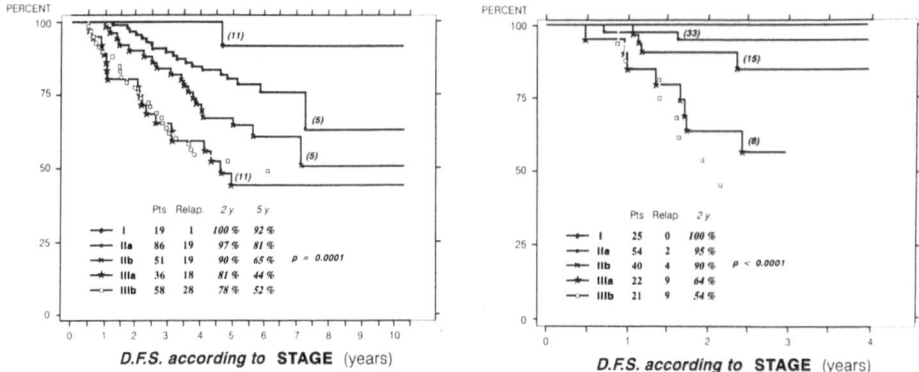

Fig. 3   **Fig. 4**

Table 5. Cox regression model DFS 03 SR 80

Significant variable	β coefficient	P. value	Exp. β
SBR or CPI	1.1306	0.002	3.0976
Clinical T	0.6176	0.006	1.8544
Tumor regression			
	- 0.9312	0.03	0.3941

We found a significant difference between grade I on one hand, grade II and III on the other hand. The absence of difference between grade II and grade III emphasizes the requirement for other techniques to assess the biological prognosis of breast cancers. Although it is still a matter of contest, hormone receptors seem to be an important predictive parameter. For 80 patients who are ER and/or PR positive the 2 years DFS is 94 % whereas it is 64 % in 19 ER and PR negative patients (p = 0.0007). It is too early to provide data on the cathepsine level study.

Table 6. 03 SR 80 pattern of relapses

	No of Pts	No of Metastases	No of Loco-regional	No of Loco-regional + Metastases
T1	23	0	1 (7)	0
T2	112	12 (12)	17 (14)	3 (2)
T3	57	15 (32)	8 (15)	1 (3)
T4	58	18 (32)	7 (16)	3 (7)
TOTAL	250	45 (19)	33 (14)	7 (3)

( ) = 5 year actuarial rate

For 03SR80, the pattern of relapses according to T is shown on Table 6. Among 85 relapses, there were 45 distant metastases, 33 locoregional recurrences and 7 locoregional and distant relapses. The actuarial 5 year rate of local recurrence is 14 %. The actuarial 5 year rate of breast preservation is 94 %.

In protocol 02SR86, we observed 24 relapses 15 distant metastases, 2 locoregional and distant relapses and 7 locoregional recurrences (2 T3 — 5 T4). The 5 year overall survival for 03SR80 are 95 % (I), 94 % (IIa), 80 % (IIB), 60 % (IIIA), 58 % (IIIB).

Tolerance and cosmetic results

Some degree of hematological toxicity was almost constant and it necessitated delaying some treatment. Thus, the induction treatment was spread in the first protocol and in the second protocol 30 % patients had 7 induction doses instead of 8. Mild symptoms of neurotoxicity were frequent and they were impaired by the rescue protocol because of the cisplatinum (14 grade 1 and 2).

Despite the application of cold cap, alopecia is observed in 65 % of patients. We have not observed any clinical or subclinical cardiotoxicity. Performance status was mildly or moderately impaired in most patients.

The cosmetic results depend on tumor size and/or breast size. They are always excellent or good for small tumors, good for large tumors in small breast and may be fair for large tumors in large breast.

Discussion

Our study dealing with 412 patients treated between 1980 and 1990 confirms that the tumor regression induced by neo-adjuvant chemotherapy allows to propose breast preservation to most patients with breast cancer whatever their initial tumor size. In stages I and II when compared to lumpectomy and irradiation, our strategy improves survival and also local control in T2 tumors [16-18].

In operable T3 tumors, our strategy allows breast preservation in 94 % patients with equivalent locoregional control as mastectomy. The actuarial 5 years distant relapse rate although not satisfactory compares favorably to the literature data for such tumors [19, 20].

In non operable T3 and T4 tumors most investigators recommand primary chemotherapy but in most studies the breast sparing management if planned at all is limited to complete responders. Despite the extension of breast preserving management to almost all patients the local control that we observed is as good as that achieved by mastectomy [21-23]. The definitive improvement in DFS and in survival in these stages will come from chemotherapy intensification, from drugs modulation, from circumvention of resistance, from better adjustement of hormonotherapy and even perhaps in the near future from quite new methods based on the progress of advance in biology.

Conclusion

These studies which show that intensive neo-adjuvant chemotherapy combined to hormonotherapy improves the prognosis of many patients with infiltrative breast cancer, and which establish the validity of management with breast preservation and a feasible and convenient schedule for radiation, confirm the proposals of Claude Jacquillat.

Acknowlegedments to Brigitte Cédreau.
This study is sponsored by CRAC, Comité de Paris de la Ligue contre le Cancer.

References

1. Nissen-Meyer R, Kjellgren K, Malmio K, Mansson B, Norin I (1978) Surgical adjuvant chemotehrapy : results on one short course with cyclophosphamide after mastectomy for breast cancer. Cancer 41 : 2088-2098
2. Fisher B, Carbone P, Economou SG et al (1975) Phenylalanine mustard (L-PAM) in the management of primary breast cancer : a report of early findings. N Engl J Med 292 : 117-122
3. Early Breast Cancer Trialist's collaborative Group (1988) Effects of adjuvant tamoxifen and cytotoxic therapy on mortality in early breast cancer : an overview of 61 randomized trials among 28,896 women. N Engl J Med 319 : 1681-1692
4. Fisher B, Redmond C, Dimitro NV et al (1989) A randomized clinical trial evaluating sequential methotrexate and fluorouracil in the treatment of patients with node negative breast cancer who have estrogen receptor negative tumors. N Engl J Med 320 : 473-478
5. Bonadonna G, Valagussa P (1988) The contribution of medicine to the primary treatment of breast cancer. Cancer Res 48 : 2314-2324
6. Mansour EG, Gray R, Shatila AH et al (1989) Efficacy of adjuvant chemotherapy in high risk node negative breast cancer. N Engl J Med 320 : 485-490
7. The Ludwing Breast Cancer Study Group (1989) Prolonged disease-free survival after one course of perioperative adjuvant chemotherapy of node negative breast cancer. N Engl J Med 320 : 491-496
8. Jacquillat Cl, Baillet F, Auclerc G, Maylin Cl, Weil M (1982) Initial chemotherapy + conservation radiotherapy in stages I, II and III breast cancer. In : Proceeding of the 13th International Cancer Congress, Seattle, Washington (abstract), September
9. Jacquillat Cl, Weil M, Auclerc G, Auclerc MF, Khayat D, Baillet F (1987) neoadjuvant chemotherapy in the conservative management of breast cancer : A study of 205 patients. In : Salmon SE (ed) Adjuvant Therapy of Cancer, vol. 5. Grune and Stratton, New York, pp 403
10. Jacquillat Cl, Weil M, Auclerc G et al (1985) neo-adjuvant chemotherapy in the conservation management of breast cancers : study of 205 patients. In : Jacquillat Cl, Weil M, Khayt D (eds) neo-adjuvant Chemotherapy. John Libbey Eurotext, Paris, pp 197
11. De Vita VT (1988) On the value of response criteria in therapeutic research. In : Jacquillat Cl, Weil M, Khayat D (eds) neo-adjuvant Chemotherapy. John Libbey Eurotext, Paris, p 3

12. Calle R, Pilleron JP, Schlienger P, Vilcoq JR (1978) Conservative management of operable breast cancer. Cancer 42 : 2045-2053

13. Pierquin B, Raynal M, Otmezguine Y et al (1988) Le traitement conservateur des cancers du sein : résultats à 13 ans. In : Baillet F (ed) Le traitement Conservateur du Cancer du sein. Cedem, Langres, p 67

14. Jacquillat Cl, Weil M, Baillet F, Borel Ch, Auclerc G et al (1990) Results of neo-adjuvant chemotherapy and radiation therapy in the breast conserving treatment of 250 patients with all stages of infiltrative breast cancer. Cancer 66 : 129

15. Jacquillat Cl, Baillet F, Weil M et al (1988) Results of a conservative treatment combining induction (neo-adjuvant) and consolidation chemotherapy, hormonotherapy and interstitial irradiation in 98 patients with locally advanced breast cancer (IIIA-IIIB). Cancer 61 : 1977

16. Delouche G (1988) Le traitement conservateur des petits cancers du sein opérables. 30 années d'expérience. In : Baillet F (ed) Le traitement Conservateur du Cancer du sein. Cedem, Langres, p 51

17. Montbardon X, Gérard JP, De Laroche G et al (1988) Cancer du sein : traitement conservateur du cancer du sein à Lyon : a propos de 1 000 cas de 1950 à 1986. In : Baillet F (ed) Le traitement conservateur du cancer du sein. Cedem, Langres, p 61

18. Fowble B, Gray R, Gilchrist K, Goodman RL, Taylor S, Tormey CD (1988) Identification of a subgroup of patients with breast cancer and histologically positive axillary nodes receiving adjuvant chemotherapy who may benefit from post-operative radiotherapy. J Clin Oncol 6 : 1107-1117

19. Klefstrom P, Grohn P, Heinonen E, Holsti L, Holsti P (1987) Adjuvant postoperative radiotherapy, chemotherapy and immunotherapy in stage III breast cancer ; 5 years results and influence of levamisole. Cancer 60 : 36-42

20. Chauvergne I, Durand M, Mauriac L et al (1988) Traitement combiné de 270 cancers mammaires localement étendus ; résultats d'un programme thérapeutique contrôlé. In : Jacquillat Cl, Weil M, Khayat D (eds) neo-adjuvant Chemotherapy. John Libbey Eurotext, Paris, p 225

21. Lippmann MR, Swain SM, Egan EF et al (1988) neo-adjuvant chemotherapy in the combined modality approach of locally advanced non metastatic breast cancer. In : Jacquillat Cl, Weil M, Khayat D (eds) Neo-Adjuvant Chemotherapy. John Libbey Eurotext, Paris, p 225

Results of Cisplatin (CDDP)/Etoposide (VP16)/5-FU and alternatively Adriamycin or Mitomycin C (PEFAM) combination in primary resistant breast cancer and in heavily pre-treated metastatic breast cancer

D Khayat, Ch Borel, M Weil, G Auclerc, E Vuillemin, Cl Jacquillat

In spite of the activity of chemotherapeutic agents, metastatic breast cancer remains an incurable disease.

Combination chemotherapy will induce an objective response in about two-third of the patients, but complete response rate remains below 20 % and median survival is about 24 months. In order to increase response rate, more especially in heavily pretreated patients resistant to most classical drugs, a chemotherapy regimen combining VP16, Cisplatin, 5-FU, Mitomycin C in alternance with Adriamycin (PEFAM) was tested in a phase II pilot study.

VP16 is active as a single drug in the treatment of breast cancer, a response rate of 20 % has been reported with pretreated patients [1]. The combination VP16 and CDDP is synergistic in murine tumors [2, 3] ; it is one of the most efficient combination for treating lung small cell carcinoma and in germ cell tumor where responses have been observed even in case of resistance to Cisplatin. The interaction of VP16 with topoisomerase II inhibits DNA repair of CDDP damage [4]. 5-FU and CDDP in combination have been shown to have synergistic cytotoxicity against both murine and human neoplasms. Cisplatin can increase the availibility of the reduced folate necessary for tight binding of FdUMP to dTMP synthase, thus enhancing the cytotoxicity of the Cisplatin and 5-FU combination [5].

Adriamycin has been kept in the regimen because of its major activity in the treatment of breast cancer, and this in spite of the frequency of a previous chemotherapy including an anthracyclin. Although usually incorporated in second line regimen, there is considerable evidence that Mitomycin C is an effective agent against tumors resistant to Adriamycin and Cyclophosphamide.

This regimen activity was first evaluated for patients with metastatic disease or experiencing locoregional recurrence. These patient form group A.

In our first protocol (03SR80) we have treated 250 patients with all stages of infiltrative breast cancer with neo-adjuvant chemotherapy. Response to induction chemotherapy by VTMFA (Vinblastine, Thiotepa, Methotrexate, 5-FU, Adriamycin), is a significant independant pronostic factor [6]. Therefore, in our second protocol (02SR86), patients with no clinical tumor regression after three courses of VTMFA received then the PEFAM regimen [7]. Those patients constitute group B.

Service d'Oncologie Médicale, Hôpital de la Salpétrière, 47 boulevard de l'Hôpital, 75013 Paris, France

Group A

Patients and methods

Between june 1987 and september 1990, 61 patients experiencing metastatic breast cancer and/or a locoregional recurrence have been treated by the PEFAM regimen. Main characteristics of these patients are shown in Table 1. Fifty-seven percent of patients experienced liver metastasis. Only 23 % had never been treated by chemotherapy. Pretreatment investigations consisted of chest CT-scan, abdominal CT scan and baseline bone scan.

Table 1. Patients characteristics - Groups A

Characteristics	No (%)
No of patients	
Age (years)	
median	54
range	31-75
Loco-regional recurrence only	15 (25)
Distant metastasis	46 (75)
soft tissues	15 (33)
bones	27 (49)
lung	16 (35)
liver	26 (57)
others	7 (15)
Prior chemotherapy	
none	14 (23)
adjuvant	30 (49)
metastastic first line	17 (28)

The regimen combines a continous infusion of 1,000 mg/m^2 of 5-FU from day 1 to day 3 and 35 mg/m^2 of Cisplatin from day 1 to day 3 also, 100 mg/m^2 of VP16 on day 1 in 1 h infusion, and either 10 mg/m^2 of Mitomycin C (cycle 1, 3, 5) or 45 mg/m^2 of Adriamycin (cycle 2, 4, 6) every 21 to 28 days as count permitted.

Response is assessed after 2 cycles of chemotherapy by clinical examination, chest radiographs, liver ultrasound and repeated scans where appropriate. Complete response (CR) was defined as disappearance of all symptoms and signs of disease with normalization of the CT scan, and bone scan. Partial response was defined as greater than 50 % reduction in the sum of the maximum perpendicular diameters of mesurable lesions. Toxicity was evaluated using world health organization (WHO) criteria.

Results

Median follow-up is 13 months (range : 0-37). Patients received on average 5 cycles (range : 1-12). Response rate to chemotherapy is shown on Table 2. Five patients with metastatic disease are not evaluable : 3 because of major toxicity in the first 2 cycles and 2 lost to follow-up after 1 cycle. Response rate is 62 % including 16 % of complete response. The incidence of previous treatment by chemotherapy on the response rate to PEFAM is significant as shown on Table 3. Patients having never been treated by chemotherapy show a response rate of 73 % including 25 % of complete response, whereas for second line metastatic treatment response rate falls to 40 % including 7 % of complete response. Most responsive sites of metastatic disease are soft tissues, lung ; it is especially interesting to notice a 53 % response rate for liver including 24 % of complete response (Table 4).

Table 2. Maximum response to chemotherapy

	Metastatic disease*		Loco-regional recurrence		Disease	Total
	No	%	No	%	No	%
Complete response	7	17	2	13	9	16
Partial response	19	46	7	47	26	46
Stable disease	7	17	5	33	12	22
Progressive disease	8	20	1	7	9	16

(*) 5 patients are note evaluable

Table 3. Response to chemotherapy according to prior treatment

	Prior chemotherapy					
	None		Adjuvant		Firt metastatic line	
	No	%	No	%	No	%
Complete response	3	25	5	17	1	7
Partial response	7	58	14	48	5	33
Stable disease	2	17	6	20	4	26
Progressive disease	0	0	4	15	5	33

Table 4. Response to chemotherapy according to disease sites

	Soft tissue		Bone		Lung		Liver	
	No	%	No	%	No	%	No	%
Complete response	4	16	2	10	6	50	5	24
Partial response	12	48	8	38	3	25	6	29
Stable disease	8	32	5	24	2	16	7	33
Progressive disease	1	4	6	29	1	8	3	14

In locoregional recurrence without distant metastases, 11 patients out of 15 experienced complete remission. After 3 cycles of PEFAM, locoregional control was achieved by radiotherapy and/or surgery. Six of these patients experienced recurrences within an average of 10 months (range : 4-14). Five patients are still in complete remission with a median follow-up of 14 months (range : 7-29).

For the 26 responsive patients with metastatic disease, an alternative treatment was often administered after 6 cycles of PEFAM regimen consisting of VTMFA or Vinovelbine and Epirubicin in order to avoid cumulative toxicities due to Cisplatin. Median survival without progression for these responsive patients is 23 months (3 + - 35).

For the 46 patients with metastatic disease median survival computed since the onset of PEFAM treatment is 23 months (Fig. 1). For responsive patients actuarial survival rate is 65 % at 24 months whereas median survival of non responsive patients is only 9 months (p = 0.0001) (Fig. 2). Last median survival computed since onset of metastatic disease is 37 months (Fig. 3). Four patients are still in complete remission 24 to 36 months after beginning of treatment.

Group B

Patients and methods

Between january 1988 and november 1990, 27 patients with primary breast cancer without metastases and resistant to neo-adjuvant chemotherapy have been treated by the PEFAM regimen. Main characteristics of these patients are shown on Table 5. Fifty-two percent are stage III patients. All patients are resistant to previous Anthracyclin containing neo-adjuvant chemotherapy. Twenty of them have received the VTMFA regimen : Vinblastine 6 mg/m^2, Thiotepa 6 mg/m^2, Methotrexate 25 mg/m^2, 5-FU 350 mg/m^2, Adriamycin 25 mg/m^2, 3 weekly cycles according to protocol 02SR86 [7]. At the end of these three cycles there was no objective clinical response. These patients received then

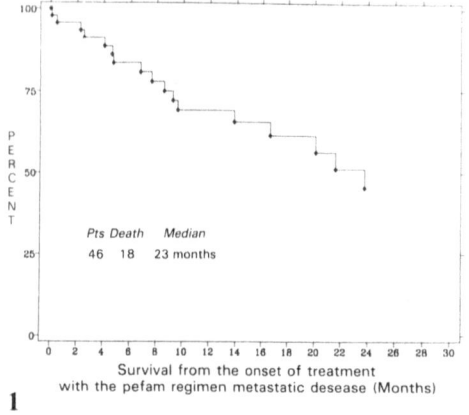

1

Survival from the onset of treatment
with the pefam regimen metastatic desease (Months)

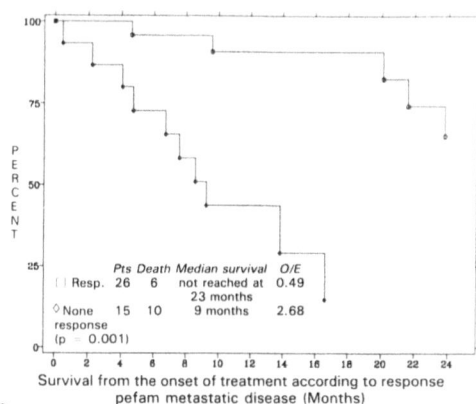

2

Survival from the onset of treatment according to response
pefam metastatic disease (Months)

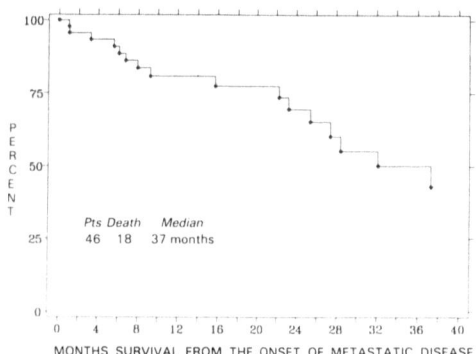

3

MONTHS SURVIVAL FROM THE ONSET OF METASTATIC DISEASE

Fig. 1. Survival from the onset of treatment with the PEFAM regimen metastatic disease

Fig. 2. Survival from the onset of treatment with the PEFAM regimen metastatic disease

Fig. 3. Survival from the onset of metastatic disease

Table 4. Response to chemotherapy according to disease sites

	Soft tissus		Bone		Lung		Liver	
	No	%	No	%	No	%	No	%
Complete response	4	16	2	10	6	50	5	24
Partial response	12	48	8	38	3	25	6	29
Stable disease	8	32	5	24	2	16	7	33
Progressive disease	1	4	6	29	1	8	3	14

3 cycles of PEFAM every 21-28 days according to procedure already established for group A. After 3 cycles of PEFAM, the response is assessed clinically and local control from then on is achieved exclusively by radiotherapy according to protocol 02SR86. Patients received then 2 to 3 cycles of PEFAM regimen for consolidation.

Results

Twenty-five patients have effectively received 2 to 3 cycles of PEFAM before radiotherapy and on average a total of 5 cycles (range : 2-8). Two patients were lost to follow-up after one cycle of PEFAM and are therefore not evaluable for response and for toxicity.

After induction chemotherapy and before radiotherapy, response rate is 64 % including 16 % of complete response (Table 6). After radiotherapy, 21/25 patients are in complete remission (84 %). For 4 patients, a clinicaly detectable residual tumor led us to have a mastectomy performed in order to achieve local control. Two of these 4 patients have infortunately developed liver and bone metastasis 2 to 6 months after mastectomy. The other 2 are still in complete remission, 3 and 12 months after surgery.

Table 5. Patients characteristics Group B

Characteristics	No (%)	
No of patients	27	
Age (years)		
median	48	
range	27-79	
Stage (AJC, 1988)		
IIa	1	(4)
IIb	12	(44)
IIIa	7	(26)
IIIb	7	(26)
Prior chemotherapy	27	(100)
VTMFA*	20	(74)
Other anthracyclin containing regimen	7	(26)

(*) VTMTA = Vinblastine, Thiotepa, Methorexate, 5-Fluorouracil, Adriamycin

With a median follow-up of 18 months (3-35) 2 patients developed metastatic disease out of a total of 21 patients in complete remission after radiotherapy.

Toxicity

Hematologic toxicity assessable for 82 patients is shown on Table 7.

Table 6. Response after induction chemotherapy

	No	%
Complete response	4	16
Partial response	12	48
Stable disease	8	32
Progressive disease	1	4

Table 7. Worst hematologic toxicities experienced in any cycle of chemotherapy (82 evaluable patients)

Toxicity	WHO GRADE									
	0		1		2		3		4	
	No	%	No	%	No	%	No	%	No	%
Anemia	19	23	19	23	21	26	20	24	3	4
Leukopenia	0	0	0	0	36	44	30	37	16	19
Thrombocytopenia	32	39	10	12	8	10	18	22	14	17
Infection	68	83	4	5	6	7	4	5	0	0
Hemorrhage	69	84	4	5	8	10	0	0	1	1

Anemia stage III or IV has been observed for 28 % of patients and have led to repeated red blood cells transfusions. One patient developped after the fifth cycle an hemolytic and uremic syndrom. She died from this rare but severe complication probably due to Mitomycin C.

Nineteen percent of patients developed a grade IV leucopenia and 12 % had to be admitted for IV antibiotic treatment of neutropenic fever.

Seventeen percent of patients have developped a grade IV thrombocytopenia and 11 % developped bleeding episodes requiring platelets transfusion. One patient died from a cerebral hemorrhage.

Non hematological toxicities, besides almost constant nausea, vomiting and alopecia are renal, neurological and at times cardiac toxicities (Table 8).

Three patients have developed renal failures : one acute renal failure associated with an hemolytic and uremic syndrom already mentioned and 2 chronic renal failures which had to be treated by hemodialysis.

Twenty-six percent of patients developed moderate sensitive polyneuritis, most often regressive after Cisplatin discontinuation. Five percent of patients experienced non regressive severe polynevritis essentially observed after cumulative doses of 600 mg/m² of Cisplatin.

Five percent of patients developed chest pain without either coronary insufficiency or myocardial infraction. Such pains have regressed rapidly after discontinuation of treatment and may have been caused by continuous infusion of 5-FU.

Two elderly patients have developed an acute cardiac failure. These two cases have been observed during the first cycle and were not Anthracyclin related.

One of the patient responded favorably to diuretic therapy, which led us to suspect hyperhydration required by Cisplatin administration. The other patient however died rapidly in spite of symptomatic treatment.

Table 8. Worst non hematologic toxicities experienced in any cycle of chemotherapy (82 evaluable patients*)

Toxicity	WHO GRADE									
	0		1		2		3		4	
	No	%	No	%	No	%	No	%	No	%
Renal	57	70	19	23	2	2	1	1	3	4
Polynevritis	52	63	21	26	5	6	4	5	0	0
Cardiac	79	93	4	5	0	0	1	1	1	1

(*) 84 patients are evaluable for cardiac toxicity

Discussion and conclusion

In the treatment of metastatic breast cancer or locoregional recurrence, PEFAM regimen will induce a 62 % response rate including 16 % of complete response. For patients having never received previous chemotherapy, response rate is 73 % including 25 % of complete response and for second line metastatic treatment response rate is 40 % including 7 % of complete response. In the case of liver metastasis interesting results were obtained, response rate being 53 % including 25 % of complete response. Median survival without progression for responsive patients is 23 months. Median survival after onset of metastatic disease is 37 months. These results are comparable to best results published. Indeed, in most publications response rate varies from 43 % to 82 % including 4 % to 27 % of complete response with a median response duration of 6 to 13 months and a median survival of 15 to 33 months [8]. The PEFAM regimen is also a good second line protocol, a 20 % to 35 % response rate being usually reported in these cases [8].

In our series, we observed complete remissions of long duration which are still continuing to this date. This underlines rare but possible cure of metastatic breast cancer by chemotherapy. Hortobagyi reports, on a series of 1,424 patients treated for metastatic breast cancer, a 16 percent complete response rate achieved by a combination of AC ± FVM. Treatment is discontinued after two years. Twelve percent of complete responders patients are still in complete remission after 5 years and 9 % after 10 years [9]. Complete response seems to be the major criteria for extended survival.

A higher complete response rate is achievable by increasing dose intensity such as defined by Hryniuk [10]. This way, Marschner using doses of 120 mg/m² every three weeks of Epirubicin combined with 600 mg/m², Cyclophosphamide achieves 35 % of complete response [11]. Very high doses of single agents or drug combinations have been used with autologous bone marrow transplantation (ABMT) and will induce a response rate of up to 100 % including 30 % to 100 % of complete response [8].

Recombinant growth factors availability (GMCSF and GCSF) could also enable to increase dose intensity without having to resort to ABMT which is a very heavy treatment modality. We could therefore increase and split VP16 doses in the PEFAM regimen which would be more in accordance with its possible action mechanism. Renal and neurological toxicities associated with the PEFAM regimen are essentially observed after the sixth cycle ie after cumulative doses of 600 mg/m^2 of Cisplatin. But a maintenance chemotherapeutic treatment seems to be beneficial to most patients : Muss reports a significant increase of response duration when a maintenance treatment with CMF follows induction chemotherapy with FAC [12]. Thus, treatment is then continued through an alternate chemotherapy where Vinovelbin combined either with a continuous infusion of 5-FU or an anthracyclin seems to be an interesting procedure.

In primary resistant breast cancer, PEFAM regimen will induce a 64 % response rate including 16 % of complete response. After radiotherapy 84 % of patients are in complete remission with a median follow-up of 18 months, 2/21 of patients relapsed with a metastatic disease. First line neo-adjuvant chemotherapy failure is associated with not as good a prognosis as if there had been a response : 5 years disease free survival is then 46 % whereas it is 69 % in the case of response (p = 0.02) [6]. In a multivariate analysis according to the Cox model, the three independant prognosis factors are SBR or CPI, clinical T and tumor regression after induction chemotherapy [6]. Thus, we think that we must achieve more complete clinical remissions before radiotherapy.

It is a fact that the PEFAM regimen increases the rate of complete clinical remission. However, whether these « second hand » complete clinical remissions have the same good prognosis as the « first hand » complete clinical ones requires more time to be assessed.

Lastly, the activity of PEFAM regimen suggests that this combination may be used as a first line neo-adjuvant chemotherapy in locally advanced breast cancer.

References

1. Schell FC, Yap HY, Hortobagyi GN, Buzdar AV, Blumenschein GR, Issel B and Esparza L (1981) Phase II study of VP16-213 (etoposide) in refractory metastatic breast carcinoma. Proc AACR Washington : 357
2. Mabel JA, Little AD (1979) Therapeutic synergism in murine tumors for combinations of Cis-diamine-dichloroplatinum with VP 16-213 or BCNU. Proc AACR New Orleans : 230
3. Schabel FM, Trader MW, Laster WR, Corbett TH, Griswold DP (1979) Cis-dichlorodiamine platinum (II) : combination chemotherapy and cross-resistance studies with tumor of mice. Cancer Treat Rep 63 : 1459-1473
4. Tschopp L, Von Fliedner VE, Sauter C et al (1986) Efficacy and clinical cross-resistance of a new combination therapy (AMSA/VP16) in previously treated patients with acute non lymphocitic leukemia. J Clin Oncol 4 : 318-324
5. Scanlon KJ, Newman EM, Lu Y and Priest DG (1986) Biochemical basis for cis-platin and 5-Fluorouracil synergism in human ovarian carcinoma cells. Proc Natl Acad Sci USA december 83 : 8923-8925

6. Jacquillat Cl, Weil M, Baillet F, Borel C, Auclerc G, de Maublanc MA, Hous-setM, Forget G, Thill L, Soubrane Cl and Khayat D (1990) Results of neo-adjuvant chemotherapy and radiation therapy in the breast conserving treatment of 250 patients with all stages of infiltrative breast cancer. Cancer 66 (1) : 119-129
7. Jacquillat Cl, Weil M, Auclerc G, Borel Ch, Soubrane Cl, Baillet F et Khayat D (1991) Ten years of breast preserving management in infiltrative breast cancer : results in 412 patients treated by neo-adjuvant chemotherapy and radiation therapy with or without hormonotherapy. Proc 3rd International Congress on neo-adjuvant Chemotherapy, Paris Springer-Verlag
8. Henderson IC (1987) Chemotherapy for advanced disease. In : Harris Jr, Hellman S, Henderson IC, DW Kinne (eds) Breast disease. JB Lippincott, Philadelphia, pp 428
9. Hortobagyi GN, Freye D, Buzdar AU, Hug V, Fraschini G (1988) Complete remissions in metastatic breast cancer : A thirteen year follow-up report. Proceeding ASCO, New Orleans : 143
10. Hryniuk KW, Bush H (1984) The importance of dose intensity in chemotherapy of metastatic breast cancer. J Clin Oncol 2 : 1281-1288
11. Marscher N, Nagel GA (1989) High-dose epirubicin in combination with cyclophosphamide in advanced breast cancer. Final results of a dose finding study and phase II trial. Adv Clin Oncol 1 : 127-141
12. Muss H, Case D, Read S et al (1990) Induction chemotherapy followed maintenance or observation in women with metastatic breast cancer : a randomized trial of the piedmont oncology association (POA). Proceeding ASCO, Washington : 78

Primary chemotherapy for breast cancer — MD Anderson experience

GN Hortobagyi*, SE Singletary**, AU Buzdar*, MD McNeese***, MI Ross**, FA Holmes*, E Strom***, RL Theriault*, N Sneige****

Primary chemotherapy (PCT) was introduced as an experimental approach for the treatment of locally advanced (LABC) and inflammatory breast cancer (IBC) at this institution in 1973. It was our hypothesis that PCT would simultaneously downstage the patients and control micrometastases [1].

Methods and results

Our first protocol was designed for all patients with T4 lesions, or patients with primary tumors of any size, with matted, fixed axillary lymph nodes, or palpable supraclavicular node involvement. Patients with IBC were treated with the same strategy, but are reported separately. All patients were treated with 3 cycles of Fluorouracil, Adriamycin and Cyclophosphamide (FAC) [2]. Response to FAC was evaluated at a combined modality planning clinic where local therapy (radiation therapy (RT) alone for patients with an excellent response and minimal residual disease, or a combination of RT and surgery for those with a larger volume of residual tumor) was planned. After completing local/regional therapy, FAC was continued until reaching 450 mg/m^2 of Adriamycin. Subsequently, chemotherapy with a CMF combination completed two years of therapy. Patient characteristics and initial response data for this trial were presented previously at this meeting [3]. The updated 5, 10 and 15 year survival data are shown on Table 1. With a maximum follow-up of 16 years we have confirmed that 30 % of patients have remained disease-free without maintenance therapy for extended periods of time. This was accomplished without resorting to radical local or systemic procedures.

Table 1. Results of Primary Chemotherapy Trials at MD Anderson Cancer Center

| | Protocol | | |
	I	II	III
No. of pts.	174	193	88
No. rendered NED	168	190	82
Percent breast conservation	15	2	27
5-year DFS %	66/32*	56/37	NA
10-year DFS %	48/31	NA	NA
15-year DFS %	48/28	NA	NA
5-year OS %	80/45	82/46	NA
10-year OS %	64/28	NA	NA

* Patients with stage IIIA/patients with stage IIIB + IV. NA = not available

The University of Texas, MD Anderson Cancer Center, Departments of Medical Oncology, Breast Medical Oncology*, General Surgery**, Clinical Radiotherapy***, Anatomic Pathology****, 1515 Holcombe Boulevard, Houston, Texas 77030 USA

The experience obtained from this first PCT program was used to design the next generation of protocols. In the second trial, we investigated whether the extent of tumor regression following PCT could be utilized to plan the postoperative adjuvant treatment regimen [4]. 5-FU was omitted from the FAC program to allow dose intensification of A and C. The length of the treatment program was reduced to 9 months, both to improve tolerance and compliance, and because there was no convincing data to continue treatment for a longer time. One hundred and ninety-three patients with stage IIB, stage III, and stage IV (supraclavicular lymph node involvement only) breast cancer were treated with 3 cycles of Vincristine, AC and Prednisone (VACP) as PCT, followed by a total mastectomy with axillary dissection. Postoperative adjuvant therapy was determined by the extent of residual disease found in the surgical specimen. Patients with a histologically confirmed complete remission, and those with < 1 cm^3 of residual tumor received 5 additional cycles of VACP ; those with no response to PCT were crossed over to receive 5 cycles of Methotrexate, F and Vinblastine (MFVb). All other patients were randomly allocated to receive 5 additional cycles of VACP or MFVb. All patients received RT at the completion of all systemic treatment. Those patients who were still inoperable after PCT were treated with preoperative RT, surgical resection and MFBb. The response to PCT was excellent. Seventeen surgical specimens had no evidence of residual tumor and 54 additional patients had < 1 cm^3 of residual tumor in the breast. In this protocol, we confirmed the prognostic value of initial tumor volume, response to PCT, and extent of residual disease. Assessment of the randomized groups showed 4 year disease-free survival rates of 63 % and of 30 % for patients treated postoperatively, with the MFVb and VACP regimens, respectively. Although this trend favored the MFVb regimen, the difference does not reach statistical significance (p = 0.23). Similarly, the projected 4 year survival rates were 75 % and 58 % for MFVb and VACP treated groups, respectively (p = 0.64). The results also demonstrated that the majority of patients treated with PCT underwent considerable downstaging. Thus, many patients unresectable at diagnosis became excellent surgical candidates. In addition, many patients, whether unresectable or resectable at diagnosis, were downstaged sufficiently to become candidates for breast conservation procedures. Applying strict criteria of eligibility for breast conservation to the pathology reports obtained from each mastectomy specimen, we calculated that approximately 30 % of patients in this high risk group would have been good candidates for breast conservation, employing criteria similar to those one would apply to a group of patients with stage I or early stage II breast cancer at diagnosis.

Our third trial of PCT was designed to test the hypothesis that PCT produces sufficient downstaging to permit breast conservation for many patients with LABC. Over 130 patients have been registered on this protocol, which calls for 4 cycles of FAC as PCT, followed by either breast conservation, surgery or a total mastectomy with axillary dissection. Eligibility for breast conservation surgery is determined by a multidisciplinary planning clinic. Those patients who are considered ineligible for breast conservation, and those who prefer a mastectomy, are treated with a total mastectomy and axillary dissection. Eighty-six patients with stages IIB, IIIA, IIIB, and IV (supraclavicular lymph node involvement only) have completed 4 cycles of PCT and the initial local treatment. Breast conservation was possible in 27 % of these patients, in 50 % of the patients with an initial T2, and in 100 % for those patients with T1. However, the breast conservation rate for patients with T3 or T4 lesions was only 19 %. Reasons for ineligibility included skin edema at the time of diagnosis, multifocal lesions, extensive *in situ* carcinoma in the breast, diffuse calcifications, and patient preference for a total mastectomy. While our group recognized that these were all *relative* contraindications to breast conservation, we preferred to limit breast conservation to those patients who can be treated optimally with moderate doses of RT. Our long-term experience with high-dose RT to the breast shows that the late sequelae of this approach are severe and, therefore, unacceptable to us.

Conclusion

Our next generation of trials will concentrate on increasing the rapidity and completeness of regression with PCT, optimization of breast conservation procedures, and intensification strategies for optimal remission maintenance.

References

1. Hortobagyi GN, Buzdar AU (1990) Locally advanced breast cancer : The MD Anderson Experience. In : Ragaz J, Ariel IM (eds) High-risk breast cancer II. Springer-Verlag, Heidelberg, p 382
2. Hortobagyi GN, Ames FC, Buzdar AU, et al (1988) Management of stage III primary breast cancer with primary chemotherapy, surgery, and radiation therapy. Cancer 62 : 2507
3. Hortobagyi GN, Buzdar AU, Ames FC, McNeese MD (1988) neo-adjuvant chemotherapy in the management of advanced primary carcinoma of the breast. In : Jacquillat C, Weil M, Khayat D (eds) neo-adjuvant chemotherapy. Colloque INSERM John Libbey Eurotext Ltd, vol. 169, p 137
4. Hortobagyi G, Holmes F, Frye D (1990) Comparison of two adjuvant chemotherapy programs for locally advanced breast cancer : a prospective randomized trial. Proceedings of the 26th Annual Meeting of the American Society of Clinical Oncology, 9 : 21 (abstract 77)

Intensive and prolonged first line chemotherapy in breast cancer

F Burki*, J-L Misset*, M Musset*, F de Vassal*, R Despax**,
E d'Hubert***, R Hagipantelli*, S Brienza*, C Regensberg****,
M Itzhaki*, F Kemeny***, M-A de Maublanc*****, G Mathe*

One hundred and eleven patients presenting a breast cancer were treated with intensive and prolonged chemotherapy from 1980 to 1990. Medium age is 50, 2 patients have less than 20 and 5 more than 70. All fulfill selection criteria: no countra-indication to chemotherapy with anthracyclines, cancer diagnosis made with cytology, unmetastasied breast tumor, tumor diameter larger than 2 cm or associated with clinical lymphnode extent. All diagnoses are made with cytology, with cytoprognosis grading and hormonal receptor dosage. If possible, lymphnode punction is performed.

Therapeutic strategy rests on 6 cycles of chemotherapy with Pirarubicine[1] (20 mg/m^2 day 1 to day 3), Vindesine (3 mg/m^2) day 3, Fluorouracil (400 mg/m^2 from day 2 to day 5), folinic acid (200 mg/m^2 from day 2 to day 5), Cyclophosphamide (300 mg/m^2) from day 2 to day 5, all 4 weeks (THPVCF). In 23 cases Cyclophosphamide is replaced by Thiotepa (THPTTPVF), and in 4 cases Pirarubicine replaced by Adriamycin (AVCF). Treatment can be less than 6 cycles if complete response is obtained after 3 cycles or if disease is progressing under treatment. Chemotherapy is followed by mastectomy, quadrantectomy, lumpectomy, whether residual tumor is less than 3 cm or intracanalar compound dominating. All patients are informed of this schedule before treatment. If indicated, treatment is kept on after surgery with chemotherapy (Novantrone, Velbe, Methotrexate), or hormonal therapy, if there is axillary involvement.

Prognosis factors are the following : 5 % patients are T1n1b, 46 % T2, 34 % T3, 16 % T4. Cytoprognosis grade distribution is : grade 1 17 %, grade 2 46 %, grade 3 37 %. Forty-six % have positive hormonal receptor, 43 % negative.

Eighty-four patients receive THPVCF association, 23 THPTTPVF, 4 AVCF. All treatments have a dose escalation period guided by medullary toxicity. Alopecia is the main toxicity, while neutropenia justifies, in 2 cases, early treatment stop. In 1 case, treatment is withdrawn for possible cardiac toxicity. Mean number of cycles is 5, mean dose of Pirarubicine is 300 mg/m^2.

Local treatment is mastectomy in 62 % cases, quadrantectomy in 15 %, lumpectomy in 19 %, radiotherapy alone is performed in 2 cases.

Clinical evaluation : complete clinical remission is observed in 68 % cases, partial response in 16 %, stable disease in 4 %, and progressive disease in 12 %.

* DMSIT, hôpital Paul-Brousse, 94800 Villejuif ; ** clinique Pasteur, 31000 Toulouse ; *** hôpital Louise-Michel, 91 Evry ; **** clinique de Gentilly, 94 Gentilly ; ***** 49, rue du Ranelagh, 75016 Paris. France

[1] Theprubicine, laboratoires Roger Bellon, France

Pathological evaluation is performed in all patients and complete pathological remission observed in 13 (including 3 patients having positive nodes cytology before treatment). Characteristics of these patients are the following. Mean
age : 52, cytoprognosis grade : 1 (0), 2 (5), 3 (8). TNM and hormonal distribution is the same as general study population. Three relapses and 2 deaths
are observed in this population. Mean DFS is 23 months and mean survival
39 months, for a mean follow-up of 49 months (36 to 105 months). It is notable
that complete pathological remissions happen with highest cytoprognosis grades.

For the whole studied population, survival results are the following : in the
node negative patients we record 17 relapses (3 local) with a mean DFS of
26 months, 6 deaths with a mean survival of 37 months. In the node positive
population 17 relapses are recorded (8 local) with a mean DFS of 28 months
and mean survival of 41 months (12 deaths). The high rate of local relapse
in this last population explains results.

Median survival is not reached at 90 months (Fig. 1), while median DFS
is reached at 66 months. This last result can be explained by high rate of limited
surgery without local radiotherapy. Most of local relapses are the fact of infiltrating carcinoma with dominating intracanalar component. These relapses don't
influence survival curve.

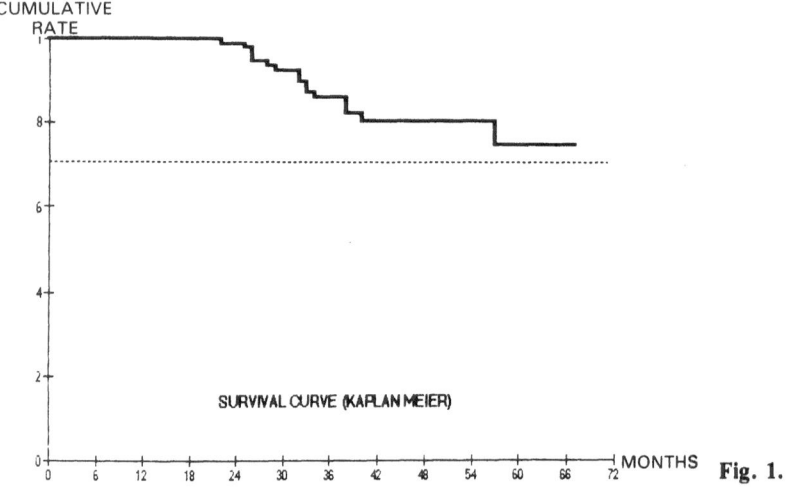

Fig. 1.

Our strategy can achieve a high rate of pathological remissions in high grade
tumors and good survival curve with a well tolerated chemotherapy schedule.
Low toxicity of Pirarubicine will allow more intense chemotherapy in bad prognosis breast cancer.

Surgical techniques for breast conserving surgery after pre-operative chemotherapy. The NSABP Experience

RG Margolese and L Begin

Pre-operative adjuvant chemotherapy in breast cancer is currently being evaluated with 2 objectives. One is the reduction of bulky tumours to enable conservative breast surgery where mastectomy might otherwise be required. The second is aimed at increasing disease free survival (DFS) and overall survival (S) by exploiting the possibility that micro-metastases might be more susceptible to chemotherapy before the primary tumor is perturbed. While a clinical trial evaluating either of these as its primary objective could also evaluate the other as a secondary objective, it is doubtful that tumor reduction, in the absence of increased DFS or S, would be pursued since it preempts access to all of the histo-biological evaluations that are now being explored as prognosis and treatment selection factors.

Methods and results

The main consideration in selecting patients for breast conserving surgery is that of local control of tumor. Although the original NSABP trial [1] evaluating lumpectomy vs mastectomy accepted patients $\leqslant$ 4 cms, later NSABP protocols accepted patients $\leqslant$ 5 cms.

In the Milan trial [2] of pre-operative tumor shrinkage, 79 % of the patients treated would have been accepted by NSABP surgeons for primary lumpectomy without preoperative cyto-reduction. Protocol B-06 showed that local recurrence rates were high in the absence of post-operative breast radiation but were quite low when such treatment was given. Examination of recurrence patterns according to tumor size suggests that any question about the appropriateness of present patient selection and local management arises in the arena of the smallest tumors, but for the larger clinical sizes there is no apparent difference in local recurrence rates. Furthermore, the likelihood of recurrence, especially in the non-irradiated patients, goes on at a steady rate for several years, yet there is no difference in disease free survival or overall survival (Fig. 1) whether or not total mastectomy was performed or radiation has been used [1]. This means that viable tumor cells not adequately controlled at the first operation, can grow slowly or lie dormant in the breast for up to 8 years after primary surgery, but have no apparent impact on long term outcomes. Therefore local control of tumor, while eminently desirable, can be considered simply as a local or regional problem. The use of adjuvant chemotherapy therefore should be directed at improving long term survival. The later NSABP protocols accepted patients up to and including 5 cms in diameter.

Sir Mortimer B. Davis, Jewish General Hospital, 3755 Cote Ste Catherine, Montreal, Quebec H3T 1E2, Canada

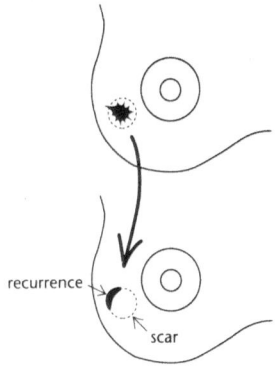

Fig. 1. Residual tumour

All of these protocols had adjuvant hormone therapy, chemotherapy, or hormonal-chemotherapy and all showed substantially low local recurrence rates. These recurrence rates cannot be expressed in a single table because of different selection factors in each protocol. Protocol B-13 and B-14 accepted only negative node patients and differed from each other in ER receptor levels. Protocols B-15/16 accepted only women with positive nodes but again there were important differences in ER levels and in average ages for the two protocols.

Despite these differences, local recurrence rates, expressed as average annual breast recurrence, run between 0.5 and 1.5 % per year with follow-ups ranging from 2 1/2 to 9 years.

Importance of local recurrence

There are 2 patterns to local recurrence. The first is a local tumor at the site of the original tumor resection and suggests residual disease which was not completely removed at primary surgery. The second type suggests hematogenous metastases with the breast as one of the sites for clinical appearance of tumor (Fig. 2). The tumor is extensive throughout the breast and skin and often extends on to the adjuvant chest wall suggesting again that it is not localized. Therefore, breast cancer treatment strategies should be aimed simultaneously at two end points : one is local control and the second is systemic control which requires systemic adjuvant treatments.

Protocol B-18 has, as its primary aim, an increase in disease free survival and overall survival and has a secondary aim of reducing tumor volume to make lumpectomy more successful. In this type of program, many patients will have initial tumors much smaller than those reported in the Milan study and it is not surprising that complete clinical responses occur, causing some difficulties in technical management of such patients for lumpectomy. The NSABP has held workshops to deal with these issues.

It is important to realize that tumors do not shrink in the fashion of a melting ice cube but may regress irregularly, leaving islands of tumor separated by bands of fibrosis or necrosis (Fig. 3). In treating such patients with conservative breast surgery it is important to excise the original tumor volume and to be sure that the excision is directed at the appropriate site. With com-

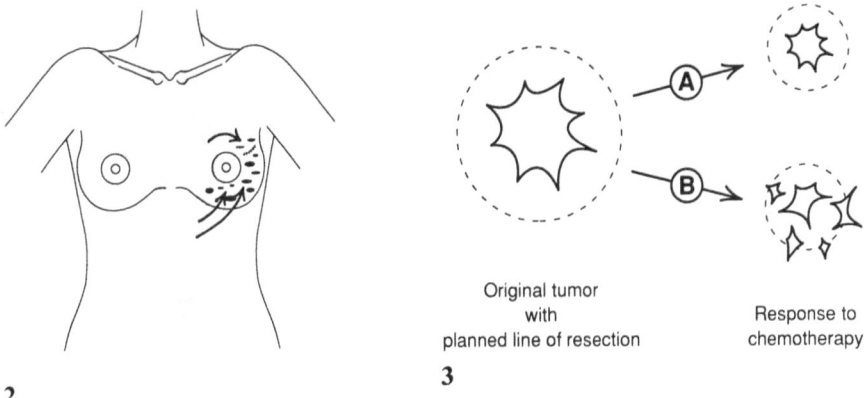

Fig. 2. Hematogenous spread   Fig. 3.

plete clinical response it is possible to relocate those tumors that have micro-calcifications by use of the pre-operative needle mammographic localization technique. Those patients without calcifications will require careful mapping of the tumor. This can be accomplished by actually drawing a diagram showing the relationship of the tumor to the areola as one anchor point and to nevi or other skin blemishes which are usually present so that a reconstruction of the map of the tumor site can be made at the time of surgery several months later.

Another technique is to use a transparent grid which can be overlaid on the breast at the time of surgery to relocate the site of the original tumor. In many patients, tumor shrinkage is accompanied by a discoloration of the overlying skin which instantly attracts the surgeon's eye and allows for accurate placement of the incision. The skin can also be tattooed or marked with the indelible pen used by radiation therapists but this must be renewed by the patients and many patients do not like this responsibility. Any of these techniques will suffice to ensure that the surgeon returns accurately to the site of the original tumor and care must be taken to completely excise the original tumor volume in order to ensure that local tumor control is achieved.

Conclusion

Patients who can be successfully treated with breast conserving surgery will be grateful, but ultimately, improvements in long term survival for breast cancer patients will come from the systemic effects of adjuvant therapy.

References

1. Fisher B (1985) Five-year results of a randomized clinical trial comparing total mastectomy and segmental mastectomy with or without radiation in the treatment of breast cancer. New Eng J Med 312 (11) : 665-673
2. Bonadonna G (1990) Primary chemotherapy to avoid mastectomy in tumors with diameters of three centimeters or more. J Natl Cancer Inst 82 : 1539-1545

Neo-Adjuvant chemotherapy in 101 non inflammatory breast cancers : treatment results

E Belembaogo, M Vernis, P Chollet, H Curé, P Verrelle,
P Kauffmann, JL Achard, G Le Bouëdec, V Feillel, J Chassagne,
YJ Bignon, M de Latour, C Lafaye, J Dauplat, R Plagne

Neo-adjuvant chemotherapy has at least the same effect on systemic metastasis prevention than an adjuvant treatment with the same protocol ; with the great advantage of decreasing tumor and metastatic node size before surgery, resulting in a lower rate of total mastectomy.

Anthracyclin-based combinations appear to be a treatment of choice in first line chemotherapies for breast cancer. Among them, FAC protocol (5-Fluorouracil, Adriamycin, Cyclophosphamide) and its homologue with Epirubicin, FEC, have been widely used, resulting in a median survival of about 18 months for metastatic patients in most papers [1]. AVCF protocol (Adriamycin, Vincristine, Cyclophosphamide, 5-Fluorouracil) is very similar ; with the same drugs, administered on 4-6 days, resulting in a higher dose intensity for 5-Fluorouracil and Cyclophosphamide, this treatment led, in our experience on metastatic patients, to a median survival of at least two years. We have been using this protocol for several years in adjuvant or neo-adjuvant situations [2, 3]. For 47 node-positive premenopausal patients, overall survival was about 80 percent at 3.420 days with 65 percent of these patients still being in complete remission ; these results were significantly better than those of 26 patients treated with CMF combination (oral Cyclophosphamide, Methotrexate, 5-Fluorouracil) [3]. In another study with 110 inflammatory breast cancer [4, 5] median overall survival was 69.2 months with a median disease-free survival of 41.9 months.

Therefore, we decided to test this AVCF protocol in a neo-adjuvant situation for non-inflammatory breast tumors ; 54 patients were treated with an interval period reduced from 3 to 2 weeks, with a good tolerance. To maximize the result, we then treated 47 patients with addition of Methotrexate to the AVCF protocol.

Patients and methods

Between january 1988 and december 1989, 101 patients without metastatic disease were treated by induction chemotherapy for non-inflammatory and non-T4 breast cancer : tumors were $\geqslant 3$ cm in diameter, or situated in the central area of the nipple (20 cases), or with a bulky suspicious lymph node in the axilla, indicating complete mastectomy (7 T1, 70 T2, 24 T3 ; whose 44 were

Centre Jean-Perrin and INSERM U71, place Henri-Dunant, boîte postale 392, 63011 Clermont-Ferrand cedex, France

N1 and 4 N2). Before treatment, every patient had a local and general assessment, and pathologic or cytologic probe of malignancy. Most patients were menopaused (67 out of 101) (range : 27-70 yr). All patients were fully evaluable for locoregional response after this ambulatory treatment. They received every 3 weeks the same induction chemotherapy with Doxorubicin 30 mg/m² D1 ; Vincristine 1 mg/m² D1 ; Cyclophosphamide 300 mg/m² and 5-Fluorouracil 400 mg/m² D2 to D5. When Methotrexate was added, patients received 20 mg/m² on D2 and D4. After 6 cycles, locoregional treatment was : radiotherapy, if a complete or nearly complete response had been obtained ; and surgical resection with postoperative radiotherapy in most other cases (Fig.1). Results were assessed clinically, with mammography and echography after 3 and 6 cycles. Clinical response was either complete or partial (> 50 % reduction in volume), otherwise the patient was considered as stable.

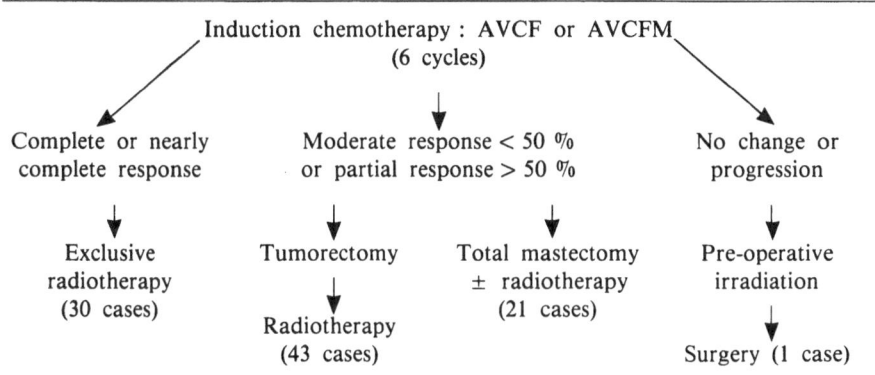

Fig. 1. Treatment schedule

Initial staging comprised complete clinical examination, bilateral mammography and echography, cyto and/or histological diagnosis by cytology or drill-biopsy, for primary tumor and nodes. Cytologic or SBR (Scarff-Bloom-Richardson) grading, modified SBR, hormone receptors, and cell cycle study by flow cytometry (EPICS, Coulter), were obtained for most patients. Every patient was proven to be devoid of metastasis by chest X-ray, liver biology and echography, bone scintigraphy, CEA and CA 153.

Assessment of response

Clinical and echographic responses were evaluated on the regression in the volume of tumor, and apparent lymph node involvement, and classified as follows : complete response (CR), partial response > 50 % reduction in volume (PR), no change (NC). For mammographic response, PR was ⩾ 33 % reduction in the main diameter of the X-ray detected opacity.

Results

A good correlation was obtained between the responses observed in the 3 methods. Responses were higher at the 6th cycle than after 3 treatments. For example, clinical responses were 8.7 % CR, 54.3 % PR, and 37 % NC after 3 cycles. They were higher with MTX, however, to an unsignificant level (Table 2). Mammographic and echographic responses are indicated in Table 3.

Table 2. Clinical results of treatment (MTX : Methotrexate)

Patients	complete	partial	stable disease
Global response (101)	20	71	10
Subgroup 1 (54 without MTX)	6	43	5
Subgroup 2 (47 with MTX)	14	28	5 $p < 0.10$

Table 3. Mammographic and echographic responses

Responses percent	Mammographic		Echographic	
	3 cycles	6th cycle	3 cycles	6th cycle
Complete (CR)	3.4	18.7	0	15.8
Partial (PR)	20.5	29.7	47.7	57.9
No change (NC)	76.1	51.6	52.3	26.3

Clinical and mammographic responses were not different in premenopausal *vs.* menopausal patients, however with a slighly, unsignificant higher level of CR in premenopausal. Echographic response was better ($p < 0.03$) in premenopausal women.

Mammographic response was lower ($p < 0.04$) in the 26.8 % of patients that were positive for both oestrogen and progesterone receptors.

A positive correlation was observed between S phase percentage in the cell cycle study and mammographic response at the 6th treatment : this response increased with S phase level ($p < 0.05$). When patients were separated in 2 subgroups ($<$ and $\geqslant 10$ percent S phase) significance level increased to $p < 0.02$. The presence of an aneuploid cell population had not a clear influence on response *per se* ; however, response was better with AVCFM than with AVCF, when aneuploid cells were present, by clinical ($p < 0.05$), mammographic ($p < 0.01$), and echographic ($p < 0.02$) evaluations. Conversely, SBR and MSBR had no significant influence.

Thirty patients were treated by radiotherapy alone after complete or subcomplete response ; 44 had a residual tumor that was treated by conservative surgery and radiotherapy. Only 19 had total mastectomy and radiotherapy, 2 a total mastectomy alone (Table 1). Tolerance was acceptable, without major toxicity. Febrile aplasia was uncommon, and treatment was generally resumed on day 21, rarely on day 28. Median survival is not yet reached ; until now we observed 2 local, 3 local and metastatic, and 9 metastatic failures whose

7 have died of their disease. The local recurrence rate until now has been 3/30 for radiotherapy alone, 2/19 for complete mastectomy.

Conclusion

This study shows that neo-adjuvant chemotherapy allowed a conservative approach of locoregional treatment in about 80 % of the patients with exclusive radiotherapy or with surgery plus radiotherapy.

References

1. French Epirubicin Study Group (1988) A prospective randomized phase III trial comparing combination chemotherapy with cyclophosphamide, fluorouracil, and either doxorubicin or epirubicin. J Clin Oncol 6 : 679-688
2. Misset JL, De Vassal F, Jasmin C, Musset M, Schwarzenberg L, Belpomme D, Plagne R, Le Mevel B, Guerrin J, Jeanne C, Mosice V, Delgado M, Hayat M, Machover D, Ribaud P, Mathé G, Chollet P, Metz R, Fumoleau P, Fargeot D, Schneider M, Gaget G (1984) Five-year results of the French adjuvant trial for breast cancer, comparing CMF to a combination of adriamycin, vincristine, cyclophosphamide and fluorouracil. In : Jones SE, Salmon SE (eds) Adjuvant therapy of cancer IV. Grune and Stratton, New York, p 243
3. Misset JL (1990) Actualization of survival of the precedent trial, personal communication
4. Attia J, Curé H, Ferrière JP, Achard JL, Kwiatkowski F, Dauplat J, Chollet P, Plagne R (1989) Effectiveness of an induction adriamycin-based chemotherapy (AVCF) on inflammatory breast cancer : prognostic factors allowing a longer survival under treatment. International Association for Breast Cancer Research, International Breast Cancer Research Conference, Tel Aviv, Israel, March 5-9
5. Attia-Sobol J, Ferrière JP, Chollet P, Curé H, Verrelle P, Bignon YJ, Achard JL, Legros M, Feillel V, De Latour M, Lafaye C, Dauplat J, Rozan R, Plagne R (1990, submitted article) Treatment results, survival and prognostic factors in 110 inflammatory breast cancers : univariate and multivariate analysis. Cancer (in press)

Flow cytometric DNA analysis and Samba computer assisted image analysis in the evaluation of breast carcinoma chemosensitivity

M Briffod, F Spyratos, M Tubiana-Hulin, C Pallud, J Rouëssé

Preoperative chemotherapy for operable breast carcinoma permits a new approach for studying in vivo tumor cell behaviour during the course of chemotherapy (CT). We have previously demonstrated [1, 2], using sequential cytopunctures, that before treatment small nuclei, flow cytometric (FCM) diploid DNA content and low S-Phase (S %) seemed to be indicators of tumor chemoresistance. In tumors with initial large nuclei and non-diploid DNA content, cytomorphological changes in malignant cells (especially increased nuclear surface) and changes in FCM DNA profiles during CT were early indicators of tumor cell chemosensitivity. In this report, we completed our study using a cell image processor analysis on cytological samples obtained before treatment and after the first cycle of CT on 24 carcinomas.

Material and methods

We selected 24 cases from our group of patients with large primary carcinoma (T3, N0-N1, M0). All patients received 3 cycles of preoperative AVCMF chemotherapy.

For each patient, morphological, Samba and FCM DNA analyses were done on samples from fine-needle cytopunctures before treatment and after the first cycle. Part of the extracted material was ejected onto slides for cytological examination (including evaluation of cytomorphological changes on malignant cells) and for Samba analysis. The remaining material in the needle was ejected in buffer and stored for FCM DNA analysis.

Partial clinical regression, not inconsistent with mammographic and histological findings, and complete histological regression were considered as objective regression. In other cases we considered that there was no regression.

Samba Image Processor analysis

For each case, slides before and after the first cycle were stained together by the Feulgen reaction. For 21 cases, Feulgen reaction was done on previously MGG stained slides. For each slide, 100 malignant nuclei were selected by the pathologist, and lymphocytes of the slide were used as an internal standard. Rat hepatocytes, stained at the same time, were used as an external standard.

Cell image analyses were performed on a Samba 2005 (TITN). For this purpose, we selected IOD parameter (integrated optical density) for DNA histograms.

Centre René-Huguenin de Lutte Contre le Cancer, 35, rue Dailly, 92211 Saint-Cloud, France

FCM DNA analysis

For each patient, samples before and after the first cycle were processed the same day on an Epics C Flow-cytometer.

Regarding ploidy index, tumors were classified in diploid and non-diploid tumors. Changes in DNA content and in kinetic parameters were eventuelly corrected taking into account the ratio between benign and malignant cells evaluated on cytologic smears. Only changes > 15 % were taken into account.

Results

Ten carcinomas had shown an objective regression (including 3 cases of complete histological regression) and 14 carcinomas did not show regression.

When comparing FCM and Samba DNA profiles before and after the first cycle, it appears that tumors can be divided into three groups.

In group 1 (10 cases), DNA profiles were identical before and after the first cycle. Before treatment, these tumors had either a single DNA peak (3 diploid and 1 non-diploid) without cells in S phase (S%) and in G2M, or a major peak (2 diploid and 4 non-diploid) with a small G2M peak but no cells in S%.

The group 2 (6 cases) showed some changes in DNA profiles with an increased G2M peak without additionnal values. Before treatment, these tumors (5 non-diploid and 1 diploid, all with large nuclei) had a small S% and a small G2M.

In group 3 (8 cases), after the first cycle all showed obvious changes in DNA profiles with a decrease of the major peak and an increase of cells in S% and G2M. Futhermore, dispersed additionnal values along the scale in (G2M) × 2 and (G2M) × 4 regions were observed, but these changes were only detectable on Samba DNA histograms. Before treatment, all these tumors were non-diploid with high S% and G2M peak. Furthermore, all had initial large nuclei and all had shown obvious cytomorphologic changes after the first cycle. When changes were compared to regression, in the first and second groups respectively, only 1/10 and 1/6 cases were evaluated as objective regression. In the third group, all had objective regression ; 5 had partial and 3 complete histological regression. (Khi 2 with Yates' correction, p = 0.0002)

Discussion

In most cases, regarding changes in DNA histograms, a good correlation was observed with both methods. Nevertheless, peak position definition was better with FCM than with Samba. But, by visual elimination of inflammatory, connective and benign epithelial cells, Samba permits a better estimation of changes in DNA in DNA patterns induced by chemotherapy.

Furthermore, Samba analyses give some additional information on kinetic effects of CT on malignant cells. Indeed, where FCM analyses showed a blockade of cells in G2M in groups 2 and 3, it appears with Samba analyses that, in group 3 where all tumors showed an objective regression, part of the cells are not really blocked in G2M. In this group, even if cell division, either nuclear (corresponding to enlarged nuclei) or cytoplasmic (corresponding to multinucleated cells) Lookes blocked, cells seem able to enter a new cycle explaining values in (G2M)2 or (G2M)4 regions and then probably die.

Conclusion

FCM and Samba give additionnal information on the early effect of CT on primary tumor cells and could help to select responsive tumors.

References

1. Briffod M, Spyratos F, Tubiana-Hulin M et al (1989) Sequential cytopunctures during preoperative chemotherapy for primary breast carcinoma. Cytomorphologic changes, initial tumor ploidy, and tumor regression. Cancer 63 : 631-637
2. Briffod M, Spyratos F, Tubiana-Hulin M et al (1990) Évaluation de la chimiosensibilité tumorale par cytoponctions séquentielles lors de la chimiothérapie des cancers du sein opérables d'emblée. A propos de 74 cas. Bull Cancer 77 (suppl 1) : 65-71

Application of dose intensity to Neo-Adjuvant therapy

WM Hryniuk

In animal model systems, where the success of treatments depend on drug dose, tumor sensitivity, and tumour burden it is simple to determine optimum chemotherapy by exploring various schedules and doses beyond lethal toxicity. However, deliberately administering doses beyond lethal levels is not permissible in human oncology. Therefore, many schedules, combinations, and schemes have been introduced to control toxicity while retaining antitumour effect. In some measure, these schedules and schemes have obscured dose-response relationships and have arrested progress.

Dose-response relationships can be rediscovered by simply stating how much drug is given per unit time. This is called dose intensity [1] and we have arbitrarily expressed it as mg/m²/wk.

Dose intensity can be calculated from intended drug dose (« projected dose intensity ») or doses received after reductions and delays (« received dose intensity »).

Dose intensity correlates with outcome for a variety of single agents in various malignant diseases [2]. For example, in randomized trials of first-line chemotherapy of advanced breast cancer using Adriamycin alone, or Adriamycin combined with ineffective doses of vincristine, the relationship between received dose intensity of Adriamycin and response rate is linear, the slope is very steep, and there is little scatter to the data (Fig. 1).

Two of the points in figure 1 are from a prospective randomized trial comparing two dose intensities [3] of Adriamycin. The response rates were 58 % and 25 % ($p < 0.02$), and the median survival times were 20 mo. and 8 mo. respectively ($p < 0.01$).

For regimens which contain more than one active drug, dose intensity can still be calculated provided one makes several assumptions : that the drugs in the combination are of approximately equal activity ; that drug interactions are not important ; and that the route of administration or the schedule do not directly determine the antitumour effect.

In certain situations we know these assumptions are not correct, and in such situations we avoid making dose intensity calculations. However, for most situations these assumptions are safe to make [2]. In any case, the question of equality or inequality of drug activity should not prevent the calculations because when a significant degree of inequality exists, it can be detected [4].

The number which results from calculation of dose intensity for combination regimens is termed « average relative dose intensity », and this correlates with treatment outcome in several situations [2].

Chief Executive Officer, Hamilton Regional Cancer Centre, Department of Medicine, McMaster University, 711 Concession Street, Hamilton, Ontario, Canada, L8V 1C3

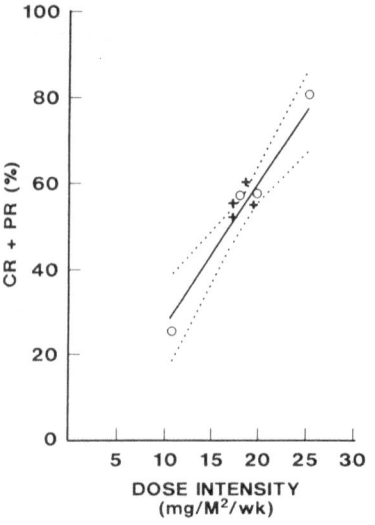

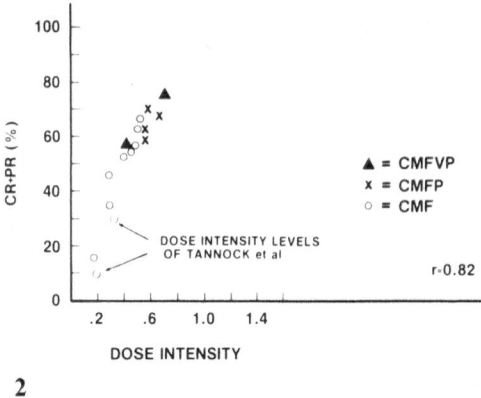

2

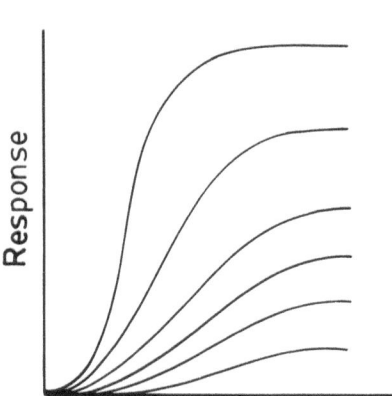

3

Fig. 1. Relationship between received dose intensity and response to first-line Adriamycin chemotherapy of advanced breast cancer. The dotted lines are the 95 % confidence limits about the regression line. o = Adriamycin alone ; + = Adriamycin plus sub-threshold dose-intensities of Vincristine

Fig. 2. Response rate vs average relative dose intensity of CMF-containing chemotherapy in advanced breast cancer. Calculations are from doses delivered after reductions for toxicity. Dose intensities are relative to the Cooper regimen [2]. Tannock et al [6] study results are superimposed on results from a retrospective analysis [5]

Fig. 3. A family of hypothetical curves relating response to dose intensity

For example, in a retrospective analysis of first-line CMF combination therapy of advanced breast cancer one can demonstrate that response rate correlates very well with received dose intensity [5]. In addition, in a prospective randomized trial testing dose intensity at 2 levels Tannock et al [6] supported the hypothesis by showing that their results firmly anchor the lower end of the dose response line derived from the retrospective analysis (Fig. 2).

In such analyses, we are locating results on a family of curves which relate response to dose intensity (Fig. 3). For some diseases (testicular cancer and lymphoblastic leukemia) we may have already reached the plateau with present-day chemotherapy after producing initial high rates of response. For non-small cell lung cancer we may still be on a very shallow dose response line with currently available drugs. However, for several diseases we could be working on the relatively steep portion of an intermediate dose-response line. In such situations, further improvements might be expected from increases in dose intensity. This could be the case for small cell lung cancers and for carcinoma of the ovary and breast and in lymphomas.

Application of dose intensity analysis may also be useful in neo-adjuvant chemotherapy. Consider, for example, adjuvant chemotherapy of stage II breast cancer with CMF-containing regimens.

In Figure 4 are shown the results pooled from 17 randomized trials involving over 6,000 patients [7] and considering all 4 categories of patients together : over and under age 50 and with 1-3 or more than 3 nodes positive. The 3-year relapse-free survival correlates with projected average relative dose intensity. Not included in this analysis were the results of the Nissen-Meyer study where 1,200 mg/m² of cyclophosphamide were given over the 6 days immediately following mastectomy [8]. The Nissen-Meyer treatment produced a 10 % increase in 3-year relapse-free survival.

The data in Figure 4 suggest that such a 10 % increase might also have been obtained from a CMF-containing regimen of .24 dose intensity relative to 6 months of the Cooper or Bonadonna regimens.

Could the full effect of 6 months of a Bonadonna-type CMF regimen be reproduced simply by increasing four-fold the Nissen-Meyer dose of Cyclophosphamide ? That is, could an increase in Cyclophosphamide dose from 1,200 mg/m² to 4,800 mg/m² given over 6 days produce the same results as .96 CMF over 6 months ? It would have been frivolous to ask such a question 26 years ago when Dr Nissen-Meyer first started his study. Even today the question is provocative. However, we are in the era of minimal breast surgery, cytokines, stem cell rescue, H3T inhibitors, Mesna and WR-2721. It might now be possible to do the study to answer the question.

In that connection, the Ludwig group has demonstrated that in node positive breast cancer, a single perioperative cycle of an attenuated variant of the Bonadonna CMF is inadequate compared to 6 cycles of CMF with Prednisone and Tamoxifen added [9]. However, a single perioperative cycle of the attenuated variant of CMF might be much less effective than the suggested dose of 4,800 mg/m² of cyclophosphamide given over 6 days.

Additional questions in neo-adjuvant therapy which could be approached by dose intensity analysis are : what is the optimum treatment according to disease burden ; and what is the best method of combining radiotherapy and chemotherapy ?

To answer these questions it may be useful to refer to Figure 5 which compares results in women under 50 with 1-3 nodes positive, with those with 4 or more nodes positive. Consider Figure 5A. When women under 50 with 1-3 nodes positive are given CMF-containing chemotherapy, their disease-free survival rises steeply to an early plateau of dose intensity. More CMF chemotherapy would not appear advantageous if given in this plateau region. Furthermore, if radiotherapy were given on the plateau the dose intensity of chemotherapy could be reduced somewhat, yet, there would be little influence on outcome. In contrast, if radiation were given with chemotherapy regimens of low dose intensity such as on the steeply rising portion of the curve, radiation-induced reductions in dose intensity could have much more significant effects on disease-free survival.

Consider the 4 or more node positive group (Fig. 5B). There is a continuous improvement in disease-free survival with increasing dose intensity. Thus, more dose intensity chemotherapy might further improve results in this subgroup of patients. Conversely, a radiotherapy-induced reduction in received dose intensity would operate with equivalent negative effect on all regimens.

Dose intensity analysis also helps us identify the most active drugs within combinations and gives an indication of how to best use the agents.

For example, as shown in Figure 6 reproduced from reference 10, in salvage chemotherapy of ovarian cancer the response line for regimens which do not contain Cisplatin has a low slope (line 3), the response rate for combinations which do contain Cisplatin has an intermediate slope (line 2), and for regimens using Cisplatin alone the dose-response line has the most steep slope (line 1). These data indicate Cisplatin is the most active drug in ovarian cancer and adding other drugs only diminishes the effect of Cisplatin.

Two randomized trials have been recently reported each comparing two different dose intensities of Cisplatin as single agent in front-line therapy [11, 12]. These permit a new analysis of dose intensity in ovarian cancer chemotherapy. In each trial there was a higher response rate for the higher dose intensity arm. However, the steep slope of the Cisplatin dose response line (line 1 in Fig. 6) was not continued at the higher dose intensities employed in the recent trials. Thus, there is a strong suggestion that a plateau is being reached for the relationship between dose intensity and response rate of Cisplatin therapy of advanced ovarian cancer.

This introduces the concept of an *inflection dose intensity* : the dose intensity at which the rate of increase in response rate falls off to the point where different active drugs should be introduced rather than pushing to higher dose intensities of the single drug.

For treatment of ovarian cancer the *inflection dose intensity* for Cisplatin may be between 30-40 mg/m^2/wk.

It is necessary to distinguish between the effects of total dose from those of dose intensity. Undoubtedly, both dosage parameters are important, depending upon the drug and the tumor growth rate, but there are insufficient data from preclinical or clinical studies to allow a judgement to be made as to the relative importance of either.

Nevertheless, the concept of dose intensity is useful because at least it gives us a paradigm within which to study dosage questions and suggest ways to try to improve treatment results with presently available drugs.

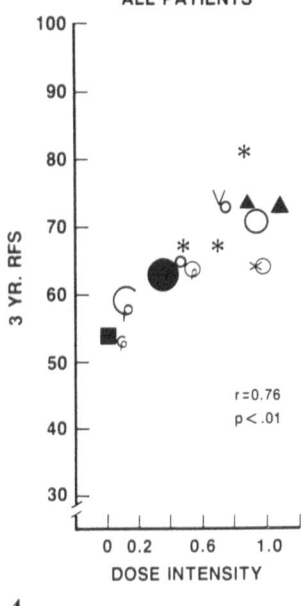

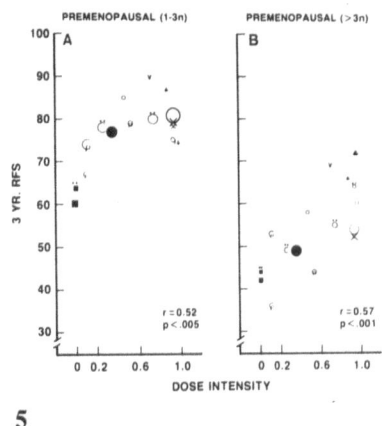

5

Fig. 4. Relationship between 3-year relapse-free survival and average relative dose intensity for adjuvant chemotherapy trials containing all four prognosis groups (< 50, one to 3 and more than 3 positive nodes ; < 50, one to 3 and more than 3 positive nodes). The size of the symbols is proportional to the number of cases in each dose intensity subgroup. Symbols : V, CMFV ; o, CMF ; C, Cyclophosphamide ; C_p, Phenylalanine mustard ; o_p, C_pMF ; •, C_pF ; ••, trials with radiotherapy added ; *Received Dose Intensity at 3 levels of Bonadonna CMF

Fig. 5. Three-year relapse-free survival (RFS) vs average relative dose intensity for adjuvant chemotherapy in premenopausal women (< 50 years) : (A) 1-3 positive nodes and (B) > 3 positive nodes. The size of the symbols is proportional to the numbers of cases at each dose intensity. Symbols as in Figure 4

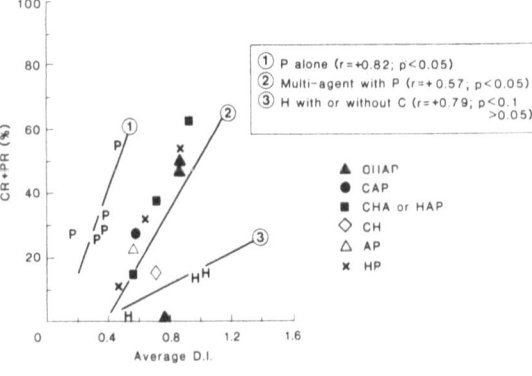

6

Fig. 6. Clinical response of ovarian cancer vs average relative dose intensity of salvage Chemotherapy : 1, Cisplatin alone ; 2, multiagent regimens containing Cisplatin ; 3, regimens without Cisplatin

References

1. Green JA, Dawson AA, Feil LF (1980) Measurement of drug dosage intensity in MVPP therapy in Hodgkin's disease. Br J Clin Pharmacol 9 : 511-514
2. Hryniuk W (1988) The importance of dose intensity in outcome of chemotherapy. In : Hellman S, DeVita V, Rosenberg S (eds) Advances in Oncology. JB Lippincott Co Philadelphia, PA, pp 121-141
3. Carmo-Pereira J, Costa FO, Henriques E et al (1987) A comparison of two doses of adriamycin in the primary chemotherapy of disseminated breast carcinoma. Br J Cancer 56 : 471-473
4. Levin L, Hryniuk W (1987) Dose intensity analysis of chemotherapy regimens in ovarian carcinoma. J Clin Oncol 5 : 756-767
5. Hryniuk W, Bush H (1984) The importance of dose intensity in chemotherapy of metastatic breast cancer. J Clin Oncol 2 : 1281-1288
6. Tannokc IF, Boyd NF, DeBœr G et al (1988) A randomized trial of two dose levels of CMF chemotherapy for patients with metastatic breast cancer. J Clin Oncol 6 : 1377-1387
7. Hryniuk W, Levine MN (1986) Analysis of dose intensity for adjuvant chemotherapy trials in stage II breast cancer. J Clin Oncol 4 : 1162-1170
8. Nissen-Meyer R, Kjellgren K, Malmio K et al (1978) Surgical adjuvant chemotherapy : results with one short course with cyclophosphamide after mastectomy for breast cancer. The Scandinavian Adjuvant Chemotherapy Study Group (SACSG) project. Cancer 41 : 2088-2098
9. The Ludwig Breast Cancer Study Group (1988) Combination adjuvant chemotherapy for node-positive breast cancer — inadequacy of a single perioperative cycle. N Engl J Med 319 : 677-683
10. Levin L, Hryniuk WM (1987) The application of dose intensity to problems in chemotherapy of ovarian and endometrial cancer. Sem in Onc 14 : 12-19
11. Colombo N, Pittelli MR, Lissoni A et al (1990) Randomized study of two cisplatin (P) dose-intensity regimens in patients with stage II/IV epithelial ovarian cancer (EOC). Proc Amer Soc Clin Oncol 9 : 160
12. Boni C, Cocconi G, Lottici R (1990) Conventional vs high dose-intensity cisplatin in advanced ovarian cancer. Preliminary report of a randomized trial. Proc Amer Soc Clin Oncol 9 : 168

Conservative management of breast cancer by exclusive radiation therapy following Neo-Adjuvant chemotherapy : results in 236 patients with a minimum 5 years follow-up

F Baillet, C Jacquillat, M Housset, BQ Hu, S Delanian, C Rozec, P Brunel, L Ucla, C Maulard

The use of exclusive radiation therapy as loco-regional treatment of breast cancer is indicated only if this approach is both effective and well tolerated. After the pioneer work of B. Pierquin [1], we began using exclusive radiation therapy including interstitial brachytherapy boosts in 1977. Treatment was begun using large field external beams to deliver 45 Gy to the breast and regional nodes in 5 fractions of 1.8 Gy per week. All portals were used each treatment day. The internal mammary nodes were irradiated using a direct beam. Interstitial implants were used to boost the dose to the primary site by 30 to 35 Gy. Guide needles implanted on the same plane were spaced 2 cm apart with a 1.5 cm separation between planes if 2 or more planes were used. Patients with palpable nodes and/or rapidly growing or inflammatory primary lesions received adjuvant chemotherapy.

Although, among 44 patients treated according to this protocol, half had tumors classified T3T4, the loco-regional failure rate was 22 %, the 5 years survival rate was 65 % and the breast conservation rate was 89 %. Considering effective loco-regional control, these results, as compared to other published series, were excellent. However cosmesis was not as satisfactory since less than half of the breast conserved showed no or minimal traces of treatment.

In 1980, taking into account the effective local control already obtained and in order to improve cosmesis, we decided to decrease the presribed dose for the brachytherapy boost to 25 Gy or 30 Gy according to the absence or presence of residual tumor prior to brachytherapy. Secondly, to decrease mechanical damage to tissues, we replaced the metal guide needles with plastic vector tubes. Thirdly, we modified B. Pierquin et al Paris system of dosimetry, which defined the reference isodose as the isodose surface equal to 85 % of the based dose rate, and we adopted, as our isodose reference, the isodose surface equal to 85 % of the first continous isodose within the radioactive set-up.

At the same time we were modifying the brachytherapy protocol, C. Jacquillat and collaborators developed a new protocol of primary chemotherapy to be used in the management of breast cancer preceding locoregional therapy. We added the « neo-adjuvant » chemotherapy to our protocol with the principal objective of decreasing the risk of metastasis as much as possible. In addition we hoped that this chemotherapy would facilitate subsequent irradiation by reducing tumor volume.

Finally, the large field external beam protocol was modified for certain patients groups, that is : patients with large (T > 7 cm) and/or rapidly gro-

Services de Radiothérapie et d'Oncologie Médicale des Hôpitaux Salpétrière et Necker, Paris, France

wing and/or inflammatory lesions and/or palpable nodes were treated using a hypofractionated protocol (IHF). A dose of 23 Gy was given in 4 fractions over 17 days with 5 Gy given days 1 and 3 and 6.5 Gy given days 15 and 17. We decided to use IHF in this prognostic group since we considered that it was extremely important to continue chemotherapy in these patients with the fewest interruptions possible. This particular protocol had been developed from clinical observations and, in non randomized studies, gave results similar to standard external beam therapy protocol (IC). We also carried out a randomized study of IHF versus IC which confirmed the equivalent effectiveness of these 2 modalities of external beam therapy [2]. This randomized study included patients in the neo-adjuvant chemotherapy protocol, patients receiving radiation therapy without neo-adjuvant chemotherapy and patients who had undergone conservative or radical surgery. We also used IHF when socioeconomic factors had to be taken into account since IHF is an easy and economical treatment modality. In 1983, for certain large tumors we began to use split course interstitial brachytherapy with a source shift (SCIBSS) at the time of the second course in order to try to decrease normal tissue damage and perhaps improve effectiveness. This novel method of brachytherapy is feasible, since it is possible to clearly define source positions for this tumor localization [3].

In 1985, since we were obtaining excellent control of primary tumor but for tumors greater than 5 cm an often less than satisfactory cosmesis, we again decided to decrease the dose prescribed for single course implants by 5 Gy.

Patients

In total, from 1980 to 1985 we treated 236 patients with breast cancer by exclusive radiation therapy following primary chemotherapy. Tumor characteristics were as follows : T1 = 16 (7 %), T2 = 94 (40 %), T3 = 84 (35 %), T4 = 42 (18 %), N palpable = 81 (34.5 %), rapid doubling time or inflammatory signs = 60 (25.5 %). Mean tumor diameter was 5.7 cm. Mean patient age was 55 years (range 24 to 87 years).

Results

We obtained the following results. Complete clinical regression of the primary tumor was observed in 21 % of patients after chemotherapy, in 73 % after external beam therapy and in 99 % after the brachytherapy boost. After chemotherapy the mean tumor diameter which measured 5.7 cm before therapy decreased to 2.74 cm ; after external beam therapy the mean residual tumor diameter decreased to 0.9 cm and after brachytherapy to 0.02 cm. There were only 2 immediate local failures amoung these 236 patients treated without surgical removal of the tumor. At 5 years, 32 patients (13.5 %) had developed locoregional recurrences : 27 T failures and 5 N failures without primary tumor recurrence. Among the 27 patients with T failures, 10 had distant metastases.

The 17 patients without distant metastases were treated for salvage. Successful local control was achieved in :

1) 4 of 8 patients managed by mastectomy,

2) 7 of 7 patients were treated by lumpectomy and perioperative interstitial brachytherapy using C. Maylin's technique [4], and

3) 1 of 2 patients managed by interstitial brachytherapy.

Among the 5 patients with N failure, 3 had distant metastases. Successful loco-regional control was achieved in the 2 patients without distant disease after salvage axillary dissection. A total of 97 % of patients conserved their breast. Cosmetic results were determined at 5 years or at the time of death or at the last normal examination preceeding recurrences. Cosmesis was defined as good (with no or minimal traces of treatment) in 78.5 % of patients. The overall 5 years survival of 78.5 % was superior to the reference date published for France in the « Enquête Permanente Cancer » [5].

We tried to determine the causes of local failure by analysing the results according to tumor size. In France, patients with small tumors (T1-T2 < 3 cm) are usually managed by lumpectomy followed by radiation therapy. We obtained excellent results for the 30 patients in our protocol belonging to the small tumor group. Only 2 patients (6.5 %) developed local recurrences. The only pertinent fact concerning these recurrences was that they were located just at the limit of the volume receiving the brachytherapy boost. These patients had successful salvage therapy, and 100 % of patients conserved their breast with good cosmetic results in 96 % cases. The 5 years survival in this group was 91 %.

A total of 82 patients with advanced tumors (40 T3 > 7 cm and 42 T4) were treated according to our protocol. Nine patients (11 %) developed local recurrences and 94 % conserved their breast with good cosmetic results in 65 % cases. The 5 years survival rate was 66.5 %. Insufficient implant volumes did not seem to be a cause of local failure in this group. Among the 62 patients receiving single course brachytherapy boosts, 6 of the 23 patients (26 %), those with residual tumor prior to brachytherapy developed local recurrences, while only 3 of the 39 (7.5 %) patients with no palpable tumor prior to implant, failed locally. Although among the 20 patients receiving split course implants with source shifts, 10 (50 %) had residual tumor at implant, none of the patients in the split course group subsequently developed tumor recurrence. It is particulary pertinent to note the difference in the mean initial tumor diameter in these two treatment groups. Patients receiving single course implants had tumors averaging 6.8 cm while patients receiving split course implants had tumors averaging 10.4 cm. The excellent tumor control obtained in the split course group was not accompanied with an improvement in cosmetic results, since only 50 % of patients in this group had good cosmesis as compared to 68 % fo patients in the single course group. It is likely that this difference in cosmetic results is due more to the difference in mean tumor size treated, than to the difference in brachytherapy technique.

Single course brachytherapy was used in all 108 patients with medium size tumors (T2 ⩾ 3 cm and T3 ⩽ 7 cm). The incidence of local failure was comparable for the large T2 group and the small T3 group (14 % versus 18 %). Other factors seem to influence local control. There were fewer local recurrences after IHF (8/69 = 11.5 %) than after IC (8/37 = 21.5 %) and fewer local recurrences when the neo-adjuvant chemotherapy regimen included Adriblastine (4/45 = 11 %) than with use of the same regimen but without Adriblastine (11/63 = 17.5 %).

If residual tumor was present before the brachytherapy boost, the prescribed boost dose was increased by 5 Gy. Among the 31 patients with residual tumor before implant, 3 (9.5 %) developed local recurrences versus 13 of the 77 (17 %) patients with no residual T before implant. The presence of residual tumor after primary chemotherapy correlated with an increased incidence of local failure.

Only 1 of 22 (4.5 %) patients without a reliquat prior to beginning radiation therapy developed a recurrent local lesion versus 15 of 86 (17.5) patients with palpable tumor at that time. Among the 108 patients treated for medium size tumors, 95 % conserved their breast with good cosmesis in 83 %. The 5 years survival was 82 %.

References

1. Pierquin B, Baillet F, Wilson JF (1979) Radiation therapy in the management of primary breast cancer. Am J Roentg 127 : 645-648
2. Baillet F, Housset M, Maylin C, Boisserie G, Bettahar R, Delanian S, Habib F (1990) The use of a specific hypofractionated radiation therapy regim versus classical fractionation in the treatment of breast cancer : a randomized study of 230 patients. J Radiat Oncol Biol Phys 19 : 1131-1133
3. Baillet F (1985) Une nouvelle méthode de curiethérapie plus efficace et mieux tolérée : la curiethérapie en 2 temps avec changement de position des sources et radiosensibilisant. Bull Acad Nat Med 169 : 231-238
4. Maylin C, Baillet F, Clot P, Mignot L (1980) Intérêt de l'association tumorectomie-curiethérapie per-opératoire dans le traitement conservateur du cancer du sein. J Eur Radiother 1 : 139-141
5. Fédération Nationale des Centres de Lutte contre le Cancer (1982) : Enquête permanente. Cancer. Résultats et analyse de survie. Doin, Paris

Abstract. We present a technique for the conservative management of breast cancer by exclusive radiation therapy with an interstitial boost following neo-adjuvant chemotherapy. We treated 236 patients (pts) from 1980 to 1985 (T1 : 7 %, T2 : 40 %, T3 : 35 %, T4 : 18 %). Locoregional failures developed in 13.5 % pts (27 T and 5 N without T). Local salvage was attemped in the 19 pts with no distant metastasis : mastectomy in 8 pts (4 developed second relapses), lumpectomy with perioperative interstitial brachytherapy (Pr Maylin technique) in 7 pts (no patient relapsed), interstitial brachytehrapy in 2 pts (1 pt relapsed), axillary dissection in 2 pts (no second relapse). The overall results at 5 years are : breasts conserved 97 %, survival 78.5 %, excellent comestic results 78.5 %. Only 2 pts developed local recurrences among the 30 T1 + T2 < 3 cm with 100 % breasts conserved, 96 % excellent comestic results, 91 % 5 years survival. Among the 82 pts with large tumors (T3 > 7 cm and T4), 62 (mean T : 6.8 cm) had single course interstitial boosts with 9/62 (14.5 %) local recurrences and 20 (mean T : 10.4 cm) had split course interstitial boosts with no local recurrences. Breast conservation for the entire large

*tumor group was 94.5 % with 65 % excellent comestic results and 66.5 %
5 years survival. Among the 108 pts with medium tumors (T2 > 3 cm
T3 < 7 cm) the 69 pts treated with hypofractionated irradiation had fewer local
recurrences (8/69 : 11.5 %) than the 37 patients treated by classical fractionation (8/37 : 21.5 %). In this medium T group, 5/45 (11 %) patients receiving
neo-adjuvant chemotherapy with Adriblastine developed local recurrences as
compared to 11/63 (17.5 %) of patients receiving chemotherapy without Adriblastine. Breast conservation in the medium T group was 95 % with 83 %
excellent cosmetic results and 82 % 5 years survival.*

Prognosis of breast cancer by state of the art laboratory techniques

WP Mulloy

The purpose of this paper is to make us aware of techniques that have been developed recently to improve the prognostic value in cancer of the breast.

These state of the art methods allow us to divide lesions into two categories: those with a more favorable prognosis which would require a less aggressive treatment approach ; and those of a more malignant nature, which would justify the use of comprehensive adjuvant chemotherapy.

The 5-year survival for localized breast cancer (Stage I) is 90 %, but this falls to only 60 % if the tumor is beyond this stage [1]. The challenge is to identify those patients who risk a recurrence of this disease within a short period of time.

Current indicators

Prognostic indicators currently used include tumor size, grade and histological type, and presence or absence of metastases.

Tumor size

The first factor to be considered is size. If the primary tumor is 2 cm or less and is unifocal at time of discovery, the current approach is to perform a « tumorectomy », and evaluate its morphology, as well as examining the ipsolateral axillary lymph nodes. This is an important indicator of its growth potential and whether early detection has indeed taken place.

For tumors of this size the above mentioned surgery has replaced the modified or radical mastectomy, and gives us the same information and prognostic value as the more comprehensive maneuver. Once this has been accomplished we can classify the tumor according to the *TNM method :*

T (tumor) : 1 to 4 with increasing size,

N (lymph nodes) : 0 : for no nodal involvement ; 1 few nodes ; 2 : many nodes,

M (metastases) : 0 : no distant metastases ; 1 : few ; 2 : many.

This is an important prognostic entity and has served us well as a first step in assigning survival rate in cancer of the breast.

Department of Medicine, Graduate Hospital, Philadelphia, PA, USA

Tumor morphology and differentiation

The next technique is to describe the tumor in terms of its cellular morphology, and to evaluate its differentiation. The cell size, nuclear-cytoplasmic ratio, inclusion bodies, and the number of mitotic figures are all considered at this point. We have here a powerful diagnostic tool, but are unable to distinguish those with a fast-growing potential from others that have less tendency to recur [2].

Estrogen and Progesterone receptors (ER and PgR)

For this reason the presence of estrogen receptors (ER) and progesterone receptors (PgR) have been measured to help predict which tumor will respond to hormonal manipulation [3]. Studies indicate that women with tumors containing ER respond favorably to endocrine therapy, either additive or ablative. This has been observed in 55 % of patients with these receptors, but in only 3 % or less in tumors lacking them. If both ER and PgR are positive, this raises the favorable response rate to 80 %.

Detection of ER and PgR can be performed by several methods, of which two important ones are here presented.

Enzyme immunoassays (EIA)

Monoclonal Antibodies (MAb) against estrogen and progesterone receptors are used in bead-based sandwich EIA [4]. This method is simple, easily reproducible, and affords excellent quality control. The main advantage is that it correlates well with results from radioligand binding assays run concurrently. For these reasons it has mostly replaced the radiolabeled steroid molecules, which were tedious procedures and had high interlaboratory variability.

However, both these assays rely on the use of cytosol preparations and cannot appreciate heterogenicity in receptor distribution among individual cells.

Immunocytochemical assays (ICA)

This method also uses Monoclonal Antibodies to estrogen and progesterone receptors with an immunoperoxidase detection system. This permits semiquantitative assessment of hormone receptor content on a single cell basis. With the use of a computer-based image analyzer, the results can be read accurately, and this is especially suitable for small, hypocellular tumors or even needle aspiration biopsies [5]. The assay has been performed on formalin fixed paraffin-embedded material as well as on frozen sections.

There is an excellent correlation between EIA and ICA for both types of receptors. It is recommended that both EIA be performed for quantitation, and that ICA be run for tumor heterogenicity. Of the two methods, the latter is preferred for estrogen and progesterone receptors.

Epidermal growth factor receptor (EGF-R)

It has been demonstrated that growth factors and their receptors are involved in cell proliferation. The epidermal growth factor receptor (EGF-R) is an integral membrane protein and causes significant increase in cellular mitotic activity. The 2 known ligands for this receptor are the epidermal growth factor and the transforming growth factor-alpha (TGF-α).

Elevated levels of epidermal growth factor receptor have been identified in primary breast cancer, and correlate closely with poor prognosis. Its presence in large quantities allows the cancer cells to proliferate abundantly. While absence of EGF-R is associated with a better prognosis, and more likely response to Tamoxifen therapy.

An excellent study done by Sainsbury and his group at Newcastle upon Tyne demonstrated a significant inverse relation between EGF-R and ER status, as well as a marked association with tumor size and poor differentiation [6]. The relapse free interval and overall survival were greatly reduced for patients with EGF-R positive tumors compared to those negative for this compound.

In addition, it was noted that survival and relapse-free periods were shortened in ER negative patients who were EGF-R positive.

We are, therefore able to subdivide breast tumors into four categories :
1) ER positive, EGF-R positive,
2) ER positive, EGF-R negative (which would have the best prognosis),
3) ER negative, EGF-R positive (which would have the poorest prognosis),
4) ER negative, EGF-R negative.

It was shown in this study that ER negative tumors, which usually have a poor prognosis, have a better outcome in the absence of EGF-R. These are referred to, by Sainsbury, as « double negative » patients.

The presence of EGF-R was found to be the most important variable for predicting relapse free periods and overall survival in lymph-node-negative patients, and the second most important in lymph-node-positive ones.

DNA ploidy and cell cycle analysis

In addition to ER and PgR status, DNA ploidy and percent S-phase identify the subset of node-negative patients who have a high risk of recurrence.

To optimize the prognostic value of DNA flow cytometry, Kallioniemi et al, in Finland, has calculated several parameters of the DNA histogram [7]. These included the DNA index, the size and number of aneuploid peaks, and the S-phase and G2/M-phase cell cycle fractions. The most valuable diagnostic indices were found to be DNA index and S-phase fraction (SPF). DNA aneuploidy was associated with a three-fold risk of death as compare to DNA diploidy. The highest risk was associated with hypertetraploid DNA index, while a tetraploid DNA index gave a relatively low risk.

The SPF yielded additional significant data in both DNA diploid and DNA aneuploid tumors. By combining DNA index and SPF, 3 types of histograms emerged :

Type I : DNA diploidy together with low (< 7 %) SPF, associated with very favorable prognosis.

Type III : DNA aneuploidy with high DNA indices (> 2.20) or high SPF, had the worst prognosis.

Type II : All other tumors, intermediate.

The conclusion is that the type of histogram is an independent and powerful prognostic indicator in breast cancer. It significantly improves the prognostic value of DNA flow cytometry compared to the analysis of DNA ploidy alone.

Risk ratios obtained by DNA flow cytometry and PgR analysis offer a means to subdivide tumors of similar TNM stage into different prognostic categories.

Discussion

We may now state with confidence that the past few years have seen the emergence of specific assays in breast cancer which allow us to distinguish subgroups of patients with a favorable prognosis, and should be approached accordingly for purposes of therapy [8, 9].

All breast cancer tumors should have this prognostic profile :
— ER and PgR detection by EIA and ICA,
— EGR-R by ICA in frozen sections,
— DNA ploidy and SPF histogram.
Thank you.

References

1. American Cancer Society (1989) Cancer facts and figures. Atlanta, GA
2. Anderson W (1971) Pathology. Mosby, St-Louis, pp 1596
3. De Sombre E R (1982) Breast Cancer : hormone receptors, prognosis and therapy. Clinics in Oncol 1 : 191
4. Greene GL, Nolan C, Engler JP, Jensen EV (1980) Monoclonal antibodies to human estrogen receptor. Proc Natl Acad Sci USA 77 : 5115-9
5. McCarty KS Jr, Miller LS, Cox EB, Konrath J, McCarty KS Sr (1985) Estrogen receptor analysis. Arch Pathol Lab Med 109 : 716-21
6. Sainsbury JRC, Farndon JR, Needham GK, Malcom AJ, Harris AL (1987) Epidermal-growth-factor receptor status as predictor of early recurrence of and death from breast cancer. Lancet 1 : 1398-402
7. Kallioniemi OP, Blanco G, Alavaikko M et al (1988) Improving the prognostic value of DNA flow cytometry in breast cancer by combining DNA index and S-phase fraction. Cancer 62 : 2183-90
9. Technical notes (1989) Cytometrics, Inc. San Diego, CA

Histological and radio-clinical evaluation of locoregional response to primary chemotherapy in non inflammatory breast cancers

F Kemeny*, J Vadrot*, E d'Hubert*, MA de Maublanc**, JF Collet**, JL Misset***

Primary chemotherapy in breast cancers has for purposes to reduce the risk of metastases, to induce tumor regression and to ease local treatment. Its efficiency has been reported by many studies [2, 4].

Materials and methods

Between 1986 and 1990, 56 patients with non inflammatory primary breast carcinomas entered study combining primary chemotherapy and surgery.

According to UICC clinical stage, TNM staging was : 4 T1 (1N1b), 32 T2 (4N1b), 12 T3 (4N1b), 2 T4 (2N1b), 4 bifocal tumors (2N1b) and 2 bilateral tumors (2N1b).

Aspiration cytology with a fine needle (6/10th or 23 gauge) carried out by two experienced cytopathologists according to their sampling method described previously [5], permitted definite diagnosis in all cases. Ninety-eight percents aspiration cytologies have sufficient cellularity (one to ten million cells controlled by measurement of Desoxyribonucleic Acid) to allow in 51 cases (91 %) an evaluation of cyto-prognostic grade of malignancy according to criteria similar to those of Scarff-Bloom-Richardson in histopathology, and in 55 cases (98 %) a significant determination of hormonal receptor status.

Primary chemotherapy combination is a 5-day cycle repeated every 4 weeks with : THP Adriamycin 15 to 20 mg/m^2 days 1-3, Vindesin 3 mg/m^2, Cyclophosphamide 300 mg/m^2 days 3-5, Folinic acid 200 mg/m^2 days 3-5, 5-Fluoro-Uracil 350 to 400 mg/m^2 days 3-5.

The types of clinical and mammographic response (CMR) are expressed in percentage of regression of the tumor. Three types have been individualised : complete Radio-Clinical Regression (100 %), Good Regression (mammographic regression $\geqslant$ 50 % with a clinical regression of 100 % or $\geqslant$ 50 %) and Bad Regression (mammographic regression < 50 % with a clinical regression of 100 %, $\geqslant$ 50 or < 50 %). When a discordance between clinical and mammographic response existed, we considered the worst response which was always mammographic.

Before surgery, 35 patients (62.5 %) had 6 cycles of chemotherapy, and 21 patients (37.5 %) 3 to 5 cycles because of bad response (15 cases) or complications (6 cases).

* Hôpital Louise-Michel d'Évry, 91014 Évry Cedex. ** 49, rue du Ranelagh, 75016 Paris.
*** Hôpital Paul-Brousse, 94804 Villejuif Cedex. France

After primary chemotherapy, 2 types of surgical treatment (total mastectomy and segmental mastectomy) were performed by the same surgeon. All patients had axillary dissections.

Patients with T4, bilateral, bifocal, or retroareolar tumors had total mastectomy. Patients with T1, T2 < 3 cm tumors had segmental mastectomy. Patients with T2 > 3 cm, T3 tumors had total or segmental mastectomy according to their response to chemotherapy.

Three types of histological response (HR) have been individualised in 58 surgically resected specimens (29 total mastectomy, 29 segmental mastectomy) : complete HR without microscopic disease, good HR with a density of residual tumor cells (RTC) 30 % in comparison with the surface of the stroma and bad HR with a density of RTC > 30 %. Next, in these surgically resected specimens, cytomorphologic changes [1, 3] in malignant cells were evaluated according to the histological type of the tumor.

Results and conclusions

Histological study of 58 surgically resected specimens allowed to evaluate the locoregional efficiency of primary chemotherapy : complete HR : 6 tumors/58 (10.3 %), good HR : 12 tumors/58 (20.7 %) and bad HR : 40 tumors/58 (69 %).

There is a tight histological concordance (95 %) between the response of the tumor and the response of its axillary node metastasis.

Primary chemotherapy induced clinical and mammographic response, complete in 11 cases (19 %), good in 27 cases (46.5 %) and bad in 20 cases (34.5 %). It allowed to increase conservative surgical treatment in 7 patients among the 22 who had initially T2 > 3 cm and T3 tumors.

A good radio-clinical regression of the tumor ($\geqslant$ 50 %) corresponds to a bad histological response in 52 % of our cases.

In our study less differentiated tumors respond better than well differentiated tumor : cytopronostic grade III before treatment is predominant (66 %) in the group of tumor with HR complete, and after treatment cytomorphologic changes are more intensive in the less differentiated component of the tumor than in the well differentiated component.

Intraductal carcinomas are less chemosensitive than infiltrative carcinomas. The incidence of occult multicentric foci of carcinomas is 25.8 %.

There is no relation between the hormonosensibility of the tumor and its histological response to the chemotherapy.

These results must be confirmed in a larger series to be statistically significant.

References

1. Briffod M, Pallud C, Spyratos F, Tubiana-Hulin M, Mayras C, Filleul A, Rouesse J (1989) Cytoponctions séquentielles au cours de la chimiothérapie préopératoire des cancers du sein. Modifications cellulaires, surface nucléaire, ploidie, histologie et régression tumorale. Bull Cancer 76 : 165-173

2. Jacquillat C, Weil M, Auclerc G, Auclerc MF, Sellami M, Khayat D, Baillet F (1986) neo-adjuvant chemotherapy in the conservative management of breast cancer. Study on 205 patients. Neo-adjuvant chemotherapy. Colloque INSERM, John Libbey. Eurotext Ltd. 137 : 197-206

3. Kennedy S, Merino MJ, Swain SM, Lippman ME (1990) The effects of hormonal and chemotherapy on tumoral and non-neoplastic breast tissue. Hum Pathol 21 : 192-198

4. Mathe G, Despax R, Misset JL et coll (1989) Intensive primary (so called neo-adjuvant) chemotherapy in operable non inflammatory breast cancer : surgical and histological evaluation of locoregional response. 16th International Congress of chemotherapy, Jerusalem, Israel, June 11-16

5. De Maublanc MA, Giraud Ch, Simondon F, Collet JF, Sarmini H (1988) Récepteurs hormonaux, cyto-ponctions et cancer du sein. Neo-adjuvant Chemotherapy. Colloque INSERM/John Libbey Eurotext Ltd. 169, pp 151-156

Breast cancer cell kinetic as prognostic parameter in perioperative adjuvant chemotherapy

P Pronzato, A Alama, A Rubagotti, P Queirolo, A Gozza,
G Gardin, PF Conte, MR Sertoli, R Rosso

Breast cancer is the most common cause of cancer-related death among women of Western Countries. Notably, prognosis of breast cancer patients is much variable, ranging from indolent neoplasm cured by surgery alone to very aggressive rapidly growing incurable tumors.

Clinical research has greatly faced the issue of prognostic features possibly able to predict the patient outcome. Recently, a series of studies has emerged on the prognostic role of some biological features of the tumor, i.e. receptors for hormones and growth factors, oncogene amplification and expression, invasion proteins, DNA content [1].

In the present study we have investigated the role of TLI (Thymidine Labelling Index), a parameter related to the tumor proliferative activity, for the prediction of response to perioperative chemotherapy in a group of operated breast cancer patients.

Patients and methods

This analysis regards a series of patients who entered a study of perioperative chemotherapy. Patients $\leqslant$ 65 years old, with clinical stage I-II breast cancer and no evidence of distant metastasis, with a good performance status and a normal cardiac, hepatic and renal function may enter the trial. Patients are randomized to 1 single cycle of perioperative chemotherapy (CEF = Cyclophosphamide, Epidoxorubicin and 5-FU) or not ; then node negative patients do not receive further treatment, while node positive patients receive alternating CEF and CMF until an overall number of 12 cycles is reached.

Thymidine Labelling Index is evaluated on tumor cell suspension with the method reported elsewhere [2].

Results

For 155 out of 490 patients entered the perioperative trial the TLI evaluation is available. Median TLI is 0.7 (range 0.1-20.8).

TLI has demonstrated ability to predict the response to perioperative chemotherapy. In fact, among patients with low TLI (< 0.7) no difference has been observed in terms of 3-year relapse rate between patients who had or had not received the perioperative chemotherapy (6/36 versus 5/43). High TLI

Istituto Nazionale per la Ricerca sul Cancro, Viale Benedetto XV, 10, 16132 Genova, Italy

patients in the perioperative chemotherapy arm did significantly better (3/40 relapses versus 10/36 relapses ; p = 0.03).

Discussion and conclusion

Perioperative chemotherapy has been considered as a tool to improve efficacy of conventional chemotherapy on the basis of theoretical and experimental findings.

Based on the mutational hypothesis, longer the interval between mastectomy and chemotherapy beginning, higher the probability of having drug-resistant cells in the micrometastases. Moreover, in some animal models, the removal of the primary mammary tumor results in a transient TLI increase of metastases [3]. Since chemotherapeutics are more active on cycling cells, the higher postoperative TLI should result in a higher activity of chemotherapy if administered earlier.

The first studies on perioperative chemotherapy, although based on single drug treatment, have shown some positive results [4].

A new era of perioperative chemotherapy studies has started in the eighties : The Ludwig Breast Cancer Group, the EORTC and the Tumor Institute in Genova have planned similar studies, in which node negative patients are randomized to perioperative chemotherapy or no therapy, and node positive patients are randomized to conventional times chemotherapy with or without the perioperative cycle.

In the present study, patients with a higher tumor proliferative activity treated with perioperative chemotherapy experienced a better disease free survival compared to patients who had not perioperative chemotherapy. On the contrary, among patients with low TLI no difference was seen according to the treatment. Thus, the TLI shows its ability to predict response to perioperative chemotherapy. This result represents a confirmation of previous studies in which a correlationship between TLI and chemotherapy effectiveness has been established.

Since most patients given adjuvant chemotherapy really do not benefit of it (they are cured by surgery alone or relapse in spite of adjuvant treatment), the tools to predict the responsiveness or characterize the minority of responders are of great importance and further studies on new modalities of adjuvant chemotherapy should include TLI evaluation.

References

1. McGuire W, Tandon A, Allred D, Chamness G, Clark G (1990) How to use prognostic factors in axillary node-negative breast cancer patients. JNCI 82 : 1006-10015
2. Conte P, Fraschini G, Alama A (1985) Chemotherapy following estrogen induced expansion of the growth fraction of human breast cancer. Cancer Res 46 : 147-152
3. Gunduz N, Fisher B, Saffer E (1979) Effect of surgical removal on the growth and kinetics of residual tumor. Cancer Res 39 : 3861-3865

4. Nissen Meyer R, Kiellgren K, Malmiok (1978) Surgical adjuvant chemotherapy : results with one short course with cyclophosphamide after mastectomy for breast cancer. Cancer 41 : 2088-2089

Abstract. *The evaluation of Thymidine Labelling Index (TLI) of breast tumors has been carried out in a series of patients entering a randomized study of perioperative chemotherapy. The aim of the study was to see the impact of TLI on the effectiveness of the new treatment modality. Preliminary results indicate that patients with high TLI are more likely to benefit from perioperative chemotherapy.*

Cytotoxic or endocrine primary systemic therapy (PST) for operable large primary breast cancer

R Leonard*, E Anderson**, A Hawkins**, A Rodger*, M Dixon**, T Anderson**, A Forrest**, U Chetty**

In 1986 we reported on a technique for assessing primary tumour response to assess the impact of pre-operative systemic therapy for large operable tumours. Careful assessment of tumour response depends on a single observer seeing the patient weekly during the treatment period of 12 weeks. Measurement of primary tumour is made by clinical assessment of the lesion with 8 diameters being taken per week to give precise volumetric data. On a monthly basis, mammographs are performed to correlate against the clinical measurements. The aim of this study then was to obtain a direct objective assay of primary tumour response to systemic therapy and to evaluate the indices of that response. By such technique we hoped to be able to confirm the appropriate systemic therapy which might be used following the definitive surgical procedure performed at 12 weeks.

Patients and methods

Between 1986 and 1989, 136 patients attended the breast clinic with tumours in excess of 4cm, thus meeting the criteria for consideration to enter into the study. Eighty-eight patients were suitable on the basis of accessability for weekly assessment and so agreed to participate in the trial. The mean age of this patient group was 53 years with a range of 33-69 years. Thirty-eight of the 88 were premenopausal and 50 post menopausal. The mean tumour diameter for inclusion in the study was in excess of 4 cm and was defined as operable stage T2 or 3 disease and N0 or 1. By definition patients with distant metastases were excluded. The histology of the wedge resection of the primary tumour had to show invasive ductal carcinoma and routine oestrogen receptor (ER) data were available following biochemical assay. Patients above the age of 70 were excluded. Prior to commencement on systemic therapy and following mammography an incisional wedge biopsy of 0,6 cm³ was taken along with an axillary node sample. Following commencement of systemic therapy the primary tumour was measured using an 8-diameter assessment technique. Mammography was performed every 4 weeks and the overall response assessed at 12 weeks. Following, this definitive local surgery was performed.

* University Department of Clinical Oncology, Western General Hospital,
** University Department of Surgery, Royal Infirmary, Edinburgh, U.K

Systemic therapies

A variety of endocrine manœuvres were examined were examined comprising for the premenopausal patients, oophorectomy in 5 cases and LHRH agonist [zoladex] in 16. For the postmenopausal patients the endocrine therapy comprised Tamoxifen in 11 cases, Aminoglutethimide in 10 cases, 4-Hydroxyandrostenedione in 16 cases and Zoladex in 3 cases. The total number commenced on endocrine primary therapy was therefore 61 of whom 15 has estrogen receptor less than 20 fmol/mg and 46 ⩾ 20 fmol/mg. Twenty-seven patients, all of whom were estrogen receptor negative and premenopausal had primary CHOP cytotoxic chemotherapy without an attempt at endocrine manœuvre.

Patients not responding to initial therapy were considered for second line therapy with cytotoxic drugs or proceeded to local excision if this was feasible.

Results

Endocrine Therapy Response

Sixty-one patients commenced endocrine therapy of whom 15 were ER negative and 46 ER positive by the previous definition. For the ER negative group there were no regressions on any endocrine manœuvre although 10 were judged to have no significant change over a month of assessment and 5 had progressive disease. For the ER positive group of 46 patients there were 24 regressions [52 %], 6 had no change and 16 showed progression. Amongst the non responders, 10 patients who were ER negative proceeded to second line CHOP chemotherapy in whom 8 showed regression and 4 complete regression. Of the 10 estrogen receptor positive non responders who proceeded to receive CHOP, 3 had tumour regression including 1 complete regression.

Initial Cytotoxic Therapy Group

Twenty-three out of 27 who received initial chemotherapy had definite tumour regression and in 9 cases the regression was complete. The aggregate response to chemotherapy was 72 % (including the endocrine non-responders) and the aggregate complete response rate was 28 %.

Later follow-up

Eighty-two out of the 88 patients in the study proceeded to mastectomy and 6 had wide local excision. With a median follow-up of 42 months from start of therapy and a range of 16-74 months, 23 patients have relapsed either at loco-regional sites (8 patients), at distant sites (9 patients) or a combined local and distant relapse (in 6 cases). Thirteen of these patients subsequently died of disease. The actuarial disease free survival is estimated around 80 % and the actuarial overall survival 82 % with a maximum 6 years follow-up.

Discussion and conclusion

Initial tumour size is quite a powerful predictor of long term survival and for patients presenting with primary breast cancer > 4 cm such as those included in this study long term survival beyond 8 years is approximately 40 %. It is too early yet to be confident about long term follow-up results in the study but the early follow-up at 4 years is encouraging when the results are contrasted against the historical experience from our own institution.

There are many questions that could be addressed in a follow-up to the study reported in this paper but it was agreed locally that the appropriate way to proceed would be to compare the approach with a totally conventional management of such patients ie comprising surgery followed by adjuvant therapy based upon the patient's nodal involvement and menopausal status. Thus, in the current trial, patients have been randomised in the conventional arm to surgery plus Tamoxifen, oophorectomy or adjuvant chemotherapy and in the trial arm to preoperative chemotherapy or endocrine therapy as based upon the estrogen receptor status of the tumour. From this trial, we hope to have more accurate information on the survival benefit as well as any other possible benefits from this novel approach.

We believe the study shows that pre-operative systemic therapy does allow the direct assessment of tumour response and hence has a potential for selection of appropriate systemic therapy. We have demonstrated conclusively that estrogen receptor negative tumours do not respond adequately to endocrine therapy. However, early intervention with combination cytotoxic chemotherapy is very effective in patients with ER negative cancers. The overall survival for the group managed in this selective manner, demanding as it is of very careful and frequent monitoring during the preoperative assessment period, compares very favourably with the historical series and now is being tested in a randomised prospective trial.

Abstract. Eighty-eight patients presented with primary breast cancer tumour size in excess of 4 cm [T2/3, N0/1, M0] and agreed to participate in a study of primary systemic therapy [PST]. Tumour was confirmed by biopsy following which 61 patients were commenced on endocrine therapy [ET] and 27 inital cytotoxic chemotherapy (CT) using a 3 weekly CHOP regimen. Twenty-four other patients (all estrogen receptor, ER, ≥ 20 fmol/mg cytosol protein) responded to endocrine therapy including 1 clinical complete remission (CR). The median time to halving of tumour volume was 44 days with a range of 2.5-150 days for the ET responders. 20/27 non responders proceeded to receive chemotherapy in addition to the 27 ER negative patients who received initial CHOP chemotherapy. The overall response rate to chemotherapy was 72 % including 27.6 % complete response, incorporating 17 % pathological complete response. There were no cases of progressive disease on chemotherapy. The time to reduction of half tumour volume on chemotherapy was 20.2 days with a range of 2.6-77.3 days. The poorest responding group to che-

motherapy were those patients who had progressed on endocrine therapy and who were ER positive (30 % response). Of the 88 patients 82 eventually had mastectomy and 6 had wide local excision. At a median follow-up of 42 months (range 16-74 months) 23 patients have relapsed, 8 being loco regional, 9 metastatic and 6 mixed. The overall survival at last follow-up was 82 %. Currently, PST is being compared against conventional surgery and adjuvant therapy in a randomised trial.

Early results of the British Columbia breast cancer preoperative (Neo-Adjuvant) chemotherapy trial

J Ragaz, B Baird, P Rebbeck, J Goldie, A Coldman, V Basco

As a result of theoretical and experimental data emphasizing its rationale, the preoperative (neo-adjuvant) chemotherapy program for breast cancer started at our institution in 1979. At that time, a rising number of experimental studies documented enhanced growth fraction of the residual tumor after noncurative surgical cytoreduction, and some evidence became available that the preoperatively timed chemotherapy may be of benefit in this regard [3-7, 9-11, 28, 29]. Also, largely theoretical and some experimental data indicated beneficial impact of preoperatively timed chemotherapy on the development of resistance [8].

At the time when the British Columbia preoperative breast cancer chemotherapy program started, the conventional treatment recommended in North America was surgery alone for stage I breast cancer, postoperative adjuvant chemotherapy with or without locoregional radiotherapy for stage II, and radiotherapy, hormones, and Anthracycline-containing chemotherapy in selected stage III breast cancer cases. The preoperative chemotherapy for stage I and II disease, and routine mastectomy following preoperative therapy for stage III disease, were considered novel approaches. The term « neo-adjuvant therapy » was subsequently adopted, describing an approach, whereby systemic chemotherapy initiated the primary treatment first, followed by locoregional treatment modalities of surgery or radiotherapy [7]. Several early reports on the feasibility of preoperative chemotherapy in head and neck tumors [7], osteosarcoma [24, 25], stage III breast cancer [1, 13] and colorectal cancer [14], subsequently followed.

Stage I and II breast cancer

Pilot study

The preoperative chemotherapy program began in our region in 1979. The main points outlining the rationale and main objectives of preoperative chemotherapy as proposed by the British Columbia Cancer Agency group were reflected in our previous reports [15-23]. In the pilot trial, 43 patients were started with 1 cycle of Cyclophosphamide 600 mg/m^2, Methotrexate 40 mg/m^2 and 5-FU 600 mg/m^2 (CMF), after the establishment of breast cancer diagnosis by fine needle aspiration (FNA), open biopsy, or both. Subsequently, definitive surgery (modified radical or conservative mastectomy) was done, followed, in high risk patients, by 8 additional CMF cycles. High risk was defined as a presence of positive axillary lymph nodes, or alternatively, in node negative

The Breast Tumor Group of British Columbia Cancer Agency, Vancouver, BC, Canada

patients, as involvement of lymphangitic, vascular or nerve bundle vessels. After the fourth CMF cycle, node positive patients also received locoregional chest wall radiation with 3750 cGy over 16 fractions.

The results of the pilot study have concluded, that the rationale for preoperative chemotherapy was sound, its safety documented, but its survival impact when compared to postoperative chemotherapy not yet determined. Also, it was felt that FNA should play increasing role in primary diagnosis and in the risk assessment of breast cancer [17, 18, 26, 30].

In 1983, a randomized trial of preoperative vs postoperative adjuvant chemotherapy began for premenopausal stage I and II breast cancer patients, and until December 1989, 201 patients were randomized. The outline of the trial is provided in Figure 1.

1983-1989. Premenopausal patients (201 cases)
Tissue biopsie randomize :
1) CT*-M*-CT** × 8
2)   M-CT   × 9

---

*   CT = Chemotherapy, CMF according to Bonadonna
*   M = Mastectomy (modified radical, or partial)
**   Post-operative CT : Only for high risk subsets (+ ve axillary nodes ; or -ve nodes, but + ve lymphangitic, vascular or nerve-bundle involvement ; or -ve nodes, but ER-ve tumors > 2 cm size)

Fig. 1. Outline of the British Columbia randomized pre-operative (neo-adjuvant) trial for stage I and II breast cancer

Role of FNA in risk determination — flow cytometry

In addition to the cytology, we initiated a pilot project of flow cytometry determined from a FNA aspirate to measure the DNA index and % S-phase. Our recently published report analyzed the first 198 cases with primary and metastatic breast cancer [12]. The aspirated specimens were examined by conventional cytology, as well as flow cytometry DNA analysis [27]. Overall, 60 % of all samples had non-diploid DNA tumors. Preliminary results, as reflected in Table 1, showed that metastases to chest wall and skin displayed a lower median DNA index than either the primary tumor or the metastatic deposits to distant soft tissues, lymph nodes or visceral metastatic sites.

In view of other data indicating a positive association of aneuploidy and %-S-phase with recurrence rate and survival, the flow cytometry technique assessed from FNA, if adopted routinely at diagnosis, may offer an important risk-discriminating capability, applicable for large numbers of patients. Such an assessment may be particularly important in instances when preoperative chemotherapy is considered, as in this setting, when the axillary lymph node stage is unknown.

Table 1. Median DNA index in breast cancer as determined from FNA sample. Primary tumor vs metastatic deposits

Site	(Number of pts)	Median DNA index
Primary lesions	(143)	1.5
Metastases:		
local	(22)	1.05
visceral	(12)	1.7
other distant	(22)	1.6

Stage III breast cancer

Study objectives

In 1980, a preoperative study for stage III disease was started. At the onset of the study, it was projected, that primary chemotherapy and radiotherapy would render the majority of patients operable. It was emphasized, however, that chemotherapy was more effective for the microscopical systemic tumor component than for the more aged and frequently more necrotic primary tumor. Hence, eradicating, or at least substantially reducing, the systemic, but less so the locoregional tumor component, would be a likely outcome in a large subset of patients. In those instances, the subsequently performed mastectomy could substantially contribute towards prolonged disease free survival or even cure.

Materials and methods — eligibility

As outlined in Table 2, eligibility included all UICC classified stage III breast cancer patients. Patients with N3 tumors had identical chemotherapy, radiotherapy and hormonal treatment, but no mastectomy.

Treatment plan (Table 2)

The treatment was initiated with chemotherapy, including Adriamycin, Cyclophosphamide, Methotrexate (with Leucovorin) and 5-FU (the ACMF regimen), given for 3 months, followed by locoregional radiotherapy, and 3 additional months of chemotherapy. Consenting patients rendered operable had modified radical mastectomy. All patients with estrogen receptor positive or unknown tumors had hormonal treatment with tamoxifen.

The combined modality program, with the chemotherapy — radiotherapy — chemotherapy — mastectomy sequence became an institutional treatment policy in 1981 (Group 1 : CT-XRT-CT-M). A group of similarly staged

Table 2. British Columbia stage III breast cancer protocol

1) Biopsy (FNA, Open biopsy or both)
2) ACMF* × 3 months
3) XRT** × 3 weeks
4) ACMF × 3 months
5) Mastectomy*** (Modified radical)
6) Tamoxifen****

*ACMF =	Adriamycin 40 mg/m², 15 mg/m² i.v.d.1 ; Cyclophosphamide 200 mg/m² p.o. d 3-6 ; Methotrexate 350 mg/m² i.v. d 14 ; 5-FU 1000 mg/m² i.v. d 14 ; Leucovorin 15 mg/m² p.o. q 6 hours × 6 d 15 ; Courses repeated q 4 weeks
**XRT =	4000 cGy/16, following the 3rd cycle of ACMF
***Mastectomy =	in consenting patients rendered operable, followed 7-21 days the last ACMF chemotherapy course
****Tamoxifen =	20 mg/day, starting the day following the last ACMF course, and continued indefinitely, or until relapse

patients was identified, where, despite the stage III classification, mastectomy was performed as a first treatment modality (Group 2 : M-CT-XRT-CT). Because a subset of physicians refused to comply with the policy of performing mastectomy routinely in all patients rendered operable (particularly in instances of complete or partial response), a third group of identically staged and treated patients was identified who had no mastectomy at the end of their chemotherapy (Group 3 : CT-XRT-CT), and compared with the first group. Tumor stage, age, and receptor status were comparable in all 3 groups. Also, responses to preoperative treatment between groups 1 and 3 were comparable. Details of the study design are displayed in Tables 2 and 3.

Results

I. Comparison of preoperative vs postoperative chemotherapy.
   Group 1: CT-XRT-CT-M vs Group 2 : M-CT-XRT-CT.

Table 3. TNM classification of stage III breast cancer. Eligibility and treatment outline for the British Columbia locally advanced breast cancer study

Eligibility	T3-4, NO-2, MO; or
	TO-4, N2, MO;
	(i.e. stage III pts, excluding N3).
Treatment design	1) CT-XRT-CT-M*; or
	2) M-CT-XRT-CT**; or
	3) CT-XRT-CT***

*   Pre-operative therapy, chemotherapy and radiotherapy, followed by mastectomy = BCCA Institutional policy
**   Mastectomy first, followed by chemotherapy and radiotherapy
*** Chemotherapy and radiotherapy, and no additional surgery

As displayed in Table 4, at 4 year follow up, there was a statistically non-significant trend for improved DFS, and OS, favouring the preoperative group. Furthermore, as a result of downstaging by preoperative chemotherapy, a substantially larger proportion of patients from group 2 compared to group 1 had more than 3 positive axillary lymph nodes at mastectomy.

Table 4. Comparison of stage III Breast cancer patients treated with pre-operative (CT-XRT-CT-M) vs post-operative (M-CT-XRT-CT) therapy

Groups: Number of patients:	CT-XRT-CT-M 69	M-CT-XRT-CT 30	p
4 Year DFS:	57%	47%	0.5
O/E	0.9	1.1	
4 Year OS:	69%	60%	0.3
O/E	0.8	1.3	
Nodes at mastectomy:			
0:	64%	17%	
1-3:	20%	17%	0.009
4+:	16%	66%	
Delayed wound healing >21 days	0%	0%	

II. Comparison of mastectomy vs no mastectomy — Group 1 : CT-XRT-CT-M vs Group 2 : CT-XRT-CT.

Both groups had a comparable objective response (clinical CR + PR) to the preoperative therapy (90 % vs 86 % in groups 1 and 2 respectively). All pts with objective response were rendered operable. Comparison of patients with and without mastectomy showed a significantly improved DFS in patients with the surgery (p = 0.02). While a marked reduction of the recurrence rate as a result of mastectomy was documented, OS was improved only marginally (p = 0.9). Despite a high clinical complete and partial response, the majority of patients (77 %) had residual disease at mastectomy.

Conclusion

This report outlines the rationale and early results of the British Columbia Preoperative Chemotherapy Program for stages I, II and III breast cancer. Our data have confirmed, since 1980, the safety of not only 1 cycle of preoperative CMF chemotherapy for stage I and II disease, but also of a more dose-intensive and prolonged 7-8 month Anthracycline containing chemotherapy-radiotherapy regimen in stage III disease. For stage I and II disease, we have documented tha a randomized trial of preoperative vs postoperative chemotherapy can be conducted by practicing surgeons when coordinated through a research centre — an important observation, as despite the appeal and scientific rationale favouring preoperative chemotherapy, its final impact on survival will have to be proven in a randomized trial. The leading questions requiring clarification in this subset of patients is the duration and intensity of the preoperative chemotherapy, whether a more routine practice of conservative surgery will become possible, and whether the surgery, at all, will be required. The significance and advantage of FNA as a primary diagnostic and risk-assessing procedure are also considered to be of major importance.

In stage III disease, we have shown that leaving large primary tumors unresected for as long as 7-8 months while receiving Anthracycline containing chemotherapy-radiotherapy regimen is not only safe, but may confer disease free and overall survival advantage, when compared to mastectomy first followed by postoperative therapy. The downstaging of inoperable tumors by primary chemotherapy may render a significant number of large tumors operable, and may also increase the proportion of patients to become candidates for conservative instead of radical mastectomy, as reflected in recent publications by other groups [2].

Finally, we have shown, that mastectomy performed after intense chemotherapy-radiotherapy treatment improves significantly disease free survival, but its impact on overall survival will have to be determined from a randomized trial, testing mastectomy as the only variable.

References

1. Aisner J, Morris D, Elias EG et al (1982) Mastectomy as an adjuvant to chemotherapy for locally advanced or metastatic breast cancer. Arch Surg 117 : 882-887
2. Bonadonna G, Veronessi U, Brambila C et al (1990) Primary chemotherapy to avoid mastectomy in tumors with diameters of 3 cm or more. J Natl Cancer Inst 82 : 1539-1545
3. De Wyss WD (1972) Studies correlating the growth rate of tumor and its metastases providing evidence for tumor related systemic growth retarding factors. Cancer Res 32 : 374-379
4. Fisher B, Gunduz N (1983) Influence of the interval between primary tumor removal and chemotherapy on kinetics and growth of metastases. Cancer Res 43 : 1488-1492
5. Fisher B, Gunduz N, Coyle J et al (1989) Presence of a growth stimulating factor in serum following primary tumor removal in mice. Cancer Res 49 : 1996-2001
6. Fisher B, Saffer E, Rudock C et al (1989) Effects of local systemic treatment prior to primary removal on the production and response to serum growth stimulating factor in mice. Cancer Res 49 : 2002-2004
7. Frei E (1982) III. Clinical Cancer Research. An embattled species. Cancer 50 : 1979-1992
8. Goldie JH, Coldman HA (1979) A mathematical model for relating the drug sensitivity of tumors to the spontaneous mutation rate. Cancer Treat Rep 63 : 1727-1733
9. Gorelik E, Segal S, Feldman M (1978) Growth of local tumor exerts a specific inhibitory effect on progression of lung metastases. Int J Cancer 21 : 615-617
10. Gunduz N, Fisher B, Saffer EA (1979) Effects of surgical removal on the growth and kinetics of residual tumor. Cancer Res 39 : 3861-3865
11. Lange PH, Hekmat K, Bosl G et al (1980) Accelerated growth of testicular cancer after cytoreductive surgery. Cancer, 45 : 1498-1506
12. Le Riche J, Atiba J, Ragaz J et al (1989) The role of fine needle aspiration in determining the risk of breast cancer. In : Ragaz J, Ariel IM (eds) High risk breast cancer. Springer-Verlag, Heidelberg, New York, pp 120-139

13. Papaioannou AN. (1981) Preoperative chemotherapy for operable solid tumors. Eur J Cancer 17 : 263-269
14. Papaioannou AN, Polychronis AP, Kozonis JA et al (1986) Chemotherapy with or without anitcoagulation as initial management of patients with operable colorectal cancer : a prospective study with at least 5 years followup. In : Ragaz J, Band PR, Goldie JH, (eds) Preoperative (neo-adjuvant) chemotherapy. Recent results in cancer Res pp 135-142
15. Ragaz J, Baird R, Goldie JH et al (1983) Neo-adjuvant (properative) adjuvant chemotherapy for breast cancer — new approach for the management of breast cancer. Proc Am Soc Clin Oncol 2 : 111
16. Ragaz J, Baird R, Goldie JH (1984) Neo-adjuvant (preoperative) chemotherapy for breast cancer. In : Jones V, Salmon SE, (eds) Adjuvant therapy for cancer. Grunne and Stratton, Orlando, Florida, pp 425-432
17. Ragaz J, Baird R, Rebbeck P et al (1985) Neo-adjuvant (preoperative) chemotherapy for breast cancer. Cancer 56 : 719-724
18. Ragaz J (1986) Emerging modalities for adjuvant therapy of breast cancer : neo-adjuvant chemotherapy. NCI Monogr 1 : 145-152
19. Ragaz J (1986) Preoperative (neo-adjuvant) chemotherapy for breast cancer. Outline of the British Columbia Trial. Recent results. Cancer Res 106 : 85-95
20. Ragaz J, Band PR, Goldie JH (1986) Preoperative (neo-adjuvant) chemotherapy. Recent results in cancer Res 103 : 1-160
21. Ragaz J (1990) Comments on kinetics and biology of the residual cancer, and on relevant therapeutic strategies based on these phenomena. In : Ragaz J, Simpson-Herren L, Lippman M, Fisher B (eds) Effects of therapy on biology and kinetics of the residual tumor, Part B : Clinical aspects. Wiley-Liss, New York, pp 117-139
22. Ragaz J, Manji M, Olivetto I et al (1987) Preoperative combined modality (neo-adjuvant) therapy for locally inoperable breast cancer. In : Patterson HGA, Lees AW (eds) Fundamental problems in breast cancer. Martinus Nijihoff, Boston, pp 383-389
23. Ragaz J, Goldie JH, Baird R et al (1989) Experimental basis and clinical reality of preoperative (neo-adjuvant) chemotherapy in breast cancer. Recent results in cancer Res 115 : 28-35
24. Rosen G (1979) Primary ostoeogenic sarcoma The rationale for preoperative chemotherapy in delayed surgery. Cancer 43 : 2163-2177
25. Rosen G, Marcove RC, Huvos AG et al (1984) Primary osteogenic sarcoma : Eight year experience with adjuvant chemotherapy. J Cancer Res Clin Oncol 106 : 68-77
26. Salter DR, Bassett AA (1981) Role of needle aspiration in reducing the number of unnecessary breast biopsies. Can J Surg 24 : 311-313
27. Taylor IW (1980) A rapid single step staining technique for DNA analysis by fluormetry. J Histochem Cytochem 28 : 1021-1024
28. Simpson-Herren L, Sanford AH, Holmquist JP (1976) Effects of surgery on the cell kinetics of residual tumor. Cancer Treat Rep 6 : 1749-1760
29. Weiss L (1980) Metastases differences between cancer cells in primary and secondary tumors. In : Joachim H (ed) Pathol Biol Annual. Raven Press, New York, 10 : 51-81
30. Zajicek J (1974) Aspiration biopsy cytology : 1. Cytology of supradiaphragmatic organs. Karger, New York

Combined modality approach in treatment of inflammatory carcinoma of the breast — MD Anderson Cancer Center experience

AU Buzdar, GN Hortobagyi, M McNeese*, D Frye, F Holmes, G Fraschini, R Theriault, E Singletary**

Inflammatory carcinoma of the breast is the most lethal form of breast cancer and has a dismal prognosis. Most of the patients die of distant metastases with or without locoregional control within the first 2 years after diagnosis. At MD Anderson Hospital, since 1973, all patients with inflammatory carcinoma of the breast were prospectively treated with a combined modality approach in three sequential studies. All patients received 3 cycles of Fluorouracil, Doxorubicin, and Cyclophosphamide (FAC) before local therapy. In the first protocol (from 1973-1977), primary radiotherapy was the local treatment modality, and chemotherapy was continued for a total of 2 years. From 1978-1981 (Protocol II), mastectomy became the primary local treatment and FAC was reinstituted within 10-14 days after surgery. After completion of the FAC, consolidative radiotherapy was given. From 1982-1986 (Protocol III), Vincristine and Prednisone were added to the FAC regimen and doxorubicin was given by a continuous infusion (Table 1).

Table 1. Treatment Scheme

Protocol I	FAC, 3 cycles → Radiotherapy → FAC → CMF
Protocol II	FAC, 3 cycles → Mastectomy → FAC × 6 → Radiotherapy
Protocol III	FACVP, 3 cycles → Mastectomy → FACVP × 8 → Radiotherapy

FAC : 5-Fluorouracil, doxorubicin, and cyclophosphamide; FACVP : FAC + vincristine and prednisone

The data were updated as of January 1991, and these results are presented in this report. The median follow-up of the entire study patient population is 80 months (range 45-203 months). The treatment details and patient characteristics have been published in a recent report [1-3]. Of 106 patients, 74 patients have developed recurrent disease and of those, 69 have died from metastatic disease. An additional 9 patients died of other causes not related to cancer and were free of disease at the time of death. The estimated 7 year disease-free and overall survival by various patient characteristics are shown in Table 2.

There was no significant difference in the disease-free or overall survival by age of the patients.

The University of Texas MD Anderson Cancer Center, Departments of Medical Oncology, Radiotherapy*, and Surgery**, 1515 Holcombe Boulevard, Houston, TX 77030, USA

Table 2. Seven-year estimated percent disease-free and survival rates according to prognostic factors

Prognostic factors	N	Overall Survival		Disease-free Survival	
		7-year	p	7-year	p
Age (yr)					
< 50	46	26	0.3	23	0.3
⩾ 50	60	46		38	
Type of protocol					
Protocol I (1973-1977)	40	33		31	
Protocol II (1978-1979)	23	30	0.5	22	0.5
Protocol III (1980-1986)	43	41		36	
Estrogen receptor					
> 10 fm/mg	18	53		44	
< 10 fm/mg	28	28	0.08	29	0.2
unknown	60	36		29	
Tumor mass on mammography					
No	58	34	0.5	30	0.4
Yes	39	38		32	
Nodal Stage					
N0	21	30		28	
N1	25	27	0.8	18	0.6
N2	41	46		41	
N3	19	37		32	
Dermal Lymphatic Invasion					
Yes	46	28	0.02	26	0.07
No	30	61		45	
Specimen not available	30	26		27	
Response to Induction Chemotherapy					
Complete remission	12	63		48	
Partial remission	61	41	0.001	36	0.003
< Partial remission	29	14		10	
Mastectomy					
No	40	34	0.6	31	0.5
Yes	66	38		32	

Patients treated in three sequential studies have similar disease-free survival except that patients treated in Protocol III have slightly better disease-free and overall survival, but these differences were not statistically significant.

The duration of chemotherapy in Protocols II and III was reduced to 11 cycles (23 weeks) and patients in group I received 24 months of chemotherapy. A small number of patients had estrogen receptor positive tumor (most were weakly positive), but these patients had better 7 year disease-free and overall survival compared to patients with estrogen receptor-negative tumors, though the differences were not significant statistically.

Patients with mass present on initial mammogram compared to patients without any dominant mass demonstrated no difference in the disease-free or overall survival. Initial nodal status also did not correlate to disease-free or overall survival.

Presence of dermal lymphatic invasion was associated with lower 7 year disease-free and overall survival.

The response to initial chemotherapy was an important prognostic feature and patients who achieved complete responses had significantly better survival rates compared to the patients who had partial or less than partial response.

These data support that response to induction chemotherapy favorably influences the course of the disease.

Patients with less than partial response had a dismal prognosis, and in this subgroup of patients, alternate systemic chemotherapy programs may offer a better chance of long-term control and survival in this disease.

Such approaches are currently being evaluated. Mastectomy following induction chemotherapy was evaluated in 2 study protocols (II and III), and disease-free and overall survival of patients treated with only radiation therapy and mastectomy followed by radiation therapy had similar estimated seven years disease-free and overall survival. However, mastectomy provided histological response data to induction chemotherapy and in patients with significant residual disease, the role of alternate treatments could be evaluated.

Surgical debulking also results in lower required doses of radiation therapy to control local disease and with this approach late sequelae of high dose irradiation can be avoided.

References

1. Koh EH, Buzdar AU, Ames FC, Singletary SE, McNeese MD, Frye D, Holmes FA, Fraschini G, Hug V, Theriault RL, Balch CM, Hortobagyi GN (1990) Inflammatory carcinoma of the breast : results of a combined-modality approach-M.D.Anderson Cancer Center experience. Cancer Chemother Pharmacol 27 : 94-100
2. Buzdar AU, Montague ED, Barker JL (1981) Management of inflammatory carcinoma of the breast with a combined modality approach — an update. Cancer 47 : 2537-2542
3. Fastenberg NA, Buzdar AU, Montague ED, Jessup JM, Martin RG, Hortobagyi GN, Blumenschein GR (1985) Management of inflammatory carcinoma of the breast : a combined modality approach. Am J Clin Oncol 8 : 131-141

Induction chemotherapy in locally advanced breast cancer : prognostic variables affecting results

G Gardin, PF Conte, P Pronzato, A Rubagotti, T Guido,
L Miglietta, L Repetto, G Addamo, A Camoriano, M Merlano,
C Naso, G Canavese, A Catturich, R Rosso

Patients presenting with clinical features of locally advanced, non-metastatic breast cancer (T3-T4, N2-N3, M0) have a poor prognosis. After loco-regional treatment by radiation therapy and/or surgery the recurrence rate is high and rapid with median survival less than three years [1-3]. Although not evaluated in randomized clinical trials, there is evidence that the combination of local and systemic treatment has produced a substantial improvement, as compared to historical controls. Five-year survivals in excess of 50 % have been reported from studies in which chemotherapy is used before and after local treatment [4]. In the present report, we review our experience with a multidisciplinary therapeutic approach in patients with locally advanced breast cancer ; moreover we have analyzed the relevance of some pretreatment and treatment-related variables in affecting the results in terms of disease-free survival and overall survival.

Materials and methods

Since 1983, 125 consecutive patients with previously untreated locally advanced breast cancer were treated at our Institution with a multimodal program. Pretreatment evaluation consisted of a physical examination, complete blood cell count, biochemistry profile, chest X-ray, bone scan and abdominal ultrasound. All patients had a biopsy-proven diagnosis of breast cancer and no evidence of distant metastases.

Patients received neo-adjuvant chemotherapy with CAF (CTX 600 mg/m² + ADM 50 mg/m² + 5-FU 600 mg/m² every 21 days, for 3 cycles. This treatment was followed by radical mastectomy and/or radiation therapy. After locoregional treatment, patients received adjuvant chemotherapy with 3 CAF alternating with 3 CMF (CTX 600 mg/m² + MTX 40 mg/m² + 5-FU 600 mg/m²), every 21 days, for a total of 6 cycles.

The following prognostic variables were studied. Age was determined at the time of diagnosis. Clinical stage was defined as stage IIIa/IIIb according to the 1978 International Union Against Cancer TNM classification. Tumor estrogen receptor determination was done by the dextran-coated charcol method and values ⩾ 10 fmol/mg cytosol protein were considered positive. Inflammatory carcinoma was defined as a diffuse erythema involving all of the mammary gland region and positive skin biopsy for tumor in dermal lymphatics.

Istituto Nazionale per la Ricerca sul Cancro Viale Benedetto XV, n° 10, 16132 Genova, Italy

Response to chemotherapy was assessed on clinical and radiological basis during induction chemotherapy at each cycle and before local treatment. The number of axillary node metastases was categorized as none (N-), 1 to 3 positive nodes (N+ 1-3), 4 or more positive nodes (N+ > 3). Residual tumor size after induction chemotherapy was determined by measuring the largest tumor diameter in the mastectomy specimen.

Survival and disease-free survival were calculated by the Kaplan-Meier method. The statistical significance of the difference between curves was calculated by the log-rank test.

Results

The main patient and tumor characteristics at diagnosis were as follows : median age was 54 yr (range 23-76 yr), 50 patients (40 %) had ≤ 50 yr, 75 patients (60 %) had > 50 yr ; tumor estrogen receptor status was known in 98 patients, 47 cases (48 %) were ER-positive and 51 ER-negative (52 %) ; there were 27 patients (22 %) with stage IIIa, and 98 patients (78 %) with stage IIIb, including 51 cases of inflammatory carcinoma (IBC) and 9 cases with ipsilateral supraclavicular lymph node involvement.

After initial cytoreductive chemotherapy with 3 cycles of CAF, 12 patients (9.6 %) achieved CR, 69 patients (55.2 %) achieved PR, while 40 patients (32 %) had SD and 4 patients (3.2 %) had progressive disease. The objective response rate was 64.8 % (95 % Confidence Interval : 55 %-73 %).

Residual tumor in the mastectomy specimen was > 1 cm in 94 patients (81.7 %), < 1 cm in 17 cases (14.8 %), while only 4 patients (3.5 %) achieved complete pathological response.

After a median follow-up period of 48 months (range 12-80 months), 60 of the 125 patients have since suffered relapses (33 loco-regional, 20 distant and 7 local + distant), while 35 patients have died at the time of this report. The 7-yr survival and disease-free survival were 53 % and 22 %, respectively. DFS and survival of patients were analyzed in relationship to various prognostic factors. Age (≤ 50 yr vs > 50 yr), receptor status (ER-positive vs ER-negative), clinical response (responders vs non-responders) and pathological response (residual tumor size ≤ 1 cm vs > 1 cm) to neo-adjuvant chemotherapy had no significant effect on DFS or survival. DFS and survival were significantly different according to stage (IIIa vs IIIb : median DFS 72 months vs 22 months, p = 0.004 ; 7-yr survival 66 % vs 49 %, p = 0.05), inflammatory carcinoma (Non-IBC vs IBC : median DFS 58 months vs 18 months, p = 0.001; 7-yr survival 61 % vs 44 %, p = 0.02), and number of involved nodes (N+ 1-3 vs N+ > 3 : median DFS 59 months vs 25 months, p = 0.01 ; 7-yr survival 90 % vs 44 %, p = 0.003).

Discussion and conclusion

Our results confirm that multimodal treatment, combining aggressive chemotherapy and locoregional therapy, has improved prognosis of locally advanced breast cancer with a considerable percentage of patients surviving after 5 years from diagnosis.

From our findings, clinical stage at diagnosis, signs of inflammation and number of involved lymph nodes, represent the most important variables in predicting results in terms of freedom from relapse and survival, whereas prognosis is not significantly related to age, receptor status, clinical and pathological response to induction chemotherapy.

References

1. Zucali R, Uslenghi C, Kenda R, Bonadonna G (1976) Natural history and survival of inoperable breast cancer treated with radiotherapy and radiotherapy followed by radical mastectomy. Cancer 37 : 1422-1431
2. Rubens RD, Armitage P, Winter PJ, Tong D, Hayward JL (1977) Prognosis in inoperable stage III carcinoma of the breast. Europ J Cancer 13 : 805-811
3. Sutherland CM, Mather FJ (1985) Long-term survival and prognostic factors in patients with regional breast cancer (skin, muscle, and/or chest wall attachment). Cancer 55 : 1389-1397
4. Hortobagyi GN, Blumenschein GR, Spanos W, Montague ED, Buzdar AU, Yap HY, Schell F (1983) Multimodal treatment of loco-regionally advanced breast cancer. Cancer 51 : 763-768

Dose response relationship with epirubicin in Neo-Adjuvant combination chemotherapy for advanced breast cancer. End results of a prospective randomized trial

C Focan, M Th Closon, JM Andrien, M Dicato, P Driesschaert, D Focan-Henrard, M Lemaire, JP Lobelle, L Longrée, F Ries

In a retrospective analysis of the literature, Hryniuk et al suggested a significant relationship between dose intensities of combination chemotherapies and tumor response rate in advanced breast carcinoma (BC) [1].

In this disease, Epirubicin both in single or combined therapy exerted antitumor activity comparable to that of the parent compound Adriamycin [2] ; those results were achieved with an overall better tolerance with reduced hematological and cardiac toxicities [3, 4].

In 1985, we initiated a prospective randomized trial aiming to evaluate the dose response relationship of an Epirubicin based combination chemotherapy (CT) in previously untreated advanced BC.

Material and methods

After adequate staging, females previously untreated with CT, aged below 70 suffering from an histologically proven advanced BC with evaluable or measurable lesions were eligible for the study. Patients with cardiac or CNS diseases as well as those with insufficient hepatic, renal or hematological reserves were also excluded.

After randomization, patients received either an intensified FEC regimen (5-FU and cyclophosphamide 500 mg/m² day 1, Epirubicin 50 mg/m² days 1 and 8, every 3 weeks — group A) or a classical FEC regimen in which Epirubicin was only given at day 1 (group B).

Results

One hundred and forty-one patients (70 : A ; 71 : B) were fully evaluable for this report. Their characteristics were well balanced for both primary locally advanced (LA) and recurrent/metastastic (RM) groups (Table 1).

Toxicity (WHO) was assessed on 361 courses in group A (mean : 4.9 ± 2.5) and 394 courses in group B (mean : 5.7 ± 2.9). Patients in group A presented a higher frequency of anemia (26.2 % vs 9.6 in group B), granulocytopenia (6.6 % grades III-IV vs 1.8 %) and stomatitis (9.9 % vs 2.9 %). No cardiac event could be related to the therapy. Nausea, vomiting and alopecia were common.

CH St Joseph-Espérance, CHU Sart Tilman, Liège ; Hop Civil, Verviers ; CH Luxembourg, Luxembourg ; Farmitalia, Nivelles, Belgium and Luxembourg

Table 1. Patients characteristics

	A	B
Mean age (± SD)	56 ± 8	59 ± 10
Menopausal status		
pre	18	18
peri	11	19
post	39	30
Disease extension		
Locally advanced	25	22
Recurrent/metastatic	45	49
Dominant site		
Soft tissue	7	4
Bone	12	14
Viscera	26	31
Disease free intervall (months ± SD)	51 ± 52	58 ± 60
Nb of sites mean ± SD – (range)	1.9 ± 1.0 (1 – 4)	2.2 ± 1.1 (1 – 5)

The relative dose intensities delivered [1] for epirubicin were 1.53 ± 0.4 in group A and 0.93 ± 0.26 in group B ($p < 0.001$).

The response rate (WHO) was significantly higher in group A (69 ± 16 % with 9 CR and 39 PR) than in group B (41 ± 10 % with 5 CR and 24 PR ; $p < 0.001$). This was observed in the LA group (76 vs 32 % ; $p = 0.018$) as well as in the RM group (64 vs 46 % ; $p = 0.01$). The median duration of response was significantly longer in group A (22.5 months-m) than in group B (14.2 m ; $p = 0.05$).

Discussion and conclusion

In a prospective randomized trial, we evidenced a dose response relationship for an Anthracycline based chemotherapy as first line treatment in advanced BC. In the Epirubicin intensified arm, patients not only could benefit from more tumor shrinkage, but they also experienced longer sustained responses.

Those achieved results clearly support the Hryniuk's hypothesis of a dose response relationship for Anthracycline derivatives in advanced BC [1]. At the time of the initiation of this trial, the mean doses recommended for Epirubicin in combination therapy ranged from 50 to 75 mg/m² [2, 3]. More recent phase I-II evaluations on the maximum tolerated Epirubicin doses revealed that doses ranging from 100 to 120-150 mg/m² could be safely administered both in single or combination treatments [2-5]. Also, in those recent analyses, most authors suggested the existence of a steep dose response curve for Epirubicin [2-5].

References

1. Hryniuk W, Bush T (1984) The importance of dose intensity in chemotherapy of metastatic breast cancer. J Clin Oncol 2 : 1281-1288
2. Hayat M, Ostronoff M, Ibrahim A (1989) Epirubicin in breast cancer. Adv. in Clin Oncol 2 : 49-63
3. Cersosimo RJ, Hong WK (1986) Epirubicin : a review of pharmacology, clinical activity and adverse effects of an adriamycin analogue. J Clin Oncol 4 : 425-429
4. Young CM (1989) Clinical toxicity of epirubicin. Adv in Clin Oncol 2 : 29-38
5. Marschner N, Nagel GA (1989) High dose epirubicin in combination with cyclophosphamide in advanced breast cancer. Adv in Clin Oncol 2 : 127-141

Continuous prolonged intra-arterial (IA) chemotherapy for extensive locally recurrent breast cancer

JF Morere, C Boaziz, JL Breau, D Goldlust, L Israël

Local regional relapse rate following surgery for breast cancer varies from 4 % to 27 % according to histological axillary nodal status and previous adjuvant therapy [1]. In most cases, recurrences remain confined to the chest wall and/or supraclavicular, or to mammary nodes, without distant metastases [2]. However, surgery or irradiation can offer only palliation for patients with massive disease [3]. Moreover, cumulative doses of systemic chemotherapy are often reached and impairment of vascularization in previously irradiated areas renders a good response to systemic chemotherapy unlikely [4]. Intra-arterial chemotherapy allows higher local concentrations of drugs with lower systemic toxicity [4]. On the basis of these observations we have tested intra-arterial chemotherapy for patients treated for recurrent breast cancer at the Oncology department of the Avicenne Hospital.

Patients and methods

Twenty patients with extensive locally recurrent breast cancer were entered into the study. Mean age was 51 years (range 38-66 years). All had confirmed thoracic skin metastases (14/20), supraclavicular lymph nodes (3/20) or inflammatory carcinoma (7/20). Sixteen patients had previous systemic chemotherapy. In 14 patients recurrences occurred in the field of previous radiotherapy.

Intra-arterial chemotherapy was delivered through a catheter placed in the subclavian artery via the femoral artery by Seldinger's method under X ray control. The correct position of the catheter was checked by arteriography and by injections of blue dye. In 4 cases vascular distribution was studied with radiolabelled albumin.

The treatment regimen consisted of Cisplatin 10 mg/day, Bleomycin 3 mg/day in combination with Vinblastine 1 mg/day, Mitomycin C 0,5 mg/day or 5-Fluorouracil 250 mg/day according to previous therapy, each infused over an 8 hour period. Mean duration of each course was 10 days (range 6-14 days). Courses were repeated every four weeks (mean number of courses : 2).

Prophylaxis of thrombosis was made with low dose heparin.

Tolerance

Hematologic toxicity was mild, leucopenia grade 2 occurred in 7/20 patients. Other side effects consisted of pain in the arm in 4 patients out of 20 and

Service d'Oncologie Médicale, Hôpital Avicenne, 93000 Bobigny, France

« skin burn » in 3 patients. In one case catheter had to be removed because of infection. Thrombosis of the subclavian artery occured in one case.

Results

In 13/20 (65 %) patients very important responses were achieved, with disappearance of most of the skin nodules and supraclavicular involvement. These results were maintained with systemic chemotherapy, hormonal therapy and subcutaneous injections of interferon. In 2 patients a moderate response was followed by extensive surgery but a relapse occurred in the chest wall and the pleura.

Discussion and conclusion

The 65 % response rate achieved with this intra-arterial schedule seems to be superior to the response rate obtained with intravenous administration of the same combination [5, 6].

These results confirmed several studies wich reported encouraging results of intra-arterial chemotherapy as first line treatment of advanced breast cancer [7-9].

Intra-arterial prolonged chemotherapy seems to be the only way to control some massive skin and intralymphatic recurrences, especially in irradiated areas.

Mild toxicity allows its use as neo-adjuvant treatment before surgery in such cases.

References

1. Henderson JC, Harris JR, Kinne OW, Heuman S (1989) Cancer principles and practice of oncology. JB Lipincott, Philadelphia, p 1197
2. Kurtz JM, Amalric R, Brandone H, Ayme Y, Jacquemier J, Pietra JC, Hans D, Pollet JF, Bressac C, Spitalier JM (1989) Local recurrence after breast conserving surgery and radiotherapy : frequency, time course, and prognosis. Cancer 63 : 1912-1917
3. Chen KK, Montague E, Oswald MJ (1985) Results of irradiation in the treatment of locoregional breast cancer recurrence. Cancer 56 : 1269-1273
4. Stephens FO (1988) Why the use of regional chemotherapy ? Principles and pharmacokinetics. Reg Cancer Treat 1 : 1-7
5. Israel L, Breau JL, Morère JF, Lepage E, Aguilera J (1985) Inhibition de la réparation de l'ADN, objectif majeur des chimiothérapies anticancéreuses. Ann Med Interne 136 (1) : 17-20
6. Israel L, Breau JL, Morère JF, Aguilera J, John M (1986) Induction de réponses objectives par une chimiothérapie anticancéreuse fondée sur l'association prolongée de bléomycine et cisplatine. Presse Med 15 : 1183-1186
7. Aigner KR, Walther H, Müller H, Jansa J, Thiem N (1988) Intra-arterial infusion chemotherapy for recurrent breast cancer via an implantable system. Reg Cancer Treat 1 : 102-107

8. Dycker RP, Timmermann J, Schaumacher T, Schindler AE (1988) The influence of arterial regional chemotherapy and the local recurrence rate of advanced breast cancer. Reg Cancer Treat 1 : 112-116
9. Stephens FO (1990) Intra-arterial chemotherapy in locally advanced stage III breast cancer. Cancer 66 : 645-650

Locoregional advanced breast cancer. Clinical response to Neo-Adjuvant chemotherapy and survival

J Cueto, I Castillo, I Martin Lopez, R Guerrero, J Garcia Puche, V Pedraza

The locoregional advanced breast cancer shows a special poor prognosis, and the percentage of patients that survive long time after conventional treatment [1] is very low. The 5 and 10 years rate of disease free survival patients oscillates between 26 % and 15 % [2]. The predominant therapeutical failure in these cases is distal metastasis (56-81 %) more than locoregional relapse (6-50 %) having a 10 years overall survival around 20 % [3]. We present in this paper the results of the therapeutic protocol tested in our institution that includes the neo-adjuvant chemotherapy (CT) as the first therapy step.

Material and methods

The evolution of 38 female patients have been studied, mean age 55 years (28-79) with locoregional advanced cancer (14 inflammatory carcinoma and 24 advanced disease) ; mean follow-up 78 months (18-142). There were 14 (37 %) premenopausal patients and 24 (63 %) postmenopausal. The therapeutic protocol is : neo-adjuvant chemotherapy 3-6 courses as FAC sheme [4], and later evaluation of response ; in case of complete remission (CR) ; locoregional treatment was radical irradiation at 70 Gy in 7 weeks and CT maintenance with 12 courses of CMF ; in case of partial remission (PR) the locoregional treatment was : modified radical mastectomy and postoperative irradiation at 50 Gy in 5 weeks and maintenance CT with 12 courses of CMF ; in case of nonresponse (NR) to neo-adjuvant CT the patient was treated out of protocol.

Results

There was complete remission to neo-adjuvant chemotherapy in 3 patients (8 %), partial remission in 20 patients (52 %). Thus, there were 23 (60 %) favourable responses, and 15 (40 %) non responders ; the clinical presentation of tumor showed that 71 % of patients with advanced disease were favourable responders to chemotherapy versus 43 % of inflammatory carcinoma patients ; difference is statistically significant, $p = 0.04$. At the end of the follow-up, 9 patients (24 %) are alive without disease and 29 (76 %) have died by tumor. Among the 23 patients with favourable response to chemotherapy, 8 (35 %) are alive versus 1 of the 15 (1 %) non responders, statistically significant difference too, $p = 0.03$. In 29 patients (76 %) disease cannot be eradicated

Service of radiotherapy and oncology. University hospital San Cecilio, Granada, Spain

(15 uncontrolled and 14 relapsed). The therapeutic failure was only locoregional disease in 3 patients (10 %) ; metastatic disease in 12 patients (41 %), and 14 patients (48 %) showed both local and distal disease.

Conclusions

The advanced locoregional breast cancer, inflammatory carcinoma and the other clinical presentations (gross tumor, cutaneous affection, skin ulceration) have a poor prognosis. There is not a satisfactoy management of disease. The reasonable good response to neo-adjuvant chemotherapy (60 % of favourable response) is followed by a short long-term survival. Only one quarter of the patients are alive without disease after five years. The bad evolution of the advanced breast cancer is particularly poor in the inflammatory carcinoma presentation and when there is no response to neo-adjuvant chemotherapy.

After five years of treatment 7 % of patients with inflammatory carcinoma are alive versus 33 % of patients with advanced disease.

In the same period 7 % of non-responders patients are alive versus 35 % of patients with favourable response to neo-adjuvant chemotherapy.

These differences are the expression of the lower response to chemotherapy of patients with inflammatory carcinoma (43 %) versus other forms of advanced breast cancer (71 %).

The patterns of failure to the treatment, local and systemic, does not show differences between the 2 considered forms, inflammatory carcinoma and advanced breast cancer. Both show a clear predominance in distal failure.

Posterior studies must be done to find a neo-adjuvant chemotherapy schedule that could have a larger number of responders, especially in inflammatory carcinoma, considering the big percentage of metastasis showed by these patients.

References

1. Haagensen CD (1971) Diseases of the breast. WB Saunders, Philadelphia
2. Valagussa P, Zambetti M, Bignami P et al (1983) T3b-T4 breast cancer : factors affecting results in combined modality treatments. Clin Exp Metastasis 1 : 191-202
3. Fracchia A, Evans JF, Eisenberg BL (1980) Stage III Carcinoma of the breast : a detailed analysis. Ann Surg 192 : 705-709
4. Buzdar AV, Blumenschein GR, Gutterman JV et al (1979) Prospective adjuvant chemotherapy with 5-Fluorouracil, doxorubicin, cyclophosphamide and BCG vaccines. JAMA 242 : 1509-1513

Gastro-intestinal tumors

Clinical outcome of intraperitoneal hyperthermo-chemotherapy for patients with refractory gastric cancer

S Fujimoto, M Takahashi, RD Shrestha, M Kokubun, K Kobayashi, S Kiuchi, C Konno

The survival time of patients with advanced gastric cancer remains short regardless of whether or not postoperative adjuvant chemotherapy is given. Intra-abdominal spread of cancer cells is inevitable since a sensitive diagnostic to detect a small volume of tumors on the peritoneal surface has not been available. Drugs can be delivered through the circulating blood to the surface of the peritoneum, mesentery, and omentum ; however, an intra-abdominal form of chemotherapy has the dual advantages of a high regional concentration of antitumor drugs and alleviation of systemic side effects [1].

To improve the clinical outcome of patients with advanced gastric cancer, Koga et al [2] and Fujimura et al [3] have made use of continuous hyperthermic peritoneal perfusion and Mitomycin C. Sugarbaker et al [4] reported that the postoperative adjuvant application of intraperitoneal chemotherapy with 5-Fluorouracil is effective in preventing peritoneal recurrence and in lengthening survival time for patients with an advanced colorectal cancer. We describe here our own clinical trials in which intra-peritoneal hyperthermic perfusion and Mitomycin C were combined with surgery to treat 41 patients with far-advanced gastric cancer. For comparative purposes, data on 40 patients without this perfusion therapy are shown.

Subjects and methods

Patients

Eighty-one Japanese patients with far-advanced gastric cancer were treated in the First Department of Surgery, Chiba University Hospital and an associated hospital. Of these 81, 41 patients underwent intraperitoneal hyperthermic perfusion (IPHP) combined with surgery, either to prevent peritoneal recurrence or to treat peritoneal seeding (IPHP group). The remaining 40 underwent surgery alone for far-advanced gastric cancer, within the same period of time (control group).

The IPHP group was comprised of 19 men and 22 women aged 53.9 ± 12.3 years (Table 1). The control group included 25 men and 15 women aged 60.3 ± 10.5 years and a total dose of 31.1 ± 9.7 mg of Mitomycin C (MMC) was given intraperitoneally and/or intravenously. The histologic findings and types of surgery are summarized in Table 1.

First Department of Surgery, School of Medicine, Chiba University, Chiba 280, Japan

Table 1. Clinicopathologic data on 81 patients

Factors	IPHP group (n = 41)	Control group (n = 40)
Age in years	53.9 ± 12.3*	60.3 ± 10.5*
Sex (male/female)	19/22	25/15
TNM classification**		
T3	15	24
T4	26	16
Peritoneal dissemination		
p_0	16	29
p_1	10	5
p_{2+3}	15	6
Type of histology		
Differentiated	12	21
Undifferentiated	29	19
Type of surgery		
Distal subtotal gastrectomy	7	8
Pancreaticoduodenectomy	1	0
Total gastrectomy	4	11
Total gastrectomy plus splenectomy	4	14
Total gastrectomy, splenectomy, oophorectomy plus AOR***	15	0
Total gastrectomy, splenectomy plus AOR***	10	7
Intra-operative antitumor treatment intraperitoneal and/or intravenous mitomycin C	—	31.1 ± 9.7 mg/ml*
IPHP treatment		
Perfusion time (min)	117 ± 17 *	—
Inflow temperature (°C)	46.4 ± 0.7*	—
Outflow temperature (°C)	45.0 ± 0.8*	—
Mitomycin C levels at the start of IPHP	10 μg/ml	—

*   Mean ± SD
** Hermanek P, Sobin LH (1987 Stomach (ICD-O 151). In: TNM Classification of Malignant Tumours, 4th fully revised ed, Springer-Verlag, Berlin Heidelberg New York, p 43
*** AOR: adjacent organs resection

Intraperitoneal hyperthermic perfusion

A detailed description of the IPHP treatment can be found elsewhere [5-7]. In brief, under hypothermic general anesthesia at about 31°C, IPHP was carried out using the IPHP system with a closed peritoneal perfusion.

Immediately after surgical excision of the primary focus and of other bulky intra-abdominal tumors, an inflow catheter was inserted toward the diaphragm and the surface of the liver and a sump catheter was inserted into Douglas' pouch (Fig. 1). Prior to the start of the IPHP, the systemic temperature was lowered to 31°C with a cooling mat and ice-bags, as mentioned above (Fig. 1). The perfusate 3,000 — 5,000 ml containing Mitomycin C (MMC) 10 g/ml circulates for about 120 min, at the inflow and outflow temperatures of 46.4 ± 0.7°C and 45.0 ± 0.8°C, respectively (Table 1). The pulmonary artery temperature, measured using a Swan-Ganz catheter (Fig. 1), did not exceed 40°C up to the end of IPHP [8].

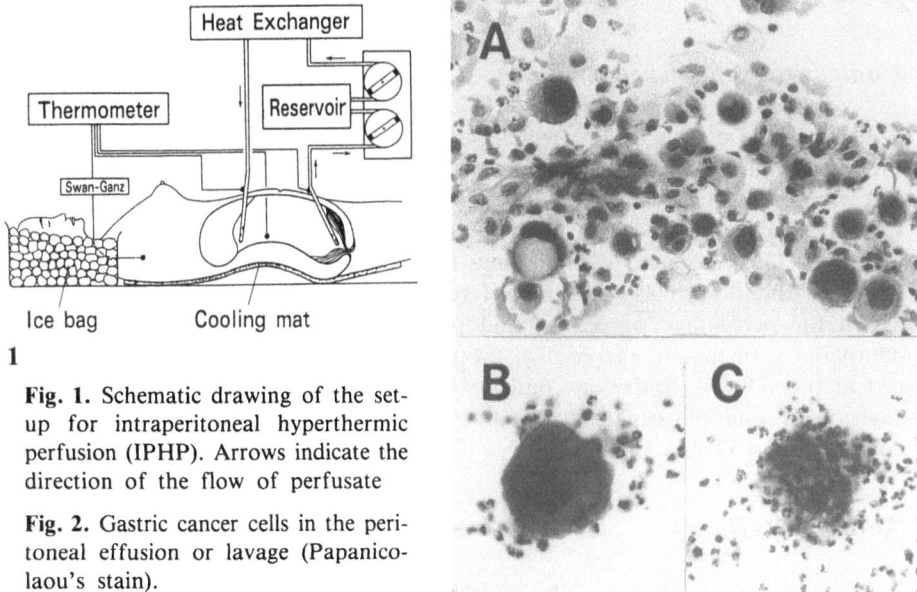

1

Fig. 1. Schematic drawing of the set-up for intraperitoneal hyperthermic perfusion (IPHP). Arrows indicate the direction of the flow of perfusate

Fig. 2. Gastric cancer cells in the peritoneal effusion or lavage (Papanicolaou's stain).
A : Typical malignant cells in cluster form (magnification × 60). B : A **2** damaged cancer cell 12 h after IPHP (magnification × 60). C : Tumor cells are surrounded by neutrophiless 24 h after IPHP (magnification × 60)

Statistical analysis

Survival time was calculated from the day of surgery to death. Survival curves were calculated using the Kaplan-Meier method [9] and survival rates were analyzed using a generalized Wilcoxon test [10]. Background factors were compared between the IPHP and control groups, and chi-square test or Student's t-test was used to determine the statistical difference.

Classification of peritoneal dissemination

Disseminating peritoneal metastasis in classified into 3 subgroups, that is p_1, p_2, and p_3, according to the clinical stage outlined by the Japanese Research

Society for Gastric Cancer [11]. P_1 is dessemination to the adjacent peritoneum (above the transverse colon and including the greater omentum), without
manifest metastasis to the distant peritoneum. P_2 is a few to several scatte-
red metastases to the distant peritoneum including the peritoneum below the
transverse colon. An unilateral ovarian metastasis without peritoneal metastasis is included in p_2. P_3 is numerous metastases to the distant peritoneum.

Results

Comparison of background factors

The mean age of the IPHP group was younger by 6.4 years compared with
the control group and the difference was significant at $p = 0.0157$ (Table 1).
The male to female ratio did not differ between the groups ($p = 0.1483$).

In the IPHP group, « undifferentiated adenocarcinoma » was more frequent
at $p = 0.0334$, compared with findings in the control group. The ratio of T3
to T4 in the TNM classification differed at $p = 0.0356$ between the groups.
When the percentage of p_0, p_1, and p_{2+3} patients in the IPHP group was
compared with that in the control group, the IPHP group was more advanced at $p = 0.00971$. Forty-one patients in the IPHPgroup underwent surgical
excision of multiple organs ($p = 8.86 \times 10^{-5}$), compared with the 40 in the
control group (Table 1).

Antitumor efficacy

In cytologic examinations of the peritoneal exudate and/or peritoneal lavage
from the 41 patients given IPHP and from the 40 in the control group, gastric cancer cells were present in 29 of 41 patients given IPHP and in 12 of
the 40 not given IPHP (Fig. 2A). In the 29 given IPHP, intra-abdominal cancer cells were not evident post-IPHP, as examined by repeated cytologic tests
of the lavage material from Douglas' pouch (Fig. 2B and 2C).

With respect to ascitic effusion, 19 patients with IPHP had effusion prior
to IPHP and no effusion post-IPHP. All the 41 patients were discharged from
hospital.

In contrast, in the 12 patients in the control group, ascitic effusion was manifest soon after surgery irrespective of 31.1 ± 9.7 mg of MMC (intraperitoneally
and/or intravenously).

Survival time

The overall survival rates for the groups are shown in Figure 3. The 1-, 2-,
and 3-year survival rates for the IPHP group were 67.9 %, 45.7 % and
38.6 %, respectively, whereas those for the control group were 30.0 %, 10.0 %
and 0 %, respectively. The survival rates for the IPHP group were superior
at $p = 8.1 \times 10^{-7}$ to those for the control group (Fig. 3).

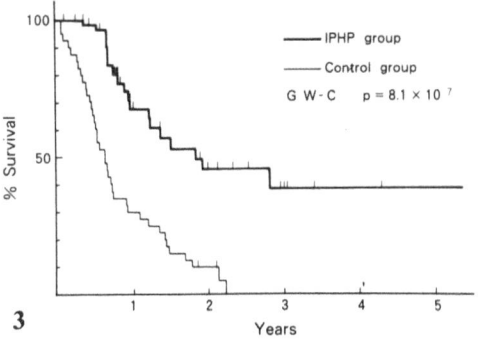

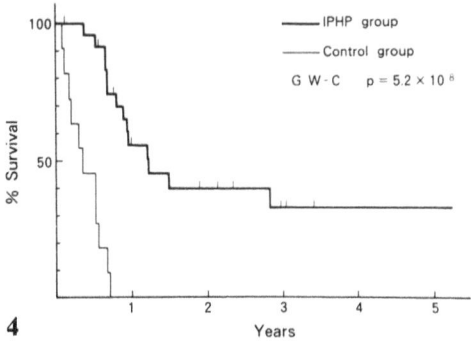

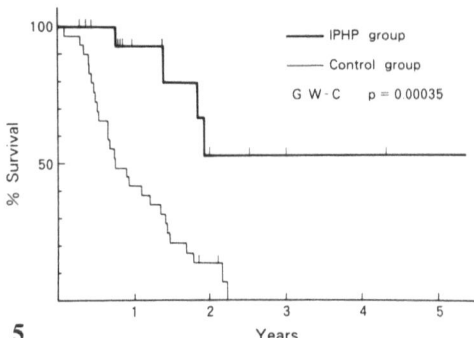

Fig. 3 Overall survival curves for the IPHP and control groups ? IPHP group (n = 41) ; ? control group (n = 40)

Fig. 4 Survival curves of 45 patients without peritoneal dissemination ? IPHP group (n = 16) ; ? control group (n = 29)

Fig. 5 Comparison of survival curves of 36 patients with peritoneal dissemination ? IPHP group (n = 25) ; ? control group (n = 11)

With regard to 45 patients with no evident peritoneal metastasis, the IPHP group included 16 patients and the control group 29 patients. As shown in Figure 4, the survival rates for the IPHP group were significantly better than those for the control group, with a statistical difference of $p = 3.5 \times 10\text{-}4$. The 1- and 2- year survival rates for the IPHP group were 92.9 % and 52.9 % respectively, whereas those for the control group were 41.8 % and 13.9 % respectively (Fig. 4).

Findings in 36 patients with peritoneal metastasis are shown in Figure 5. The 6- and 12-months survival rates of 11 patients who were not given IPHP were 45.6 % and 0 % respectively, while those of 25 patients given IPHP were 95.7 % and 55.7 % respectively. The 5 year survival rate for the IPHP group was 32.9 % (Fig. 5). Thus, the survival rates for the IPHP group were significantly higher than those for the control group, with a statistical difference of $p = 5.2 \times 10^{-8}$.

Cause of death

Outcome of the cause of death is shown in Table 2. The occurrence of death due to intra abdominal recurrence was 24.4 % (10 of 41 patients) in the IPHP group and 77.5 % (31 of 40 patients) in the control group, the difference being significant at $p = 0.0021$.

Table 2. Outcome of treatment in terms of cause of death

Cause of death	IPHP group Peritoneal seeding		Control group Peritoneal seeding	
	(+) n = 25	(−) n = 16	(+) n = 11	(−) n = 29
Peritoneal metastasis	3	0	11	17
Pleural metastasis	4	0	0	1
Intra-abdominal tumors	6	1	0	3
Hematogenous metastasis	2	3	0	6
Others	2	1	0	0
Total	17/25	5/16	11/11	27/29
	22/41		38/40	

According to data on 36 patients with peritoneal seeding at the time of laparotomy, 9 of the 25 patients given IPHP died of an intra-abdominal recurrence and 11 patients among the controls died of a peritoneal recurrence.

Side effects and complications

Transient thrombocytopenia occured post-IPHP but recovery was attained 3-5 days after IPHP, with no requirement for supportive treatment. There was a steep elevation in serum GOT and GPT levels but normal ranges were reverted to within 3 weeks post-IPHP.

The postoperative course of the 41 patients with IPHP was uneventful, except for minor leakage from the esophago-jejunostomy and ileo-transverse colostomy, in 2 patients.

Discussion and conclusion

Surgical treatment has to be given to a patient when no other choice is available or when surgery markedly surpasses the other forms of treatment. Aranha and Georgen [12] stated that patients with advanced gastric linitis plastic did not benefit from surgical treatment, because the mean survival time of the patients treated non-surgically and surgically was 6.6 months and 7.2 months, respectively. They also described that patients who underwent total gastrectomy in the presence of peritoneal metastasis survived only 4 months, therefore, alternative forms of treatment including chemotherapy and radiation therapy should be considered for such patients.

In the current study, the 50 % survival time of gastric cancer patients with peritoneal metastasis was 4.3 months in the control group, results exactly the same as those of Aranha and Georgen. Iitsuka et al [13] reported that the intraperitoneal appearance of gastric cancer cells depended upon the degree of cancer invasion to the gastric serosa and occured in almost all cases with serosal invasion exceeding 15-20 cm².

Regional therapy with antitumor drugs is more effective than systemic therapy, that is, local, higher levels of antitumor drugs and decreased systemic side effects, compared with results when the intravenous route is used. The rate at which a drug leaves the peritoneal cavity chiefly depends on its molecular weight [14]. An antitumor drug given intraperitoneally is mainly absorbed through the visceral peritoneal surface and leaves the abdominal cavity via the portal blood stream [15]. At the termination of IPHP, MMC levels in the peritoneal cavity are 10-30 times greater than those in the peripheral blood [7]. However, to secure a more enhanced antitumor efficacy, cancer cells present on the peritoneo-serosal surface need to be eradicated.

Since heat is lethal to malignant cells, particular attention has been directed to hyperthermia for treating human malignancy. The temperatures used clinically vary widely, as do the durations of treatment. Sapareto and Dewey [16] reported that « for equating a time at one temperature with an equivalent time for the same antitumor effect at another temperature, a nomogram was depicted, in which if a preselected treatment at the reference temperature is chosen, the appropriate time at any other temperature to attain the same effect can be calculated ». In the current study, the outflow temperature of the perfusate was 45.0 ± 0.8C. If 45.0°C is the lowest temparature in the abdominal cavity and the perfusion time is 117 min, an equivalent time at 43.0°C is about 500 min, based on the monogram.

CDDP, Bleomycin, MMC, and BCNU markedly enhanced antitumor efficacy when combined with hyperthermia [17-19]. The marked antitumor effects with the IPHP treatment are attributed no only to a large thermal dose (43.0°C × 500 min), but also to the concentrations of MMC present in the perfusate. However, because of the limited penetration and conduction of drug and heat into large tumor nodules, this IPHP is less effective for unresectable intra-abdominal bulky tumors.

Our study shows that intraperitoneal hyperthermochemotherapy with MMC, in combination with surgery, is an acceptable treatment for patients with far-advanced gastric cancer with peritoneal seeding. The prognosis of gastric cancer patients with large serosal penetration is expected to improve. This IPHP treatment has dual advantages over systemic chemotherapy with respect to decreasing the systemic side effects and enhancing intraperitoneal antitumor efficacy.

References

1. Sugarbaker PH (1989) Management of peritoneal carcinomatosis. Acta Med Austriaca 16 : 57-60
2. Koga S, Hamozoe R, Maeta M et al (1988) Prophylactic therapy for peritoneal recurrence of gastric cancer by continuous hyperthermic peritoneal perfusion with mitomycin C. Cancer 61 : 232-237
3. ujimura T, Yonemura Y, Fushida S et al (1990) Continuous hyperthermic peritoneal perfusion for the treatment of peritoneal dissemination in gastric cancers and subsequent second look operation. Cancer 65 : 65-71
4. Sugarbaker PH, Gianola FS, Speyer JL et al (1985) Prospective, randomized trial of intravenous versus intraperitoneal 5-Fluorouracil in patients with advanced primary colon or rectal cancer. Surgery 98 : 414-422
5. Fujimoto S, Shrestha RD, Kokubun M et al (1988) Intraperitoneal hyperthermic perfusion combined with surgery effective for gastric cancer patients with peritoneal seeding. Ann Surg 208 : 36-41
6. Fujimoto S, Shrestha RD, Kokubun M et al (1989) Clinical trial with surgery and intraperitoneal hyperthermic perfusion for peritoneal recurrence of gastro-intestinal cancer. Cancer 64 : 154-160
7. Fujimoto S, Shrestha RD, Kokubun M et al (1989) Pharmacokinetic analysis of mitomycin C for intraperitoneal hyperthermic perfusion in patients with far-advanced or recurrent gastric cancer. Reg Cancer Treat 2 : 198-202
8. Fujimoto S, Shrestha RD, Kobayashi K et al (1989) Combined treatment with surgery and intraperitoneal hyperthermic perfusion (IPHP) for far-advanced gastrointestinal cancer with peritoneal seeding. Acta Med Austriaca 16 : 76-80
9. Kaplan EL, Meier P (1958) Non-parametric estimation from incomplete observation. Am J Statist Assoc 53 : 451-481
10. Gehan E (1985) A generalized Wilcoxon test for comparing arbitrary single-censored samples. Biometrika 52 : 203-224
11. Japanese Research Society for Gastric Cancer (1981) The general rules for the gastric cancer study in surgery and pathology. Jpn J Surg 11 : 127-139
12. Aranha GV, Georgen R (1989) Gastric linitis plastica is not a surgical disease. Surgery 106 : 758-763
13. Iitsuka Y, Kaneshima S, Tanida O, Takeuchi T, Koga S (1979) Intraperitoneal free cancer cells and their viability in gastric cancer. Cancer 44 : 1476-1480
14. Dedrick RL, Meyers CE, Bungay PM, DeVita VT (1978) Pharmacokinetic rationale for peritoneal drug administration in the treatment of ovarian cancer. Cancer Treat Rep 62 : 1-11
15. Lukas G, Brindle SD, Greengard P (1971) The route of absorption of intraperitoneally administered compounds. J Pharmacol Exp Ther 178 : 562-566
16. Sapareto SA, Dewey WC (1984) Thermal dose determination in cancer therapy. Int J Radiat Oncol Biol Phys 10 : 787-800
17. Hahn GM (1979) Potential for therapy of drugs and hyperthermia. Cancer Res 39 : 2264-2268
18. Barlogie B, Corry PM, Drewinko B (1980) In vitro hyperthermochemotherapy of human colon cancer cells with cis-dichlorodiammine-platinum (II) and mitomycin C. Cancer Res 40 : 1165-1168
19. Fujimoto S, Ohta M, Shrestha RD et al (1988) Enhancement of hyperthermochemotherapy for human gastric cancer in nude mice by thermosensitization with nitroimidazoles. Br J Cancer 57 : 42-45

Neo-Adjuvant therapy for gastric cancer

CG Leichman

Only 30 % of patients presenting with gastric cancer will be amenable to surgical cure (resection margins free of microscopic disease) at the time of diagnosis. At the time of diagnosis approximately 30 % of patients will have unresectable disease by virtue of contiguous spread, and another 30 % will have disseminated disease. Those patients which can be resected have a 5 year survival rate for 15-20 % [1].

Post-operative adjuvant chemotherapy trials have not shown a survival advantage over surgery alone [2]. Preusser et al showed that pre-operative chemotherapy with Etoposide - Adriamycin - Cisplatin produced a tumor response in 70 % (21 % complete response) of patients with locally unresectable cancers. Significant myelosuppression was encountered. As Preusser's patients were surgically inoperable, they did not strictly meet the criteria accepted for neo-adjuvant therapy. Nonetheless, the responders were rendered surgically resectable. Relapses occured in 60 % of patients with a median time to recurrence of 3 months, in spite of this apparently successful treatment [3].

A review of the gastric cancer cases treated at the University of Southern California in the years 1982 and 1988 revealed a resectability rate of 50 % with an operative mortality of 3 %. The median survival of non-resectable ones was 4 months ; that of the surgically treated patients was 5 months. Based upon this data, and the large number of patients we have with gastric cancer, in 1988 we embarked upon a neo-adjuvant protocol for gastric cancer, followed by post-operative adjuvant intraperitoneal chemotherapy.

Materials and methods

Thirty patients with gastric adenocarcinoma deemed surgically resectable have been treated on protocol. All were over 18 years of age, with no other active malignancies, and with adequate renal (creatinine < 1.5 mg %) and hematologic (WBC $> 3.5/mm^3$ and platelets > 100 k/mm^3) function.

Pre-operative therapy consisted of cisplatin 100 mg/m^2 on days 1 and 28 followed by 5-FU at 200 mg/m^2/d days 1-21 and 28-49 as a continuous infusion by Pharmacia-Deltec CADD pump and an indwelling venous access device. Surgery followed restaging during a 2 week rest break. If the patient was NED at operation, a catheter was placed for intraperitoneal chemotherapy.

Intraperitoneal adjuvant therapy started 4-7 weeks after surgery with Floxuridine (FUDR) 3,000 mg given in 2 liters of dialysate warmed to 37 ° on days 1-3 and 21-23 and Cisplatin 200 mg/m^2 with vigorous hydration and sodium thiosulfate on days 4 and 24.

Nineteen males and 11 females patients have been treated on protocol. Eleven were hispanic, 10 were oriental, 8 were caucasian, and one was black. Median age was 55 years, with a range of 31-75. Median performance status was 1 (range 0-2).

Results

Twenty-seven of 30 patients (90 %) entered were eligible. Twenty-five patients (93 %) completed pre-operative therapy. Twenty-two (81 %) completed surgery, 3 refused surgery and remain alive with disease, and 2 await surgery. Sixteen patients (73 %) were rendered NED (no evidence of disease) by their surgery. Overall, 81 % of the patients NED at surgery have completed some of the scheduled post-operative therapy. Six patients (38 %) have completed the prescribed 2 courses of intraperitoneal therapy. Five patients completed only 1 course (4 refused further treatment, and 1 died with sepsis following the first course). Three have a second course pending.

Following completion of the pre-operative chemotherapy, 17 of the 27 eligible patients (63 %) had symptomatic improvement. Nineteen patients (70 %) had objective evidence of response. Endoscopic disappearance of all cancer was seen in 4 patients (15 %).

No operative specimen was free of disease. At surgical pathology staging 1 patient has intramucosal disease only, one was stage I, 10 were stage II, 4 were stage III, and 8 were stage IV.

Twenty-three patients remain alive with a median survival of 12 + months. Included in this group are 14 of 16 patients resected for cure who remain alive 3-24 months after surgery. Seven patients have died with a median survival of 4 months.

Toxicity

No surgical mortality was encountered. Toxicity from pre-operative therapy consisted of mild (grade 1-2) nausea and vomiting, and mild stomatitis. Hematologic toxicity was also mild. Toxicity from intraperitoneal therapy has consisted of mild chemical peritonitis. One patient died of peritonitis at another institution and her hematologic parameters are not known. Catheter problems (thrombosis or infection) have occurred in 4 patients (13 %).

Conclusion

This regimen is tolerable and effective at cytoreduction. Surgery is neither prevented nor delayed, nor is surgical morbity/mortality enhanced. Incorporation of this regimen into a randomized, prospective trial against a surgical control will be necessary to determine a survival advantage for this therapy.

Supported in part by a grant from Pharmacia-Deltec Company.

References

1. MacDonald JS, Steele G, Gunderson L (1989) Cancer of the Stomach. In : DeVita V, Hellman S, Rosenberg S, (eds) Cancer : principles and practice of oncology. JB Lippincott Co, Philadelphia, p 769
2. Douglass HO (1988) Western surgical adjuvant trials. In : Douglass HO (ed) Contemporary issues in clinical oncology : gastric cancer. Churchill Livingstone, New York, pp 145-172
3. Preusser P, Wilke H, Achterrath W et al : Phase II study with the combination of etoposide, doxorubicin, and cisplatin in advanced measurable gastric cancer. J Clin Oncol 7 : 1310-1317

The effects of Verapamil in potentiating the action of Doxorubicin in recently derived pancreatic carcinoma cell lines

D Alderson, CMP Collins*, T Lai, MO Symes

Multidrug resistance (MDR) to a variety of anti-cancer drugs may be exhibited by tumour cells expressing the MDRI gene product P170 glycoprotein [1, 2]. A number of agents, eg Verapamil, Quinidine and Cyclosporin A, compete with P170 for receptors on the plasma membrane vesicles active in drug transport and thus inhibit drug efflux from cells [3].

The 5 year survival rate following potentially curative resection for carcinoma of the pancreas varies from 3-13 % [4] and treatment with cytotoxic drugs does not improve the prognosis [5, 6]. As normal pancreatic ductal cells express P170 [2] it seems reasonable that MDR reversal agents, administered in conjunction with appropriate cytotoxic drugs, may increase tumour sensitivity. We have investigated this in vitro, using 4 recently derived pancreatic carcinoma cell lines.

Materials and methods

Carcinoma cells were separated from 4 pancreatic carcinomas P_2, P_3, P_5 and P_6, using Nycodenz columns [7, 8]. Cells were cultured in RPMI 1640 with 10 % v/v newborn calf serum, 1 % v/v glutamine and antibiotics.

Carcinoma cells were identified by morphology, expression of cytokeratins and ability to grow as multiple layers [8].

Aliquots of 2×10^4 tumour cells were cultured with Doxorubicin (0.1, 0.5, 1.0 μg/ml) alone or in combination with racaemic Verapamil. Inhibition of protein synthesis was determined by inhibition of [^{75}Se] Selenomethionine uptake as described previously [9].

Results

The percentage inhibition of isotope uptake following exposure to increasing concentrations of Doxorubicin is shown in Table 1. All 4 tumours showed a dose dependent inhibition of isotope uptake when exposed to Doxorubicin alone. Tumour P_2 showed an increased sensitivity to Doxorubicin in the presence of Verapamil, a concentration of 3.3 μ M being more effective than 1.0 μ M. Sensitivity to Doxorubicin alone was much greater for tumours P_3, P_5 and P_6, so that potentiation by Verapamil was only seen at the intermediate con-

University Departments of Surgery and Pathology*, Bristol Royal Infirmary, Bristol BS2 8HW, Great Britain

Table 1. Effects of increasing dose

TUMOR	P2					P3				
DAY	25	34	118	175	203	21	34	98	111	146
DOX 1µg/ml	*45.9	47.5	21.6	22.8	30.5	84.7	82.3	59.1	32.6	44.5
DOX & VERAP										
1.0µM				19.4	33.4			62.8	39.0	33.4
3.3	85.9+++	82.7+++	17.2	34.0	43.8++	85.5	83.2	68.1	42.5	54.1
5.0				39.9	48.9			63.8	42.5	61.2+
10.0				50.3++	54.3+++			67.3	50.0	62.1+
20.0				47.6++	44.5++			58.8	49.5	65.1++

* % inhibition of isotope uptake. +>0.05; ++>0.01; +++>0.001

centration of Doxorubicin (0.5 μg/ml) for tumour P_3 and the lowest concentration (0.1 μg/ml) for the day culture of tumour P_6.

The effect of prolonged culture on the sensitivity of tumours P_2 and P_3 to doxorubicin alone, and the potentiation thereof by increasing concentrations of verapamil is shown in Table 2.

Table 2. Effects of increasing culture periods

TUMOR		P2		P3				P5	P6
DAY		25	34	18	34	73	120	21	72
Concent of Dox µg/ml									
	0.1	NIL+	NIL	7.0	NIL	38.6	7.6	27.6	6.1
	0.5	14.3	8.3	54.1	38.8	59.8	80.6	80.7	83.7
	1.0	45.9	47.5	83.7	82.3	78.2	86.6	83.6	83.2
*1.0µM	0.1	15.9+++	9.3+	NIL	NIL	27.9	12.6	38.5	24.0+
VERAP	0.5	10.1	34.1+++	76.8++	41.1	61.2	85.2	80.0	88.6
	1.0	67.8++	74.3+++	85.3	82.9	82.4	85.7	83.9	81.8
*3.3µM	0.1	10.4++	16.3++	NIL	NIL	23.0	12.5	33.9	16.7
VERAP	0.5	36.6	41.9+++	72.0+	56.7++	64.3	85.3	83.7	85.9
	1.0	85.9+++	82.7+++	85.0	83.2	71.9	82.0	82.5	71.3

* % inhibition of isotope uptake. +<0.05; ++<0.01; +++<0.001

Discussion

Potentiation of doxorubicin sensitivity by verapamil was seen when the initial tumour cell inhibition by doxorubicin alone was low, tumour P_2, or when it declined on prolonged culture in tumours P_2 and P_3. The spontaneous decline in responsiveness to doxorubicin alone is of interest. Previous demonstrations of increased drug resistance on prolonged tumour cell culture have required the addition of a low concentration of drug to the culture medium [10]. That the present decline in sensitivity to Doxorubicin represented the development of multidrug resistance is suggested by its reversal in the presence of increasing concentrations of Verapamil.

References

1. Kessel P, Botterill V and Wodinsky I (1968) Uptake and retention of daunomycin by mouse leukaemic cells as factors in drug response. Cancer Res 28 : 938-941
2. Van der Blick AM and Borst P (1989) Multidrug resistance. Adv Cancer Res 52 : 165-203.
3. Cornwell MM, Pastan I and Gottesman MM (1987) Certain calcium blockers bind specifically to multidrug resistant human KB carcinoma membrane vesicles and inhibit drug binding to P-Glycoprotein. J Biol Chem 262 : 2166-2170
4. Andren-Sandberg A and Ihse I (1983) Factors influencing survival after total pancreatectomy in patients with pancreatic cancer. Ann Surg 198 : 605-610
5. Harvey JH and Schein PS (1984) Chemotherapy of pancreatic carcinoma. World J Surg 8 : 935-939
6. O'Connell MJ (1985) Current status of chemotherapy for advanced pancreatic and gastric cancer. J Clin Oncol 3 : 1032-1039
7. Ford TC, Lai T and Symes MO (1987) Morphological and functional characteristics of mouse mammary carcinoma cells separated by nycodenz columns. Br J Exp Path 68 : 453-460
8. Lai T, Angus RL, Alderson D, Collins CM, Morgan AP, Smith PJ and Symes MO (1991) Culture of renal and pancreatic carcinoma cells separated from an enzymatic digest of the solid neoplasm using a nycodenz column. J Pathol (submitted)
9. Ferro MA, Heinemann P, Smith PJB and Symes MO (1988) The effect of stilboestrol and testosterone on the incorporation of [^{75}Se] Selenomethionine by prostate carcinoma cells. Br J Urol 62 : 166-172
10. Twentyman PR, Fox NE, Wright KA and Bleehan NM (1986) Derivation and preliminary characterisation of adriamycin resistant lines of human lung cancer cells. Br J Cancer 53 : 529-537

Preoperative 5-Fluorouracil in resectable colorectal cancer. Preliminary results of a prospective randomized trial

R Cellerino, A Piga, L Latini, V Saba, E Cesini, GL Cetto,
R Bascioni, G Corradini, A Fianchini, E Landi

As many as 40 % to 50 % of patients undergoing surgery for resectable colorectal cancer will eventually relapse and, in the majority of cases, die from their disease. There is virtually no systemic treatment of real efficacy for metastatic disease ; adjuvant therapy has recently forecasted interesting perspectives but does not appear, in the near future, able to substantially affect the course of disease.

Preoperative chemotherapy has been suggested of benefit in resectable colorectal cancer ; after a first report by Avgoustis et al in 1979 [1], who treated 5 patients with a single course of chemotherapy immediately before surgery, and obtained at least a 50 % reduction in the size of the tumor, there have been some confirmations, on a slightly larger scale, of a possible benefit of preoperative chemotherapy [2-7]. The most interesting results come from the study by Gentile (1985) [5], in which 20/21 patients receiving preoperative, perioperative and postoperative adjuvant treatment were free of disease after a minimum follow-up of 2 years.

Following these encouraging reports, we have started in 1987 a prospective, randomized trial of 5-Fluorouracil followed by surgery vs surgery alone in colorectal cancer. The study is still open to accrual and we report here some preliminary results.

Patients and methods

Eligibility criteria included : histologically proven colorectal cancer ; no distant metastases ; local eradicability ; age lower than 75 yrs ; good general functions (renal, hepatic, cardiac and haematopoietic) ; good performance status (Karnofsky 70 or better) ; absence of a second tumor and general contraindications to surgery ; informed consent. Preoperative staging procedures included chest X-ray, CT or US of abdomen and bone scintigraphy. Patients were randomized to preoperative 5-Fluorouracil, 600 mg/sqm/ in 2 hrs, days -5 to -1 followed by surgery on day 0 (Arm A) or to surgery alone (Arm B). Randomization was stratified by centre only. Survival and disease free survival were the endpoints of this study, and 65 patients per arm were calculated as necessary to establish the significance of an increase of 25 % in the 5-years figures of survival and disease free survival. In the present report, disease free survival curves were calculated by the method of Kaplan and Meier [8].

Clinical Oncology, University of Ancona, 60020 Ancona, Italy

Results

Ninety-six patients have been randomized so far, 89 of which are presently evaluable. Fourty-four patients have received preoperative 5-Fluorouracil (Arm A), 45 surgery only (Arm B). The 2 arms appear well balanced for age, sex and site of the tumor. Patients in Arm A appeared distributed at surgery in more favorable staging categories : 28/44 of them were staged A-B2, versus 20/45 of Arm B. Twenty-one patients have relapsed and 9 have died : there were 10 relapses and 5 deaths in Arm A, and 11 relapses and 4 deaths in Arm B. Disease free survival curves show a limited advantage in favor of the treated group, restricted to the first 12 months of observation. No toxic effects were reported, and in no instance did chemotherapy affect surgery or influence the postoperative course.

Discussion and conclusion

Surgery represents in colorectal cancer the only effective treatment modality ; a cure rate as high as 60 % is obtainable in patients whose disease is judged eradicable at onset : the remaining 40 % of patients will present, within months or years from surgery, a relapse which will eventually lead them to death in the majority of cases.

Preoperative chemotherapy is a new treatment modality with a sound biological rationale and clinical positive results limited to tumour types which are known to respond to chemotherapy. In colorectal cancer, the poor responsiveness to chemotherapy is an obvious limit to our attempts of influencing the course of disease, but also a stimulus to experiment therapeutic alternatives.

Clinical studies of preoperative chemotherapy in colorectal cancer are limited in number and include small numbers of patients. Positive results reported in pilot trials include a shrinkage of the tumour, reduced blood losses during surgery, a prolonged disease free interval and a prolonged relapse-to-death interval [1-7]. However, these studies often include combined modalities of treatment, and it is difficult to assess what the real contribution of preoperative chemotherapy is. In addition, none of these studies have appeared yet as regular papers, and even the most favorable reports have remained at the stage of abstract after more than 5 years.

We have started this prospective, randomized study to assess the effectiveness of preoperative chemotherapy in resectable colorectal cancer. The choice of a treatment with mild toxicity was dictated firstly by the necessity of not interfering with surgery, the only therapeutic modality with established curative potential. In addition, 5-Fluorouracil is the most active drug when used as single agent in this disease, and chemotherapy is known to induce better tumor responses when given in the preoperative setting than in advanced disease [9, 10] ; furthermore, in all the pilot studies in colorectal cancer the favorable results have been obtained with a single course of preoperative chemotherapy. A less encouraging study has appeared recently, in which a single course of preoperative doxiflurine (5'-DFUR) showed a histologic therapeutic effect only in one out of 16 cases [11].

The results thus far obtained in our patients may suggest a trend in favor of preoperative chemotherapy, as shown by analysis of postoperative staging and disease free survival curves. However, the distribution of 5-Fluorouracil treated patients, in the most favorable staging categories, may be due to chance rather than to treatment ; stage distribution was not an endpoint of this study and an accurate preoperative staging was not required for inclusion of patients. Relapse and death rates are comparable in both arms.

More patients in the study, and a more prolonged follow-up, are required to establish the effectiveness of this therapeutic approach. At the moment the only firm conclusion which can be drawn regards the total absence of toxicity from chemotherapy : this was in all cases well tolerated and the age limit was therefore moved from the initial, too restrictive, 70 yrs up to 75 yrs, this leading to an improved accrual rate ; in no case the surgical act or the postoperative course were influenced by chemotherapy.

References

1. Avgoustis A, Stathopoulos G, Polychronis A, Papaioannou AN (1979) Preoperative chemotherapy of gastrointestinal tumors : a feasibility study. In : Fox BW (ed) Basis for cancer therapy. Pergamon Press, Oxford, pp 263-268
2. Papaioannou AN (1981) Preoperative chemotherapy for operable solid tumors. Europ J Cancer 17 : 263-269
3. Polychronis A, Plataniotis G, Papaioannou A, Coca H, Tsamouri M, Kalapothaki V, Trichopoulos D (1983) Pre- intra and postoperative chemotherapy (CH) with or without anticoagulation in colorectal cancer. Proc Am Soc Clin Oncol, abstract C512
4. Schnetzer G, Brickner C, Stone W, Sexauer J, Ellis R, Keller A, Young J, Newcomer L (1984) Adjuvant preoperative chemotherapy and radiation therapy in moderately advanced adenocarcinoma of rectum. Proc Am Soc Clin Oncol, abstract C519
5. Gentile JM (1985) Neo-adjuvant chemotherapy in the treatment of colo-rectal cancer. First Internat Congress on Neo-Adjuvant Chemotherapy, Paris, abstr. G70
6. Lokich J, Rich T, Chaffey J (1985) Protracted infusional 5-Fluorouracil (5-FU) as neo-adjuvant and radiation sensitizor in gastrointestinal cancer. First Internat Congress on Neo-Adjuvant Chemotherapy, Paris, abstract G68
7. Papaioannou A, Polychronis A, Plataniotis G, Tsamouri M, Kozonis J, Nomicos J (1985) Chemotherapy as initial management of patients with operable colorectal cancer. Prog Clin Biol Res 201 : 317-338
8. Kaplan EL, Meier P (1958) New parametric estimation from incomplete observation. J Am Statist Assoc 53 : 457-481
9. Corbett TW, Griswold DP, Roberts BJ, Peckham JC, Schabel FM (1978) Biology and therapeutic response of a mouse mammary adenocarcinoma (16/C) and its potential as a model for surgical adjuvant chemotherapy. Cancer Treat Rep 62 : 1471-1488
10. Fisher B, Gunduz N, Saffer EA (1983) Influence of the interval between primary tumor removal and chemotherapy on kinetics and growth of metastases. Cancer Res 43 : 1488 1492

11. Sakatoku M, Kikkawa H, Hirano M, Matsu T, Harada T, Saito H, Tatsuzawa T, Masuda S (1990) A study on preoperative administration of doxifluridine in carcinoma of the colon and rectum. Gan To Kagaku Ryoho 17 : 1039-1043

Abstract. In resectable colorectal cancer effectiveness of preoperative chemotherapy has been recently suggested by pilot studies with limited numbers of patients. We started in 1987 a prospective randomized trial of preoperative 5-Fluorouracil, 600 mg/m²/die in the 5 days preceding operation, vs surgery alone. Eligibility criteria included histologically proven, untreated, resectable colorectal cancer, age 75 or less, absence of other neoplasms or general contraindications. Eighty-nine patients have been included in the study, 44 randomized to preoperative 5-Fluorouracil (arm A) and 45 to surgery (arm B). Chemotherapy was well tolerated and of no influence on the surgical management. At surgery, patients in the treated group (Arm A) appeared distributed in the most favorable staging groups. Twenty-one patients have relapsed, 10 of whom in Arm A, and 9 have died, 5 of whom in Arm A. Disease free survival curves show a limited advantage in favor of the chemotherapy-treated group. More patients and a more prolonged follow-up are required in order to assess whether this modality of treatment may have a role in resectable colorectal cancer.

Double 5-FU modulation with folinic acid and recombinant alfa2b-Interferon : a phase I-II study in metastatic colorectal cancer patients

I Brunetti*, A Falcone*, A Vigani*, P Giannessi*, C Cianci*, M Bertuccelli*, E Baldini*, PC Giulianotti**, A Pietrabissa**, R Di Stefano**, F Mosca*, E Rovini***, PF Conte*

5-Fluorouracil (5-FU) is the most widely employed chemotherapeutic agent for patients with metastatic colorectal cancer (MCC) and objective response rates (ORR) are achievable in approximately 10-20 % of treated patients [1]. Folinic acid (FA) has been tested in combination with 5-FU on the basis of preclinical evidencies indicating that an excess of intracellular reduced folates enhances 5-FU cytotoxicity by stabilizing the binding of Thymidilate Synthetase (TS) and Fluorodeoxiuridine Monophosphate (FdUMP) [2]. At least 7 out of 9 randomized studies have demonstrated the superiority for 5-FU + FA in terms of ORR, and 3 trials also a statistically significant survival advantage [3].

Recombinant alpha-Interferon (IFN) has no antitumor activity in patients with MCC, but in vitro data have shown that IFN can enhance the cytotoxic effect of 5-FU against colon cancer cell lines [4]. A possible explanation may be its ability to inhibit the uptake of thymidine and the activity of thymidine kinase [5, 6].

Based on these preclinical data Wadler et al conducted a phase II study testing the combination of 5-FU and IFN in patients with MCC [7]. An ORR of 76 % in patients not pretreated with chemotherapy was observed.

Because of these and previous clinical results with FA we started a phase I-II clinical trial to determine the toxicity and activity of a double 5-FU modulation with FA and escalating dosages of IFN in MCC patients.

Patients and methods

Patients' characteristics

From Sept. '90, 17 patients entered the study. All of them are evaluable for toxicity and 12 are evaluable for response. Median age was 58 years (range 45-73) ; 11 were male and median ECOG PS was 1 (range 0-2). The primary was colon in 11 patients, rectum in 5 and pancreas in 1. Sites of metastases were : liver in 7 patients, lung in 4, pelvis in 4, lymph nodes in 2, bone in 1, vagina in 1 and pancreas in 1. Two were previously treated with CT (5-FU), and 1 with radiotherapy.

* Unita' Operativa Oncologia Medica, Ospedale S. Chiara, Pisa, Italy
** Istituto di Chirurgica Generale e Sperimentale Universita', Pisa, Italy
*** Istituto Nazionale per la Ricerca sul Cancro, Genova, Italy

Study design

5-FU was administered at the daily dose of 450 mg/m² iv bolus for 5 consecutive days and from day 28 weekly. FA was administered at the dose of 200 mg/m² just before 5-FU. IFN was given i.m. 3 times a week, starting the first day of 5-FU administration. The starting dose was 3×10^6 I.U. and escalated to 6, 9, 12, 15 etc. $\times 10^6$ after at least 3 patients were treated at the previous dose level. Doses were escalated until ECOG grade 3-4 toxicity occured in at least 2 out of 3 or 2 out of 5 patients if grade 3-4 toxicity had occurred in 1 of the first 3 patients.

Response and toxicity

Standard ECOG criteria were used. Toxicity was monitored weekly with clinical examination and biweekly with blood cells counts and biochemistry. Clinical responses (OR) were determined monthly by instrumental measurements of neoplastic lesions.

Results

Responses

Of the 12 evaluable patients (3 treated with IFN 3×10^6 IU, 6 with 6×10^6 IU and 3 with 9×10^6 IU) 3 had a Partial Remission (PR) (25 %), 4 had a stable disease and 5 progressed. All patients that obtained a PR were previously untreated with CT (30 % ORR in untreated ones). Of responding patients one had lung metastases, 1 pelvic disease and 1 lymph nodes metastases. Two had received IFN at 3×10^6 IU and 1 at 6×10^6 IU. The Progression Free Survival (PFS) is 3+, 2+ and 1+ respectively.

Toxicity

Toxicity is listed in Table 1. Diarrhea and mucositis were the most frequent 5-FU related toxicities and were severe ($\geqslant$ grade 3) in 35 % and 24 % of treated patients respectively. Severe hematological toxicities were not observed. Fever, chills and myalgias, related to IFN administration, were nearly universal (77 %), but patients generally developed tachyphylaxis to these symptoms during the initial 2 weeks of therapy. Sixty-five percent of patients experienced moderate and 18 % severe fatigue, and a consequent decrease in performance status. No neurotoxicity was observed. No patient required hospitalization because of toxicity. Until now ; 3 have received IFN at 3×10^6 IU, 7 at 6×10^6 IU, 6 at 9×10^6 IU and 1 at 12×10^6 IU. 5-FU related toxicities were not increased in patients receiving higher IFN dosages. Instead IFN-related toxicities, mostly fatigue and worsening in PS were more common in those receiving the highest IFN doses and 4 out of 7 patients receiving doses higher of 6×10^6 IU required IFN dose reduction and suspensions after 1 month of therapy.

Table 1. Toxicity (17 evaluable patients, pts)

Toxicity		ECOG grade (% pts)			
		1	2	3	4
Mucositis		24	29	24	—
Diarrhea		29	12	29	6
Nausea/Vomiting		59	18	—	—
Leukopenia		24	29	—	—
Anemia		24	12	—	—
Fever		53	24	—	—
Fatigue {	Moderate	65			
	Severe	18			
Anorexial {	Moderate	18			
	Severe	/			

Discussion

On the basis of the results reported by Wadler et al [7] and the conclusions of previously mentioned randomized studies with 5-FU + FA [3], that obtained a RR of 76 % in patients with MCC treated with 5-FU and IFN, we tested in a phase I-II trial the triple drug combination of 5-FU + FA + escalating dosages of alfa2b-IFN in MCC patients. As in the study reported by Wadler et al [7], many of our patients experienced mucositis and diarrhea, but, in contrast, no one experienced grade 3-4 leukopenia (13 % in Wadler's study). Escalating IFN doses in ours did not cause a parallel increase of 5-FU related toxicities. Instead IFN induced fatigue increased while increasing IFN dosage and after 1 month of therapy 4 out of 7 patients treated with single doses higher of 6×10^6 IU required dose reductions and treatment interruptions. In terms of activity 3 out of 10 untreated ones (30 %) had a partial response. Even if our preliminary results do not seem to confirm the high RR reported by Wadler (76 %), but instead is similar to the RR reported in more recent trials with 5-FU + IFN where a RR from 26 to 36 % has been observed [8, 9], our study so far indicates :

1) IFN doses higher of 6×10^6 IU at the schedule we used is too toxic for a long term treatment in most of MCC patients ;

2) The combination of 5-FU + FA + alfa2b-IFN at the dose and schedule we used has activity in MCC patients, but RR appear not to be very different from what is generally achievable with 5-FU + FA without IFN.

References

1. Choen AM, Shank B and Friedman MA (1989) Colorectal Cancer. In : De Vita VT, Hellmann J and Rosenberg SA (ed) Cancer. JP Lippincott, New York

2. Evans RM, Laskin JD and Hakala MT (1981) Effect of excess folates and deoxyi-nosine on the activity and site of action of 5-Fluorouracil. Cancer Res 41 : 3288-3295
3. Arbuck SG (1989) Overview of clinical trials using 5-Fluorouracil and leucovorin for the treatment of colorectal cancer. Cancer 63 : 1036-1044
4. Elias L and Crissmann HA (1988) Interferon effects upon the adenocarcinoma-38 and HL-60 cell lines. Antiproliferative responses and synergistic interactions with alogeneted pyrimidine antimetabolites. Cancer Res 48 : 4868-4873
5. Gewert DR, Moore G, Clemens MJ (1983) Inhibition of cell division by Interfe-rons. The relationship between changes in utilization of thymidine for DNA synthe-sis and control of proliferation in Daudi cells. Biochem J 214 : 983-990
6. Gewert DR, Shah S, Clemens MJ (1981) Inhibition of cell division by Interferons. Changes in the transport of thymidine in human lymphoblastoid cells. Eur J Bio-chem 116 : 487-492
7. Wadler S, Swartz EL, Goldman M, Lyver A, Rader M, Zimmermann M, Itri L, Weinberg V and Wiernik P (1989) Fluorouracil and recombinant alfa-2A Interfe-ron : an active regimen against advanced colorectal carcinoma. J Clin Oncol 7 : 1769-1775
8. Kemeny, Kelsen, Derby S, Sanmarco P, Adams L, Mrray P (1990) Combination 5-Fluorouracil and recombinant alfa-Interferon in advanced colorectal carcinoma : activity but significant toxicity. Proc Am Soc Clin Oncol 9 : 109
9. Pazdur R, Ajani JA, Patt YZ, Winn R, Jackson D, Shepard B, DuBrow R, Cam-pos L, Quaraishi M, Faintuch J, Abruzzese JL, Guttermann J, Levin B (1990) Phase II study of Fluorouracil and recombinant Interferon alfa-2a in previously untreated advanced colorectal carcinoma. J Clin Oncol 8 : 2031-2077

Loco-regional

Neo-Adjuvant locoregional chemotherapy in pelvis osteosarcoma

A Tienghi, G Fiorentini, G Cruciani, C Dazzi, L Albertazzi, E Emiliani*, M Marangolo

Osteosarcoma is a very rare disease affecting young people : it is calculated not to exceed 0.2 % of all the tumors. Pelvic osteosarcoma (p.o.) is even more uncommon, representing about 5 % of all osteosarcomas reported.

Recently combined treatment with neo-adjuvant chemotherapy, plus surgery, plus adjuvant chemotherapy has dramatically improved the cure rate of high grade osteosarcoma : 5-year disease-free survival of 60-70 % are reported from many centers [1-2].

Unfortunately these successfull results are limited to osteosarcomas of the extremities and not transferable to the pelvic region which has still a very poor prognosis. The curability may be influenced by a combination of prognostic factors ; the most complete analysis of these was published by Taylor and coll [3]. It was found that the site of the primary tumor played a very important role in conditioning survival.

Materials and methods

In June 1987 we designed a pilot study for the treatment of p.o. consisting of neo-adjuvant locoregional and systemic chemotherapy, local treatment (surgery or radiotherapy) and adjuvant systemic chemotherapy. The surgical approach represents a fundamental step in the therapeutic strategy of osteosarcoma ; however, in the pelvic presentation rarely a radical dissection can be assured, in spite of aggressive and mutilating operations. Radiotherapy with Cisplatin (CDDP) as a radiosensitizer, can be an alternative treatment in non operable patients.

Our treatment consisted of 2-3 cycles of neo-adjuvant chemotherapy, with high dose Methotrexate 8 g/m^2 given in 6 hours i.v. infusion and leucovorin rescue on day 1, CDDP 120 mg/m^2 given i.a. in 72 hours on day 8, Epidoxorubicin 100 mg/m^2 in 8 hours i.v. infusion on day 10 ; every 28 days.

The patients were completly reevaluated after the neo-adjuvant phase in order to decide whether to perform surgery or radiotherapy. If surgery was excluded radiotherapy was delivered with 2 daily fractions of 1.4 Gy with CDDP 5 mg a day between the two doses, up to a total dose of 70 Gy. Adjuvant systemic chemotherapy was administered 3 weeks after the local treatment and consisted of Epidoxorubicin 50 mg/m^2 8 hours i.v. on days 1 and 2, Ifosfamide 2,000 mg/m^2 1 h i.v. on days 21-25 plus mesna, Methotrexate 8 g/m^2 6 h i.v. on day 28 plus Leucovorin rescue, CDDP 120 mg/m^2 72 h i.v. and

* Medical Oncology, Radiotherapy, City Hospital, Ravenna, Italy

Etoposide 120 mg/m^2 on days 49-50-51. Three complete cycles were delivered every 3 weeks.

We know that osteosarcomas responding to chemotherapy do not necessarily decrease in size but usually become less vascular and change degree of mineralization. To evaluate response after the neo-adjuvant phase we utilized these criteria : clinical, as relief of pain and improvement in rotary motion ; X-ray, as mineralization of lytic areas ; angiographic X-ray, as reduction or disappearance of tumor vascularity ; biochemistry, as decrease in LDH and ALP levels ; CT, as decrease in soft tissue infiltration.

Since June 1987 we observed 26 patients with p.o. : eight were excluded from the pilot study (4 received only i.v. chemotherapy and 4 surgery as first line therapy), 18 were enrolled in this clinical trial.

Results and toxicity

After the neo-adjuvant phase we obtained 8 PR, 9 SD and 1 PD with pathological fracture. Four patients judged operable, underwent hemipelvectomy : necrosis was nil in 2 and of 50 % and 70 % in the other 2. Fourteen patients not operable, received radiotherapy plus daily low dose of CDDP. After local treatment all patients received i.v. chemotherapy.

At present, 18 patients received 42 neo-adjuvant and 26 adjuvant cycles ; we evaluated the number of cycles with toxicity of grade 3 and 4, according to Miller : 10 hematological (all after radiotherapy), 2 hepatic, 1 renal due to high dose methotrexate, 3 gastrointestinal. We had no severe cardiac and neurological toxicity.

Regarding survival, among the 4 patients who underwent surgery, 2 died at 17 and 18 months, with time to lung metastases of 10 and 3 months diagnosis (both patients underwent resection of lung metastases and further chemotherapy) ; two are alive and free at 23 + and 12 + months from diagnosis. In the group treated with radiotherapy, 9 patients died with a median survival of 18 months (range 5-22) ; 5 are alive with median follow up of 11 months (range 8-31). The median time to lung metastases was 6 months (0-20).

Discussion and conclusion

High grade p.o. has a very limited cure rate also in patients who undergo amputation. One of the main points is the delay in diagnosis, so that the patient bears a very large tumor burden, probably already with disseminated disease. Besides, the mass is usually irrigated by more than one artery and so we can never optimize i.a. chemotherapy as in the extremities. That is why we have never obtained the angiographic disappearance of tumor vascularity and a histological « good necrosis ».

Pelvic resections and hemipelvectomies have a high local recurrence rate dependent on surgical margins, on tumor grade and on rate of necrosis : our

4 cases were high grade and had « poor necrosis » but none had local recurrence.

Radiotherapy plus CDDP seems to be beneficial in the local control of the disease ; systemic chemotherapy following the local treatment, probably delays the appearance of lung metastases.

In patients judged non operable, our treatment shows some benefit in terms of palliation, that is a pain relief, acceptable quality of life and prolonged survival.

References

1. Benjamin RS, Raymond AK, Carrasco CH et al (1989) Primary chemotherapy of osteosarcoma of the extremities with systemic adriamycin and intra-arterial cisplatinum. Proc Annu Meet Am Soc Clin Oncol 8 : A1251
2. Picci P, Bacci G, Avella R et al (1989) Neo-adjuvant chemotherapy (NAC) for osteosarcoma of the extremities (OS). Fourth International Conference on Advances in Regional Cancer Therapy. Berchtesgaden, FRG, 5-7 June
3. Taylor WF, Ivins JC, Unni KK et al (1989) Prognostic variables in osteosarcoma : a multi-institutional study. J Natl Cancer Inst 81(1) : 21-30

Treatment of advanced intra-abdominal or thoracic malignancies using high-dose intra-arterial chemotherapy with concomitant hemofiltration

JH Muchmor, ET Krementz, RD Carter, J Preslan, WJ George

High-dose intra-arterial chemotherapy with concomitant hemofiltration (HICCH) has potential usefulness in the pre-operative or perioperative setting of treating patients with advanced intra-abdominal or intra-thoracic malignancies. Using high-dose intra-arterial chemotherapy together with concomitant hemofiltration, the effluent blood from a tumor-bearing region can be rapidly cleared of the peak chemotherapeutic drug level. This allows then the delivery of higher drug doses to a regionally confined malignancy. The use of this type of system was originally defined by Dedrick et al [1] for the treatment of patients with primary brain tumors. Aigner et al and Muchmore et al have investigated similar systems for patients with advanced intra-abdominal malignancies [2, 3]. In a group of 25 patients with advanced intra-abdominal and intra-thoracic malignancies, some have successfully undergone 40 treatments with high-dose regional chemotherapy plus concomitant hemofiltration at the Tulane Medical Center Hospital.

Material and methods

Of the 25 patients with advanced intra-abdominal or intra-thoracic malignancies, 10 were men and 15 were women ; the average age was 55 (range : 36 to 70) years. Fourteen patients had a primary or metastatic disease localized to the liver : hepatoma (2 patients), gallbladder, (3 patients), pancreas (1 patient), breast (3 patients), carcinoid (1 patient), unknown primary (1 patient) and colon (3 patients) (Table 1). Five patients had advanced unresectable pancreatic cancer, 5 had advanced peritoneal or recurrent pelvic metastases from colon (4 patients) and melanoma, and 1 an advanced bladder carcinoma. One of the above patients with subsequent pulmonary metastases was treated by a thoracic chemofiltration.

Patients with isolated liver disease had an arterial catheter placed angiographically prior to the HICCH or surgically implanted and connected to a subcutaneous port system. Patients with a pancreatic malignancy had a celiac artery catheter surgically implanted. Patients with intra-peritoneal disease or pelvic had an aortic catheter positioned at the level of the diaphragm from the femoral artery in the groin just prior to starting the HICCH. In the patient with pulmonary disease, an aortic catheter was positioned just below the left subclavian artery with a balloon partially inflated at the level of the diaphragm. Through a saphenous venotomy, a PFM 16-Fr double lumen filtration

Tulane University School of Medicine, Departments of Surgery and Pharmacology

Table 1. Patient demographics

Primary Site	Patient	Disease Location	Treatments
Colon	8	Liver	6
		Peritoneal	3
		Pelvis	7
Breast	3	Liver	4
		Lung	1
Pancreas	5	Pancreas	4
		Pancreas/Liver	3
Hepatoma	2	Liver	3
Gallbladder	3	Liver	3
Bladder	1	Pelvis	1
Carcinoid	1	Liver	1
Unknown primary	1	Liver	1
Totals	25		40

catheter was positioned above the retrohepatic veins with fluoroscopic guidance. The filtration catheter was connected to a modified Gambro unit with a 1,2 m² hollow tube filter. A balanced hemofiltration with a flow rate of 400 ml/min and ultrafiltration rate of 150 ml/min was established. A bicarbonate-based replacement solution was returned to the patient replacing the ultrafiltrate. The patient's temperature was maintained by heating the replacement solution to 38°C. Mitomycin C (20 to 25 mg/m²) infused over 20 min followed by 5-Fluorouracil (500 to 750 mg/m²) over 10 min were commonly used for patients with metastatic breast, colon, pancreas, gallbladder and bladder cancer. Cisplatin and Adriamycin were used in treating patients with melanoma, sarcoma, and hepatoma.

Results

Three patients achieved complete responses, 1 with metastatic breast cancer to the liver following HICCH alone, who maintained a CR for more than 2 years. Two had residual tumor in the pelvis which was completely resected. Seven of the 25 patients achieved a partial response with reduction in tumor size, as shown by computed tomography (CT) scan of the tumor-bearing region following at least one treatment, even though 16 of these patients failed previous chemotherapy regimens. The best responses were achieved in patients having metastatic disease from breast, colon, and pancreatic cancer. Nine patients had stabilization of their disease, and 6 had progression. The overall response rate is apparently 50 to 60 % with the longest survivor out to 30 months. The 1- and 2-year survival was 30 % and 20 %, respectively. Complications have been limited to moderate bone marrow suppression in patients with extensive pretreatment chemotherapy. Patients with celiac artery infusions had mild to moderate gastritis and duodenitis.

Discussion

HICCH appears to have potential usefulness in treating patients with advanced intra-abdominal and intra-thoracic malignancies. As a pre-operative procedure for treating advanced regional malignancies, it will probably be most beneficial in converting unresectable tumors to resectability for cure.

References

1. Dedrick RL, Oldfield EH, Collins JM (1984) Arterial drug infusion with extracorporeal removal. I. Theoretical basis with particular reference to the brain. Cancer Treat Rep 68 : 373-380
2. Aigner KR, Muller H, Walter H, Link KH (1988) Drug filtration in high-dose regional chemotherapy. Contr Oncol 29 : 261-280
3. Muchmore JH, Preslan J, Meyer M, et al (1989) Pharmacokinetics of high-dose intra-arterial chemotherapy with concomitant hemofiltration (HICCF) Prof Ann Meet Am Assoc Cancer Res 30 : A1138

Abstract. A procedure involving extracorporeal recapture of chemotherapeutic drugs has been used for the treatment of advanced or unresectable intra-abdominal or intra-thoracic malignancies. High-dose intra-arterial chemotherapy with concomitant hemofiltration (HICCH) permits the delivery of high-dose chemotherapy to a tumor-bearing area and at the same time limits the systemic toxicity. The most appropriate use of this technique is in the pre-operative or peri-operative setting. Twenty-five patients have successfully undergone 40 treatments of HICCH at Tulane Medical Center Hospital in the past two years. Three patients achieved complete responses, 2 of whom had their residual tumor resected for cure. Seven of the 25 patients achieved a partial response, 9 had stable disease, and 6 had progression.

Technical aspects of adjuvant intraperitoneal chemotherapy

J Vidal-Jove, J Esquivel, D Buck, P Barrios, MA Steves,
PH Sugarbaker

Intraperitoneal chemotherapy has been described as a potential successful tool in the management of a variety of malignancies that occur primarily in a local regional manner [1]. The benefits of this technique may be used in ovarian carcinoma, gastrointestinal malignancies [2], and mesothelioma [1, 3]. A new approach to the treatment of peritoneal carcinomatosis has been recently developed [4]. The protocol of treatment includes cytoreductive surgery, early postoperative intraperitoneal chemotherapy and adjuvant intraperitoneal and systemic chemotherapy (Fig. 1). The objective of this manuscript is to report the author's experience with adjuvant intraperitoneal chemotherapy by repeated paracentesis.

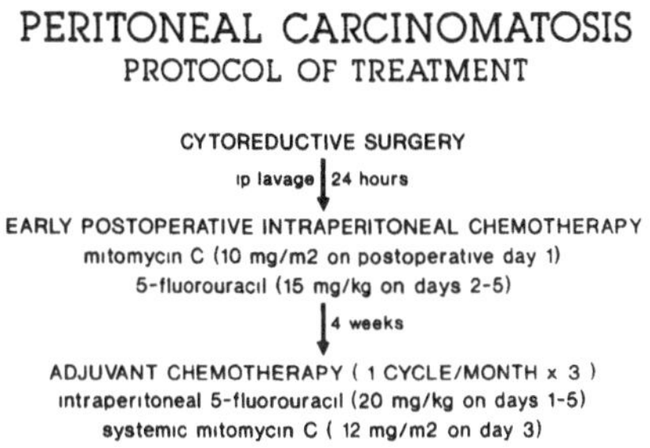

PERITONEAL CARCINOMATOSIS
PROTOCOL OF TREATMENT

CYTOREDUCTIVE SURGERY
ip lavage | 24 hours

EARLY POSTOPERATIVE INTRAPERITONEAL CHEMOTHERAPY
mitomycin C (10 mg/m2 on postoperative day 1)
5-fluorouracil (15 mg/kg on days 2-5)

| 4 weeks

ADJUVANT CHEMOTHERAPY (1 CYCLE/MONTH x 3)
intraperitoneal 5-fluorouracil (20 mg/kg on days 1-5)
systemic mitomycin C (12 mg/m2 on day 3)

Fig. 1. Peritoneal carcinomatosis. Protocol of treatment

Material and methods

At present, 23 patients (10 women and 13 men) have completed the treatment. Ages ranged between 27 and 71 (mean 49 years). Diagnosis were, in all the patients, peritoneal carcinomatosis. Eleven of them from appendiceal cystadenocarcinoma, 4 from colonic cystadenocarcinoma, 1 from cystadenocarcinoma of the Fallopian tube, 4 from colorectal adenocarcinoma and 3 from unknown primary. All the patients had previous surgery. Sixty-five percent (15 patients) had more than 3 procedures and 35 % (8 patients) had 3 or less. Procedures employed were greater and lesser : omentectomy, splenectomy, cholecystectomy, pelvic peritonectomy with sigmoidectomy and low anterior anastomosis, right and left subdiaphragmatic peritonectomies, small bowel and gastric resections, gastrojejunostomy or pyloroplasty, liver resection and hysterectomy. After com-

The Cancer Institute, Washington Hospital Center, 110 Irving St. N.W., Washington D.C. 20010, USA

plete recovery from surgery and early postoperative intraperitoneal chemotherapy, patients were included in the weekly adjuvant treatment on an out-patient basis. Intraperitoneal catheter was placed on Monday. Intra-abdominal distribution of the fluid was assessed by computerized tomography with intraperitoneal contrast. The same day, intraperitoneal chemotherapy with 5-Fluorouracil was started (20 mg/kg in 1,000 ml of 1.5 % dialysis solution). The fluid was instilled as rapidly as possible, with 23 hours dwell and 1 hour drain. This procedure was repeated in days 2, 3, 4 and 5. On day 6 the catheter was removed. On day 3, a 2 hour systemic infusion of Mitomycin C (12 mg/m^2) was administered. This cycle was repeated with a 4 week interval between treatments for a total of 3 cycles of AIPC.

Technique of placement

Catheters were placed under local anesthesia and aseptic precautions. Pre-procedure sedation with IV Demerol was usually used, at the patient's option. Entry site was either at the lateral margin of the rectus abdominous muscles or in the midline. Initial placement site was usually selected as opposite to the bulk of tumor on the pre-operative scan. An attempt was made to rotate tube site between sides on consecutive chemotherapy courses, but the review of contrast distribution from earlier studies sometimes precluded rotation of sites when peritoneal adhesions were present. In over one-half the cases, peritoneal access was obtained with a single wall 18 gauge needle. Position was confirmed with injection of Meglumine Diatrizoate 30 %, and wire exchange made for an 8.3 Fr percuflex catheter. In later patients, access was obtained with a 22 gauge Chiba needle, and two-stage wire exchange was made using the Neff introducer set (Cook, Inc.). Initially, self-retaining Cope loop-type catheters were used, but in some patients these were difficult to remove following chemotherapy, and on subsequent cases the 8.3 Fr pigtail all-purpose drain was used (Meditech, Inc.).

Final catheter position was confirmed with a small volume of 30 % contrast solution. Sufficient contrast was administered to 1 liter normal saline to represent a total of 50 ml of 60 % contrast solution between the test injections and the final infusate. This usually resulted in 1.8-2.4 % contrast in 1 liter. The entire volume was infused into the catheter via 21 gauge needle and Heparin lock under gravity ; abdominal CT scan was performed immediately using 10 mm sections from the dome of the diaphragm to the symphysis pubis.

Results

Morbidity of AIPC can be seen in Table 1. Uniform drug distribution occurred in 63 over 69 possible cycles (91.3 %). Patients tolerated oral diet during administration of the chemotherapy. No ileus was seen, nor reoperations for adhesions or for insertion or removal of catheters were needed. Two colonic

Table 1. Morbidity of AIPC after cytoreductive surgery for peritoneal carcinomatosis

Total number of patients	23	100 %
Intra-abdominal abscess	1	1.5 %
Colonic perforation	2	3.1 %
Fail to obtain peritoneal access	2	3.1 %
Bone marrow toxicity Grade III	2	3.1 %
Ileus	0	
Reoperations for adhesions	0	
Uniform drug distribution	63/69	91.3 %
Severe pain limiting instillation	2	3.1 %
Mortality	0	
Overall morbidity	9	14.2 %

perforations were observed (3.1 %) with the 18 gauge needle. No similar complications were seen in later patients with the 22 gauge Chiba needle. Two patients had severe pain that precluded complete instillation of the drug (3.1 %). Overall morbidity has been 14.2 % with 0 mortality.

Discussion and conclusion

Intraperitoneal chemotherapy is considered as an alternative route of administration in front of systemic chemotherapy. Sites with high risk recurrence rate, resection site and peritoneal surfaces, can be exposed to high doses of chemotherapy with acceptable toxicity. Also, as it has been observed in previous studies [5], portal vein levels achieved with intraperitoneal chemotherapy are 10 to 20 times greater in the portal venous blood than in peripheral venous samples. In an adjuvant setting, intraperitoneal chemotherapy may not only protect against local and regional recurrence but also minimize the incidence of liver metastases.

In our experience, adjuvant intraperitoneal chemotherapy by repeated paracentesis was used with acceptable morbidity and no mortality. To administer this chemotherapy properly to all parts of the abdominal cavity, large volumes of fluid containing drug must be administered intermittently [6]. Repeated paracentesis was a practical method to accomplish that in a large volume of patients on an out-patient basis. It was considered superior as a technique of intraperitoneal drug delivery in terms of drug distribution, low rate of complications, cost and patient acceptance [7] (Table 2).

Table 2. Clinical comparison of peritoneal access devices used for long term peritoneal access

	Burron intestoflant	Tenckboff portacate	Tenckboff catheter	Repeated paracentesis
Skin exit site	No	No	Yes	No
Insertion	Most difficulty	Moderate difficulty	Mild difficulty	Loast difficulty
Drug distribution	Deteriorates with time	Deteriorates with time	Deteriorates with time	Improve over time
Removal	Major surgery	Surgery	Minimal surgery	None
Drainage of peritoneal fluid	Usually impossible	Usually impossible	Possible 50 % of cases	Usually achieved
Intra-abdominal injuries	Rare	Rare	Rare	Uncommon
Adhesions	Frequent	Frequent	Frequent	Uncommon
Cost	High	High	Low	Low

References

1. Markman M (1986) Intracavitary Chemotherapy. Curr Prob Cancer 10 (8) : 399-437
2. Cunliffe WJ, Sugarbaker PH (1989) Gastrointestinal malignancy : rationale for adjuvant therapy using early postoperative intraperitoneal chemotherapy. Br J Surg 76 : 1082-1090
3. Vidal-Jove J, Sweatman T, Graves T, Litwin F, Davidson E, Sugarbaker PH (1991) Curative approach to malignant peritoneal mesothelioma. Case report and review of the literature. Reg Cancer Treat (in Press)
4. Sugarbaker PH (1990) Cytoreductive surgery : past accomplishment and future prospects. Acta Chirurgica Scandinavica (in Press)
5. Speyer JL, Sugarbaker PH, Collins JM, and others (1981) Portal levels and hepatic change of 5-Fluorouracil after intraperitoneal administration in humans. Cancer Res 41 : 1916
6. Jenkins J, Sugarbaker PH, Gianola FJ, Myers CE (1982) Technical considerations in the use of intraperitoneal chemotherapy delivered by Tenckhoff catheter. Surg Gynecol & Obstet 154 : 858-864
7. Sugarbaker PH (1989) Clinical experience with a new totally implanted peritoneal access device : the Burron Intestoplant. Reg Cancer Treat 1 : 140-144

Combined intravenous and intra-arterial chemotherapy using Cisplatin, Fluorouracil, Mitomycin C and Etoposide in the treatment of hepatic metastasis

D Khayat, M Weil, C Borel, G Cohen-Aloro, D Buthiau, G Auclerc, V Bassot

Hepatic metastasis is the most frequent site of treatment failure in cancer patients, reaching proportions over 50 % in the evolution of intra-abdominal tumors. Spontaneous survival, after the liver has been involved is very poor, from 2 to 6 months according to the number of metastasis and the origin of the primary tumor. Curative surgery is rarely possible, ranging from 10 to 25 % of cases mainly for solitary or very limited number of hepatic metastasis and has a 10 to 15 % post-operative mortality rate. Systemic chemotherapy, before Fluorouracil/Folinic acid combination, had a 10-15 % response rate which seems to have been improved more recently to 30-50 % with the modulation of fluoropyrimidines activity.

The reasons for such bad prognosis are multiple and complex : nature of the primary tumor, frequently from gastro-intestinal tract origin and therefore usually resistant ; heterogeneity of secondary tumors, which increases with time and disease progression along with the emergence of highly resistant clones ; possibility of secondary metastatic processes raising from the hepatic metasta- sis ; complexity and variability of the hepatic metastasis vascularization with a predominant arterial blood supply in macroscopic tumors.

However, it has been shown, in vitro, that human hepatic metastatic cells, even from pancreatic or colorectal primary tumors are in fact sensitive to stan- dard chemotherapeutic drugs but usually need higher drug concentration in order to show a significant killing of tumor cell.

The rationale for loco-regional chemotherapy is based on that goal. Indeed, by means of the local injection of cytotoxic drugs, directly with the hepatic arterial blood flow, it seems theoretically possible to circumvent drug dilution, metabolisation and elimination before it reaches its hepatic target, increasing therefore the local concentration compared to what would have been obtained after a classical intra-veinous administration. This local advantage of I.A. treat- ment over I.V. treatment is even amplified when dealing with hepatic secon- dary tumors because of relative tumor arterial preferential blood flow.

We report here the results of a pilot study using a combined treatment with 5-Fluorouracil, Cisplatin and Mitomycin C administered intra-arterially and simultaneously with VP16 by intra-venously route to patients with exclusive or predominant hepatic metastasis from various origin.

Service d'Oncologie Médicale (SOMPS) Hopital de la Salpêtrière, 47 boulevard de l'Hopital, 75013 Paris, France

Patients and methods

From 1986 till 1989, 19 patients with exclusive or predominant hepatic metastasis have been included in a pilot study aimed at evaluating the response rate
and the survival obtained with a combination of I.A. 5-FU-Cisplatin-Mitomycin
C and IV Etoposide according to the schedule described in Table 1.

Table 1. Combined IA/IV treatment - schedule

Drug	Dose	Time	Route
Cisplatin	100 mg/m²	4 h, day 1	IA
5-Fluoro-uracil	1 000 mg/m²	continuous infusion days 1, 2, 3	IA
Mitomycin C	6 mg/m²	bolus, day 1	IA
Etoposid	100 mg/m²	1 h, day 1	IV

Two patients were not evaluable for response or survival because of patient
withdrawal before the end of the first course of chemotherapy due to cardiac
(1 case) or digestive (1 case) toxicity.
The characteristics of the 17 evaluable patients are summarized in Table 2.

Table 2. Patients characteristics

Number	19	Previous treatment	
Sex		none	3
male	5	chemotherapy	16
female	14	IV	6
Age		IA	2
median	54	Both IV/IA	8
range	35-68	Extrahepatic metastasis	
Primary tumor		lung	7
breast	11	gone	9
colorectal	3	lymphnode	5
duodenal	1	peritoneal	1
ACUP	2		
Apudoma	2		

Briefly, 11 patients (64 %) had hepatic metastasis originating from breast
cancer and 23 % from gastro-intestinal tract cancer. Eighty-four percent of
them were resistant to previous chemotherapy including 10 patients (60 %) who
were resistant to exclusive or combined intra-arterial treatment. Ten patients

(60 %) had extrahepatic metastasis at the time of entry in the study representing a total of 22 metastatic sites (7 lung, 9 bone, 5 lymphnodes and 1 peritoneal). The number of treatment cycles per patient ranged from 1 to 10 (mean = 4,5) for a total of 78 analyzed cycles.

The I.A route was always administered through an I.A implanted port (Porth-A-Cath® in 12 cases and Lifeport® in 7 cases). During the surgical placement of the catheter, a prophylactic cholecystectomy was performed. Catheter thrombosis prophylaxis was based on daily oral aspirin (300 g/day) and heparin before and after each chemotherapy infusion. Responses were assessed on CT-scans every 6 weeks.

Results

Seventeen patients are evaluable for response after a total of 78 cycles of combined chemotherapy. Hepatic response rate is 52.6 % with a median duration time for response of 29 weeks. There were 1 complete and 9 partial responses.

The median survival for the 17 patients is of 47 weeks with a statistically significant benefit for responders (58 weeks) versus non responding patients (22 weeks ; p = 0.05). Four more patients were stabilized. Responses (Table 3) were seen in breast (8/10), ACUP (1/2) and apudoma (1/2) cancer patients. Extra-hepatic responses were seen in 10 patients (52 %).

Table 3. Hepatic responses

Response	Nb	Primary tumor	Duration (weeks)
RC	1	Breast	63
PR	9	Breast: 7	78, 23 +, 50, 32 +, 26, 24 +, 4 +, 44 +
		ACUP: 1	25 +
		Apudoma: 1	
ST	4	Breast: 1 Colorectal: 1 Duodenal: 1 Apudoma: 1	
PO	3	Breast: 1 Colorectal: 1 ACUP: 1	

Regarding toxicity, there were 6 episodes of grade III and IV leucopenia and 2 episodes of grade III and IV thrombocytopenia. Other toxicities include nausea and vomiting (21 %), polynevritis (5 %), creatinine elevation (15 %) and angina pectoris (5 %).

Two thrombosis of the implanted port have been observed not reversible after local injection of urokinase (5,000 UI).

Discussion

We report here the result of a prospective pilot study of a combined I.A and I.V chemotherapy of hepatic metastasis from various origin. The high response rate on hepatic and on extra-hepatic tumors (3/17 patients) seems to indicate that combined I.A and I.V treatment, using a synergistic combination of Cisplatin, Fluorouracil, Mitomycin C and Etoposide, is of interest in this type of patients. It is obvious that using this combined route, we did not observe as many extra-hepatic failures as we were used to see when using locoregional route alone.

Tolerance was rather acceptable with hematologic limiting toxicity and seems comparable to that observed after I.V chemotherapy.

Catheter thrombosis was efficiently prevented by prophylactic administration of oral aspirin with only 2 cases of thrombosis among 19 patients.

Finally, although the population of patients included in that study had a very bad prognosis because of resistance to previous treatment, including a sequential use of I.A and I.V treatment, and of the presence of extra-hepatic metastasis in the majority of patients, we demonstrated here a survival benefit for responding patients that reached statistical significance (58 weeks versus 22 weeks ; $p = 0.05$).

This is most probably due to the adjonction of an I.V component to the treatment that was able to increase the control of extra-hepatic metastasis. However, whether this combined I.A/I.V treatment is indeed one of the good treatment so far available for the treatment of hepatic metastasis needs to be confirmed on a larger study that, according to these results, seems to be worth starting.

Acknowledgment to Brigitte Cédreau for her assistance.

References

1. Jacquillat Cl, Weil M, Khayat D (1988) Proceeding of the 2nd International Congress on Neo-Adjuvant Chemotherapy. John Libbey Eurotext Ed, London, vol. 169
2. Pickren JW, Tsukada Y and Lane WW (1982) Liver metastases : analysis of autopsy data. In : Weiss L & Gilbert H (eds) Liver metastases. G.K. Hall medical publishers, Boston pp 2-18
3. Bengmark S, Hafstrom L (1969) The natural history of primary and secondary malignant tumors of the liver, I/the prognosis for patients with hepatic metastases from colonic and rectal carcinoma by laparotomy. Cancer 23 : 198-202
4. Jaffe BM, Donegan WL, Watson F, Spratt JS (1968) Factors influencing survival in patients with untreated hepatic metastases. Surg Gynecol Obst 127 : 1-11

5. Chen HSG, Gross JS (1980) Intraarterial infusion of anticancer drugs : theoretic aspects of drug delivery and review of responses. Cancer Treat Rep 64 : 31-40

6. Foster JH (1982) Treatment of metastatic cancer to liver. In : De Vita V., Hellman S. and Rosenberg S.A. (eds) Cancer : principles and practice of oncology. Lippincott JB Co. Philadelphia, pp 1553-1563

7. Khayat D, Le Cesne A, Azar N, Cour V, Vu Thi Myle C, Auclerc G, Thill L, Vallantin X, Cohen-Aloro G, Langlois P, Bousquet JC, Jacquillat Cl (1988) Intra-arterial treatment of hepatic metastases using the 5-Fluoro-Uracil, Adriamycin, Mitomycin C (FAM) chemotherapeutic regimen. Reg Cancer Treat 1 : 62-64

8. Chang AE, Schneider PD, Sugarbaker PH (1987) Hepatic arterial infusion chemotherapy : clinical trials with the implantable pump. In : Lokich JJ (ed). Cancer Chemotherapy by Infusion. Precent Press Inc Chicago pp 435-446

9. Kemeny N, Daly J, Reichman B, Geller N, Bodet J, Oderman P (1987) Intrahepatic or systemic infusion of fluorodeoxyuridine in patients with liver metastases from colorectal carcinoma. Ann Int Med 107 : 459-465

10. Holn D, Stagg R, Rayner A, Lewis B (1987) The NCOG randomized trial of intraveinous (IV) vs hepatic arterial (IA) FUDR for colorectal cancer metastatic to the liver. ICRCT, abstract B6 : 26

Drug sensitivity testing for regional chemotherapy

KH Link, R Kunz, J Ullrich, HG Beger

Non resectable solid tumors at various locations can be treated by regional chemotherapy (RC). In the various protocols a variety of drug combinations and infusion times are applied even for histologically identical tumors [1, 6]. Since most tumor types respond individually to identical regimens, their individual chemosensitivity should be considered for successful therapy. Therefore, we assessed the validity of individual chemosensitivity testing for RC in a two-step approach, using the 'Human tumor colony assay' (HTCA) [2] as in vitro test procedure.

Materials and methods

Individual tumor biopsies were taken surgically from the sites to be treated regionally. A standardized tumor cell suspension was worked up from the tissue for drug testing in the HTCA as previously described [2, 8]. Aliquots of the tumor cells were exposed to the test drugs at the concentrations of 1 and 10 μg/ml (5-FU: 10 and 100 μg/ml) for 1 h and to drug free medium (untreated control), washed, and cultured in a soft agar medium. The colony growth of treated dishes was related in [%] to the untreated control. The test was sensitive, if colony growth at the concentration relevant for regional treatment was $\leqslant$ 50 % and resistant, if growth was > 50 % of the untreated control. The test drugs used were Adriamycin, Cisplatin, 4-Epidoxorubicin, 5-FU, Mitomycin C, and Mitoxantrone.

In the prospective correlative trial (PCT), the HTCA results of 30 patients with liver metastases from colorectal cancer (N = 24), melanoma (4), breast cancer (1), and carcinoid (1) were related to the clinical outcome of RC. The HTCA was performed and patients treated according to standard protocols — without impact of the HTCA on drug selection. Clinical response was defined as a CEA reduction by $\geqslant$ 50 % or CT-scan documented tumor volume reduction by $\geqslant$ 50 %, if no tumor markers were available. In the prospective decision aiding trial (PDAT), 18 patients with primary liver tumors (N = 4) and liver metastases from colorectal cancer (4), carcinoid (3), breast cancer (3), others (2), and with peritoneal carcinosis of ovarian cancer (1) and sarcoma (1) were enrolled. Active drugs were selected according to the individual HTCA-sensitivity for intra-arterial infusion (N = 16) and intraperitoneal instillation (N = 2). 19 in vitro/in vivo correlations were obtained. Clinical response in the PDAT was defined as a CT-scan documented tumor volume reduction by $\geqslant$ 50 % or as stop of prior CT-scan proven progression (2 patients).

Department of General Surgery, University Ulm, Steinhövelstr. 9, 7900 Ulm, Germany

The RC procedures used in both trials were either intra-arterial infusion with or without concomitant hemofiltration, chemoembolization or intraperitoneal instillation. The intra-arterial infusion time was 20 min to 60 min, the intraperitoneal instillate exposure > 3 h, the chemoembolizate remained in the target for 1 month or more.

Results

The results of the individual chemosensitivity tests in the PCT and PDAT are shown in Table 1. In the PCT, in vitro sensitivity correlated correctly with clinical response in 21/21 and resistance in 6/9 cases. In the PDAT, these correlations were 12/15 for in vitro sensitivity and 3/4 for resistance. Thus, specificity of in vitro sensitivity for predicting response to RC was 100 % in the PCT, and 80 % in the PDAT. In vitro resistance specificity was 67 % in the PCT, and 75 % in the PDAT. — The clinical response rate to RC in the PDAT was 72 % (CR + PR + NC) or 61 % (CR + PR), with 17 % CR. In 2 patients, CR/PR were documented in second-look operations. Responders in the PDAT were detected by the HTCA in 12/13 patients, resulting in a test-sensitivity to detect clinical response in 92 %.

Table 1. Results of individual chemosensitivity testing with the HTCA in the prospective correlative (PCT) and decision aiding test (PDAT)

	PCT		PDAT	
Clinical	response	progression	response	progression
In vitro				
— sensitive	21*	0	12	3
— resistant	3	6	1	3
In vitro				
— sensitivity correct	100% (21/21)**		80% (12/15)	
— resistance correct	67% (6/9)		75% (3/4)	

* patients with in vitro/in vivo correlations
** correct correlations in vitro/in vivo

Discussion and conclusion

The main parameters for chemotherapeutic drug effectivity are concentration, exposure time, and individual chemosensitivity [4, 9, 11, 12]. In regional chemotherapy, concentration and time can be optimally adjusted with various techniques [1, 6]. Drug selection, however, is made empirically and not according to individual sensitivity. In order to be able to consider individual sensitivity

in our RC-programs for liver tumors and peritoneal carcinosis, we assessed
the validity of chemosensitivity testing in regional chemotherapy with the
HTCA. In previous tests for drug activities in the HTCA (in vitro phase-II
studies) we found, that regionally applicable drugs exert in vitro concentration dependent response rates that are representative for the clinically achievable remission rates in RC, indicating an acceptable relevance of the HTCA
for RC [7]. These results supported our hypothesis, that in vitro sensitivity
may be individually associated correctly with clinical response. If this was true,
the HTCA could be used for individual drug selection in RC. The reliable correlation (100 %) of HTCA-sensitivity with response to RC in the PCT confirmed our assumption and encouraged us to use the HTCA in the PDAT for
individual drug selection in RC. In this trial, in vitro drug sensitivity correlated in 80 % correctly with clinical response.

Our high specificity of HTCA-sensitivity for response to RC (80-100 %)
is in contrast to the HTCA-results in systemic chemotherapy, where prediction of response can be correct up to 60 %, of resistance, however, up to 99 %
[3, 5]. This difference in validity of the HTCA in regional vs. systemic chemotherapy may be due to the closer pharmacological relations between the drug
exposure conditions in vitro and the clinical pharmacokinetics of the regional
high concentration compartment therapy in vivo, as proposed on evaluation
of our PCT results (8). The clinical relevance of drug testing in RC is underli-
ned by our PDAT-response rate of 72 % in histologically different solid tumors.
Our PDAT results meanwhile have been confirmed by others who conducted
intrahepatic chemotherapy of colon-carcinoma-liver metastases with combinations of in vitro active drugs, inducing extremely high clinical remission rates
of 88 % [10]. In conclusion, RC should produce optimal results, if drugs were
not only applied at highest concentrations and optimal times [9] but also selected according to individual sensitivity.

References

1. Aigner KR, Patt YZ, Link KH, Kreidler J (1988) Regional cancer treatment. Karger, München
2. Hamburger AW, Salmon SE (1977) Primary bioassay of human tumor stem cells.
   Science 197 : 461-462
3. Hanauske AR, Hanauske U, Von Hoff DD (1986) The human tumor cloning assay
   in cancer research and therapy : a review with clinical correlations. Current problems in cancer 9 (12) : 1-66
4. Hyrniuk WM, Figueredo A, Goodyear M (1987) Applications of dose intensity to
   problems in chemotherapy of breast and colorectal cancer. Semin Oncol 14 : 3-11
5. Kern DH, Weisenthal LM (1990) Highly specific prediction of antineoplastic drug
   resistance with an in vitro assay using suprapharmacologic drug exposures. JNCI
   82 (7) : 582-588
6. Kreidler J, Link KH, Aigner KR (1988) Advances in regional cancer therapy. Karger, München
7. Link KH, Aigner KR, Kessler D (1988) In vitro chemosensitivity profiles of human
   malignancies for high-dose regional chemotherapy. Contr Oncol 29 : 28-42

8. Link KH, Aigner KR, Kuehn W, Schwemmle K, Kern DH (1986) Prospective correlative chemosensitivity testing in high-dose intra-arterial chemotherapy for liver
   metastases. Cancer Research 46 : 4837-4840
9. Link KH, Staib L, Beger HG (1989) Influence of exposure concentration and exposure time cxt on toxicity of cytostatic drugs to HT-29 human colorectal carcinoma
   cells. Reg Cancer Treat 2 : 189-197
10. Medenica S, Alonso K, Huschart T, Tyler K (1990) Tumor tissue culture for deter-
    mining efficient drug for intra-arterial, intrahepatic chemotherapy of colon carci-
    noma liver metastasis. J Cancer Res Clin Oncol 116 (Suppl) : 645
11. Odaimi M, Ajani J (1987) High-dose chemotherapy. Concepts and strategies. Am
    J Clin Oncol (CCT) 10 (2) : 123-132
12. Skipper HE (1990) Dose intensity versus total dose of chemotherapy : an experi-
    mental basis. In : De Vita VT, Hellmann S, Rosenberg StA (eds) Important advances
    in oncology 1990. JB Lippincott, Philadelphia, p 43

Abstract. *The validity of individual chemosensitivity testing in regional chemotherapy (RC) was confirmed using the « Human tumor colony assay »
(HTCA) in a prospective correlative (PCT) and decision aiding trial (PDAT).
In both trials, the HTCA- and clinical results were correlated. In the PCT,
the drugs for RC were chosen according to the standard protocols, while in
the PDAT drugs were individually selected for RC according to the HTCA-
results. In vitro sensitivity correlated correctly with clinical response in 100 %
in the PCT and 80 % in the PDAT, respectively. The HTCA is helpful in
selecting active drugs for RC based on individual chemosensitivity.*

Preoperative intra-arterial chemotherapy of advanced breast cancer. Response rate as prognostic factor for overall survival

RP de Dycker, J Timmermann, T Schumacher, RLA Neumann

The treatment of primary inflammatory mammary carcinomas has always been problematic. Inflammatory breast cancer disease represents about 1.7 % to 2.5 % of all mammary carcinomas [3, 4, 13, 14, 17].

Therapy involves irradiation and/or chemotherapy followed by surgical curing [3, 4, 10, 11, 13, 17]. The 5-year survival rate of only 15 % underlines the extremely bad prognosis of these carcinomas [15]. With the development of adjuvant cancer treatment there was a notable improvement of the global 5-year survival rate ranging from 28 % to 55 % [3, 10, 11, 13, 17]. First line radiotherapy and/or chemotherapy are usually indicated in these cases, with the aim of reducing tumor size and inflammation before surgery [4, 10].

The 2 rationales for preoperative chemotherapy are the effect of primary tumor removal on the growth kinetics of metastasis and the Goldie-Coldman hypothesis [6, 7]. Noncurative reduction of tumor results in an increase in the proliferation of residual tumor cells. Chemotherapy given prior to the operation prevents these kinetic events and suppresses tumor growth. The Goldie-Coldman hypothesis suggests an increase in the number of drug-resistant phenotypic variants in a growing cell population. Thus appropriate preoperative chemotherapy should not only destroy cells made more sensitive by their kinetic alteration, but also prevents cell proliferation and thus, prevent an increase in resistant cells.

Our objective was to identify a means of achieving operability more rapidly without additional discomfort to the patient [5, 8, 9].

Patients and methods

From May 1985 to May 1989, 45 patients suffering from primary inflammatory breast cancer were entered in this Phase II trial. All mammary carcinomas showed inflammatory features according to Haagensen's criteria (erythema, diffuse œdema, single or multiple tumors in the breast). Apart from pretherapeutic staging, a histological confirmation was obtained in all patients by means of incision biopsy. All 45 patients had T4 lesions and the axillary nodal status was clinically in all cases N1-2.

The age distribution shows clearly the tow peak values between 45-55 years and between 65-75 years of age. Twenty-one patients were premenopausal and 24 patients were postmenopausal (Fig. 1).

Dept of gynecologic oncology, Acad Marienhospital-Altenessen, University of Essen, Hospitalstr. 24, 4300 Essen 12, Germany

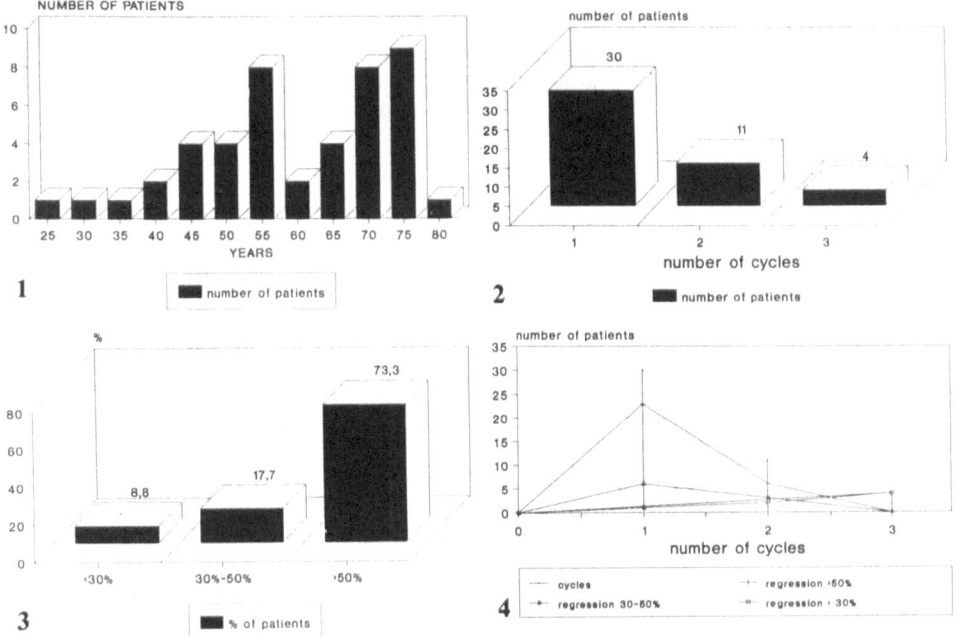

Fig. 1. Age distribution of all patients

Fig. 2. Number of cycles of intra-arterial chemotherapy

Fig. 3. Rate of regression

Fig. 4. Overall survival rate after 5 years

————— all patients N = 45
— — — premenopausal patients N = 21
— . — postmenopausal patients N = 24

The intra-arterial chemotherapy was performed supraselectively under digital subtraction angiographic guidance. Each cycle consisted of two treatments ; in the first, the intravascular catheter was inserted via the brachial or femoral a. into the lateral thoracic a., in the second, 11 days later into the internal mammary a. In each case, cytostatic agents were infused for 72 h. In the meantime, the patient was immobilized and received subcutaneous thrombosis prophylaxis of $3 \times 5,000$ IU heparin/day [5-9]. We administered 30 mg Mitoxantrone (Novantron, Lederle) through each artery at a rate of 10 mg per 24 h. A total of 60 mg/cycle mitoxantrone was applied. A new cycle was started after 4 weeks if necessary [6, 7]. The efficacy of the intra-arterial chemotherapy was evaluated by the disappearance of the inflammatory features according to Haagensen'criteria and by the regression of the tumor size evaluated by clinical and radiographic measurements. The operation was in all cases performed 4 weeks after the last infusion of mitoxantrone.

In all cases a high rate of necrosis and lymphocellular infiltration was found.

Postoperatively, all premenopausal patients were treated with 6 cycles of systemic chemotherapy (Cyclophosphamide, Methotrexate, 5-Fluorouracil) ; postmenopausal women received Tamoxifen 30 mg daily for a period of 2 years [6-9].

Results

After only 1 cycle, all 45 inflammatory mammary carcinomas responded to the intra-arterial chemotherapy with obvious regression of the tumor (Fig. 2). In 66 % of all tumors a radical mastectomy was possible after 4 weeks. All inflammatory mammary carcinomas lost the features defining them as such. Eight weeks later, 91 % of all tumors were operable. In all cases the margins of resection were histologically free of tumor or lymphangiosis carcinomatosa. During the preoperative check-up we noted objective reduction in tumor size. There was a regression of 50 % and more in almost 75 % of all cases. A complete remission with total disappearance of tumor involvement was not diagnosed. Only in 8.8 % we found a minor response of < 30 % (Fig. 3). After an observation period of 5 years 48 % of our group of patients is still alive with a median survival time of 39 months (Fig. 4).

If we examined the 2 treatment groups postoperatively, there was a clear difference between the pre- and postmenopausal women. The group of patients treated with Tamoxifen after the radical mastectomy showed a survival rate of 83 % and the median survival time had not been reached.

For the chemotherapy group the results are not as good ; a survival rate of 30 % with a median survival time of only 28.7 months. In our group of patients we found a time to progression (TTP) of 21.4 months and 25 % of all patients were totally disease-free after 5 years. The premenopausal patients treated with chemotherapy showed clearly the difference in prognostic features with a TTP of 18.2 months and only 7 % of the patients were disease-free after 5 years. In the tamoxifen group we found a median disease-free survival time of 30.4 months and after 5 years 49 % of the patients were without any symtoms of disease (Fig. 5). A very interesting correlation can be seen between the response to preoperative intra-arterial chemotherapy and the overall survival in each group of patients.

During the first treatment cycle we found a response rate of 77 % with a regression of more than 50 %. In the group of carcinomas treated with 2 cycles we found a response rate of 50 % and during the third treatment cycle the response rate was < 30% (Fig. 6). If we now examined the overall survival rate in those 3 groups of patients we found an interesting correlation : in the group of patients treated with one cycle 57 % were alive after 5 years and the median survival time had not been reached. In the group treated with 2 cycles the overall survival rate was 50 % and the median time was 28.9 months. In the group of patients treated with 3 cycles all patients deceased and the median survival time was only 9.03 months (Fig. 7).

After 5 years, all patients treated with more than 1 cycle of preoperative intra-arterial chemotherapy developed a progressive disease with a TTP of 21.4 months in the group with 2 cycles, and 9.03 months in the group with

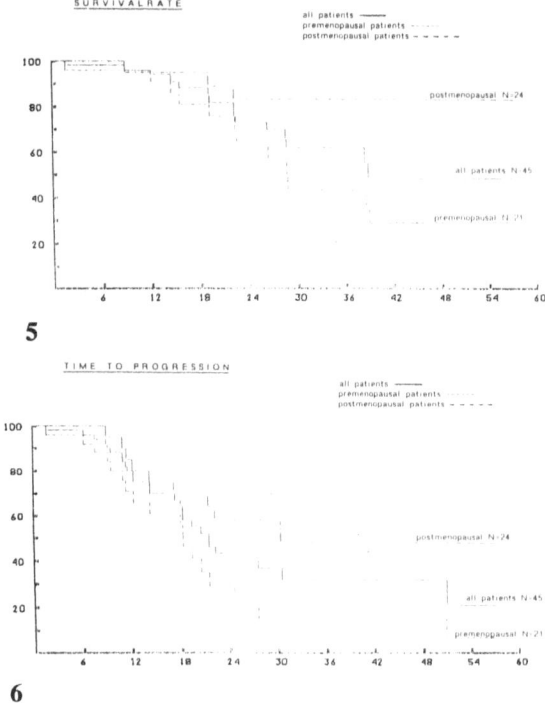

Fig. 5. Time to progression after 5 years

_____   all patients N = 45
— — —   premenopausal patients N = 21
— . —   postmenopausal patients N = 24

Fig. 6. Rate of regression after each cycle of chemotherapy

3 cycles. Only the patients treated with one cycle had a significant longer TTP
of 24.4 months and 33 % were alive without symptoms of disease (Fig. 8).

Discussion and conclusion

The diagnosis of « inflammatory mammary carcinoma » is based on clinical
features described by Haagensen as pathognomonic for this rare type of breast
tumor [3, 4, 13]. This carcinoma has a very poor prognosis : almost all those
affected die of distant metastases within 12-24 months [3, 14]. With the development of cytostatic cancer treatment there was a notable improvement of
the global 5-year survival rate ranging from 28 % to 55 % [3, 10, 11, 13, 15,
17]. Choosing a treatment regimen that enhances the patient's quality of life
is an important consideration for the patient's psychological well-being as well
as important medically. Since there are alternative treatments, it is important

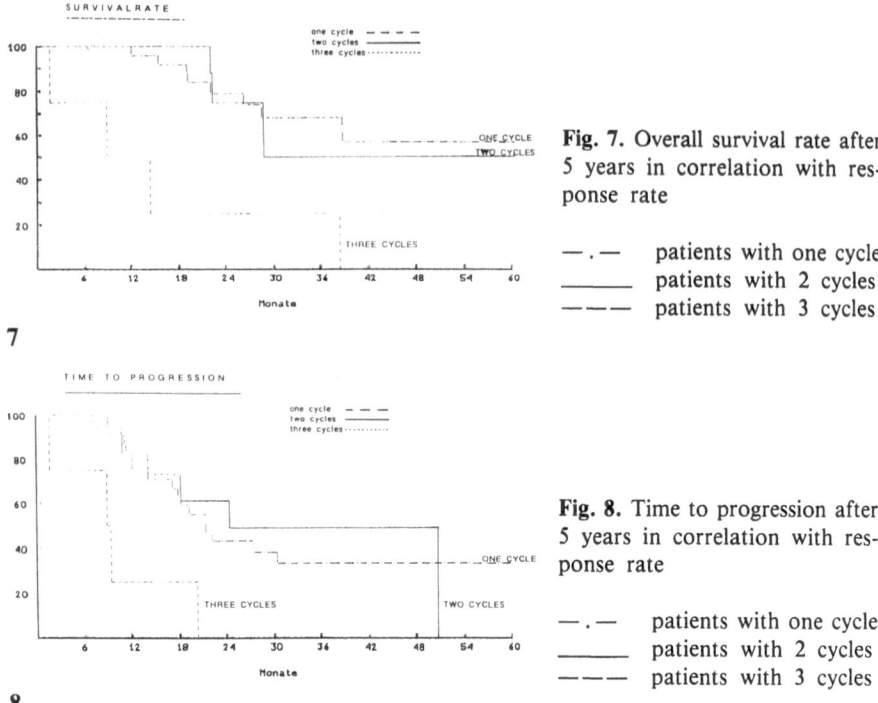

Fig. 7. Overall survival rate after 5 years in correlation with response rate

— . — patients with one cycle
——— patients with 2 cycles
— — — patients with 3 cycles

Fig. 8. Time to progression after 5 years in correlation with response rate

— . — patients with one cycle
——— patients with 2 cycles
— — — patients with 3 cycles

to select a treatment programme that the patient can accept. Otherwise compliance will be poor and even the antitumor benefits of the treatment will be compromised. In turn, quality of life will be reduced even further, because curbing or inhibiting the growth of the cancer is one of the most important ways of improving a patient's quality of life. In 1985, we looked for a new treatment modality in the management of primary locally advanced mammary carcinomas [5-9]. The benefit of the intra-arterial chemotherapy is shown by several parameters. Compared with the literature data [1, 2, 12, 14, 16] and considering the age of the patients (Fig.1), the interval between diagnosis and operation was very short (Fig. 2). The tumors were operable after 8 weeks in 91 % of all these cases. The regression of 50 % or more was noticed in almost 75 % of all cases (Fig. 3). We have observed the response rate from each treatment cycle and have noticed that after 2 cycles of intra-arterial chemotherapy no further response in regression of the tumor is to be expected from continuing this treatment modality (Fig. 4). The overall survival rate after 5 years of 83 % in the Tamoxifen group and 29 % in the chemotherapy group demonstrates the extreme difference between pre- and postmenopausal women (Fig. 5). The most appropriate assessment of palliative treatment namely the time to progression underlines this difference (Fig. 6). In the postmenopausal group we find the better prognostic features like more receptor positive tumors with a small growth fraction and a slow growth velocity. In inflammatory breast cancer the response to preoperative chemotherapy can be a new prognostic factor in the further treatment of those patients [11]. In our group of patients there is a good correlation between the response to intra-arterial chemotherapy and overall survival after 5 years (Fig. 7). All patients treated with more than 2 cycles of chemotherapy deceased and only the group of patients treated with one cycle showed a good survival rate of 57 % (Fig. 7). If we examine the time to progression curves, we do find the same correlation. After 5 years, all patients treated with more than one cycle of intra-arterial chemotherapy developed a progressive disease with a median TTP of 9.03 months for the patients with 3 cycles and a TTP of 21.4 months for the patients with 2 cycles of treatment (Fig. 8). In the group of patients with 1 cycle we observed a TTP of 24.4 months and 33 % were alive without symptoms of disease (Fig. 8).

On the basis of our results, intra-arterial regional chemotherapy of primary locally advanced breast cancer can be regarded as an alternative to preoperative systemic cytostasis with or without irradiation [1, 2, 7, 8, 14, 16]. Our 5-years survival rate and the time to progression indicate the efficacy of the intra-arterial chemotherapy. In inflammatory breast cancer the response to preoperative intra-arterial chemotherapy can be a possible prognostic factor in the further treatment of this special entity of mammary carcinomas.

References

1. Aigner KR, Walther H, Muller H et al (1988) Intra-arterial infusion chemotherapy for recurrent breast cancer via an implantable system. Reg Ca Treat 1 : 102-107
2. Carter RD, Faddis DM, Krementz ET et al (1988) Treatment of locally advanced breast cancer with regional intra-arterial chemotherapy. Reg Ca Treat 1 : 108-111
3. Chauvergne J, Durand M, Dilhuydy MH, Hoerni B, Germain T, Lagarde C (1981) Traitment des cancers du sein inflammatoires. Rev Fr Gynecol 76 : 227-235
4. Chu AM, Wood WC, Doucett JA (1980) Inflammatory breast carcinoma treated by radiotherapy. Cancer 45 : 2730-2737
5. De Dycker RP, Neumann RLA, Timmermann J (1988) Lokoregionale Chemotherapie beim fortgeschrittenen Mammacarcinom. In : Seeber S, Aigner KR, Enghofer E (ed) Die lokoregionale Tumortherapie. De Gruyter, Berlin, p 103-109
6. De Dycker RP, Neumann RLA, Timmermann J, Schindler AE (1988) Lokoregionale Chemotherapie beim fortgeschrittenen Mammacarcinom eine Alternative in der Primärtherapie. Tumor Diagn Ther 4 : 137-141
7. De Dycker RP, Neumann RLA, Timmermann J, Wever H, Schindler AE (1988) Arterielle regionale Chemotherapie fortgeschrittener Mammacarcinome. Dtsch Med Wochenschr 113 : 1229-1233
8. De Dycker RP, Timmermann J, Neumann RLA, Wever H, Schindler AE (1989) Arterial regional chemotherapy of advanced breast cancer. Journal of Chemotherapy (Vol. 1) 4 : 1193-1195
9. De Dycker RP, Timmermann J, Schumacher T (1990) Arterial regional chemotherapy of advanced breast cancer — 4-year survival rate. Recent Advances in Chemotherapy. Lewin-Epstein Ltd. 784.1-784.2
10. Hortobagyi GN, Ames FC, Buzdan AV et al (1988) Management of Stage III primary breast cancer with primary chemotherapy, surgery and radiation therapy. Cancer 62 : 2507 2516

11. Jacquillat C, Baillet F, Weil M et al (1988) Results of conservative treatment combining induction (neo-adjuvant) and consolidation chemotherapy, hormonotherapy, and external and interstitial irradiation in 98 patients with locally advanced breast cancer. Cancer 61 : 1977-1982

12. Koyama H, Wada T, Takahasi Y et al (1975) Intra-arterial infusion chemotherapy as a preoperative treatment of locally advanced breast cancer. Cancer 36 : 1603-1612

13. Kusche M, Scharl A, Reusch K, Bolte A (1987) Therapie und Prognose des inflammatorischen Mammakarzinoms. Tumor Diagn Ther 8 : 108-114

14. Noguchi S, Miyauchi K, Nishizawa Y et al (1988) Management of inflammatory carcinoma of the breast with combined modality therapy including intra-arterial chemotherapy as induction therapy. Cancer 61 : 1483-1491

15. Rubens RD, Armitage P, Winter PJ et al (1977) Prognosis in inoperable Stage III carcinoma of the breast. Europ J Cancer 13 : 805-811

16. Stephens FO (1989) Advanced breast cancer — intra-arterial induction chemotherapy. Reg Ca Treat 2 : 5-8

17. Zylbergerg B, Salat-Baroux J, Ravina JH, Dormont D, Arniel JP, Diepold P, Israel V (1982) Initial chemoimmunotherapy in inflammatory carcinoma of the breast. Cancer 49 : 1537-1543

Abstract. From May 1985 to May 1989, preoperative intra-arterial regional chemotherapy with mitoxantrone was administered to 45 patients suffering from primary inflammatory breast cancer. The aim of this phase II trial was to identify a means of achieving operability more rapidly without additional discomfort to the patient. The intra-arterial chemotherapy was performed supraselectively under digital subtraction angiographic guidance. After local operability was achieved, a radical modified mastectomy was done. All mammary carcinomas showed a good response 4 weeks after arterial chemotherapy. Eight weeks later 91 % of all tumors were operable. Mammography showed tumor regression of 50 % and more in almost 75 % of all carcinomas. After 5 years, the survival rate is 48 % with a median survival time of 39 months. The median disease-free survival time is 21.4 months for all patients and 21 % are alive without any symptoms of disease after 5 years. The response rate after preoperative intra-arterial chemotherapy shows a positive correlation with the applied number of cycles. Only the group of patients treated with one cycle of intra-arterial chemotherapy has an overall survival rate of 57 %, and 33 % are still alive without any progression. In the group of patients treated with 2 cycles, we have an overall survival rate of 50 % and all patients developed a progression. After 5 years, all patients treated with 3 cycles deceased with a median survival time of only 9.03 months.

High dose of rTNFα with interferon-g and melphalan in isolation perfusion (ILP) for in transit melanoma metastases and recurrent soft tissue sarcoma

D Liénard, F Lejeune, P Ewalenko

Experimental studies on human tumour xenografts have demonstrated that recombinant Tumour Necrosis Factor alpha (rTNFα) has a potent antitumour activity [1, 2]. In humans the antitumoral efficacy is hampered by severe systemic side effects and in these conditions a minority of clinical responses have been reported, especially in melanoma [3].

The number of rTNFα receptors increases when the cells, in culture or in human xenografts, are treated with interferon-g [4, 5]. In addition, a synergistic anti-proliferative activity of rTNFα and IFN-γ was demonstrated [6, 7]. An enhancement of the cytolytic activity of rTNFα by hyperthermia (40 °C) was shown in vivo and in vitro in experimental tumours [8, 9].

Cytotoxic activity of rTNFα in human xenografts is enhanced when alkylating agents are added [10, 11]. Melphalan is the most active agent on melanoma when used in ILP with hyperthermia [12].

For increasing the regional therapeutical efficiency of rTNFα and reducing the systemic side effects, we designed a protocol using ILP of the limbs with hyperthermia for regional in transit metastases of melanoma and recurrent soft tissue sarcoma.

Material and methods

Thirty-two patients entered the study and received a total of 35 ILP with the triple combination of rTNFα, IFN-g and melphalan. There were 25 females and 7 males, whose mean age was 61 years (range 18-83). There were 20 stage IIIa and 3 stage IIIab melanoma patients. Four patients had more than 100 in transit metastases and most of them had more than 5 tumour nodules. Thirteen of these patients had been previously treated by ILP with melphalan or rTNFα alone and had recurrences. There were 8 recurrent high grade soft tissue sarcomas including 3 MFH, 3 liposarcomas, 1 synoviosarcoma invading bone, 1 lymphangiosarcoma, and 1 spindle cell carcinoma.

One was treated by previous ILP with melphalan and Actinomycin D and the 8 patients were eligible for amputation. Twenty-eight ILP were performed through the iliac vessels, 4 through the femoral ones and 3 through axillary vessels. Priming of the membrane oxygenator consisted in Haemacel ®, heparin, bicarbonate and autologous fresh blood. The arterial blood temperature in the perfused limb was maintained at 40 °C during the whole perfusion.

rTNFRα (Genetech-Boehringer Ingelheim) was injected as a bolus in the arterial line, the total dose ranging between 2 and 4 mg — the last 25 patients received 4 mg —, under hyperthermic conditions (40 to 40.5 °C) for 90 minutes. rIFN-γ (Boehringer Ingelheim) was given s.c. on days -2 and -1 and in the perfusate, with rTNFα, at the dose of 0.2 mg. Melphalan (Alkeran ®, Well-come, England) was administered in the perfusate at doses giving a concen-tration of 40μg/ml.

rTNFα is a major mediator of septic shock and to avoid systemic side effects the patients included in this study received a prophylactic treatment con-sisting in a continuous infusion of 3 μg/kg/min of Dopamine and fluid chal-lenge starting before the injection of rTNFα and for at least 72 hours post-operatively.

Results

All the patients experienced fever and chills mainly 8 hours after the end of the perfusion. There were 16 cases with hematologic toxicity including neutro-penia (1 grade 4 and 1 grade 3) and thrombocytopenia (1 grade 4 and 3 grade 2) which were all reversible. There was no hepatic nor kidney toxicity. Only mild hypotension was observed in 4 patients and the regional toxicity attribu-ted to rTNFα was minimal in the 35 ILP. No direct toxic effect of rTNFα on the vessels has been observed.

In all cases, an early and spectactular softening of the tumours was seen within the 3 first days as the first sign of tumour response. Twenty-two out of the 23 patients are alive and a median follow-up time of 9.5 months has been obtained with a range of 1 to 31 months. One patient recurred in the perfused limb and died from disseminated melanoma 9 months after the ILP. Seven patients are alive but developed distant metastases in the liver, lungs, GI tract and skin but never recurred in the treated area. In the 23 melanoma patients there were 20 CR and 3 PR with no failure. Time to objective res-ponse was 14 days (10-20) for CR and 16 days (13-21) PR. Most of the CR occurred with bulky tumours. Complete remission was documented histologi-cally in 7 patients. Only one recurrence in the thigh of the perfused limb is observed after 8 months. Among the 8 patients suffering from recurrent soft tissue sarcoma, all of them are alive, 6 CR have been observed. Two patients treated recently are not fully evaluable. In the cases of sarcomas, tumoral hypervascularization disappeared within the first 10 days after the treatment and is correlated with complete histological response.

Conclusion

These preliminary results demonstrate a rapid and impressive response of mela-noma mestastases and sarcoma recurrences to high dose rTNFα when admi-nistered by ILP, either alone or in combination with IFN-θ and chemothe-rapy. This triple drug regimen appears to be a safe and attractive therapeutic approach in the treatment of regionally advanced melanoma and soft tissue sarcoma, especially in case of melphalan failure.

References

1. Balkwill F, Moodie E, Freedman V et al (1978) Human interferon inhibits the growth of established human breast tumors in the nude mouse. Int J Cancer 30 : 231-235
2. Balkwill F, Lee A, Aldom G et al (1986) Human tumor xenografts treated with human TNF alone or in combination with IF. Cancer Res 46 : 3990-3993
3. Retsas S, Leslie M, Bottomley D (1989) Intralesional tumor necrosis factor combined with interferon-gamma in metastatic melanoma. Brit Med J 298 : 1290-1291
4. Aggarwal BB, Eessalu TE, Hass PE (1985) Characterization of receptors for human tumor necrosis factor and their regulation by gamma-interferon. Nature 318 : 665-667
5. Ruggiero V, Tavernier J, Fiers W et al (1986) Induction of the synthesis of tumor necrosis factor receptors by interferon-gamma. J Immunol 136 : 2445-2450
6. Fiers W, Brouckaert P, Guizez Y et al (1986) Recombinant interferon gamma and its energism with tumor necrosis factor in the human and mouse systems. In : Schellekens H, Stewart WE (eds) The biology of the interferon system. Elsevier Science, Amsterdam, pp 241-248
7. Sohmura Y (1988) Antitumor effect of recombinant human tumor necrosis factor alpha and its augmentation in vitro and in vivo. In : Bonavida et al (eds) Tumor necrosis factor/cachetin and related cytokines. Karger, Basel, pp 189-195
8. Watanabe N, Niitsu Y, Umeno H et al (1988) Synergistic cytotoxic and antitumor effects of recombinant human tumor necrosis factor an hyperthermia. Cancer Res 48 : 650-653
9. Niitsu Y, Watanabe N, Umeno H et al (1988) Synergistic effects of recombinant human tumor necrosis factor and hyperthermia on in vitro cytotoxicity and artificial metastasis. Cancer Res 48 : 654-657
10. Mutch DG, Powell CB, Kao et al (1989) In vitro analysis of the anticancer potential of tumor necrosis factor in combination with cisplatin. Gynecol Oncol 34 : 328-333
11. Regenass U, Muller M, Curschellas E et al (1987) Anti-tumor effects of tumor necrosis factor in combination with chemotherapeutic agents. Int J Cancer 39 : 266-273
12. Krementz ET, Ryan RF, Carter RD et al (1985) Hyperthermic regional perfusion for melanoma of the limbs. In : Balch CM, Milton GW (eds) Cutaneous melanoma — Clinical management and treatment results worldwide. JB Lippincott, Philadelphia, pp 171-195

Testicular circulatory isolation prevents testicular exposure to doxorubicin in a rat model

H Arakawa, KJ Muller, WG Doubek, JA Stern, MC LaRegina, KC Tolman, CJ Coscia, FE Johnson

Steady progress in the treatment of cancer has increased the proportion of long-term survivors, and delayed treatment toxicity such as infertility is becoming an important consideration. Despite many reports documenting the adverse effects of cytotoxic drugs on fertility in men [1], a practical method to avoid this is not currently available. We are investigating a mechanical approach to this problem, which we have termed testicular circulatory isolation (TCI). This consists of temporarily interrupting the blood supply to the testis during drug administration. In the rat, testicular injury due to doxorubicin is reduced by TCI [1]. TCI can partially protect male rats from drug-induced infertility [2], and no long-term testicular injury results from TCI [3]. We now report an investigation of the mechanism of this protective effect.

Materials and methods

Fifty-six 8-week-old male Sprague-Dawley rats received TCI plus doxorubicin under pentobarbital anesthesia. Total arrest of blood flow in the left testicle was produced by application of a vascular clamp to the spermatic cord and a crushing clamp to the gubernaculum as described [1]. Immediately thereafter, doxorubicin was given as an IV bolus (6 mg/kg). Forty-five min after doxorubicin administration, both clamps were removed. The animals were killed by exposure to CO_S and necropsied. The time of necropsy varied from 30 min after doxorubicin administration (while the left testicular vasculature was still clamped) to 50 min after administration (5 min after clamp removal) and extended to 48 hours after clamp removal. The following organs were removed for analysis : both testes, serum, heart, liver, left kidney, and left lung. An additional 21 rats served as controls, and received an identical drug dose but no TCI. Although testicular cooling has been described as a method to increase tolerance of the testis to the ischemic injury imposed by TCI [2], no cooling was done in this work. Tissue and serum samples were assayed for doxorubicin by a modification [4] of the HPLC procedure described by Formelli et al [5].

Results

The results for testicular doxorubicin levels are depicted for both groups of rats in Tables 1 and 2. No anthracycline was detected in the left testicles of

Departments of Biochemistry/Molecular Biology, Surgery and Comparative Medicine, St. Louis University Medical Center, St. Louis, Missouri, 63110-0250, USA

Table 1. Doxorubicin levels (μg/g) in testes after IV administration of 6 mg of doxorubicin per kg BW in rats not receiving TCI

Tissue	Time after doxorubicin administration							
	30 min	50 min	75 min	4 h 45 min	12 h 45 min	24 h 45 min	48 h 45 min	
Right testis	0.55 ±0.02	0.57 ±0.01	0.63 ±0.08	0.64 ±0.12	0.74 ±0.14	0.53 ±0.04	0.61 ±0.04	
Left testis	0.63 ±0.05	0.63 ±0.08	0.59 ±0.08	0.57 ±0.10	0.53 ±0.06	0.63 ±0.10	0.61 ±0.06	

Concentrations of doxorubicin in testes of 3 rats were measured at each time point. At each time point, six separate determinations were done (duplicate assays on each of three animals). These are represented as mean ± standard deviation

Table 2. Doxorubicin levels (μg/g) in testes after IV administration of 6 mg of doxorubicin per kg BW in TCI-treated rats

Tissue	Time after doxorubicin administration						
	30 min	50 min	75 min	4 h 45 min	12 h 45 min	24 h 45 min	48 h 45 min
Right testis	0.66 ±0.10	0.61 ±0.05	0.50 ±0.06	0.56 ±0.09	0.52 ±0.04	0.59 ±0.06	0.40 ±0.04
Left testis	ND	ND	ND	ND	ND	ND	ND

Concentrations of doxorubicin in testes of 8 rats were measured at each point. At each time point, 16 separate determinations were done (duplicate assays on each of 8 animals). These are represented as mean ± standard deviation. ND, not detectable

TCI-treated rats. Drug levels in all other organs were closely comparable in the TCI group an the controls.

Discussion and conclusion

The rationale of TCI rests on an exploitation of the pharmacokinetic properties of doxorubicin, the well-defined vascular supply to the testicle, and our ability to safely interrupt it. This work, like others [6], indicates that doxorubicin levels reach a peak early after drug administration and rapidly decay. The pattern of drug levels in organs other than the left testicle in the TCI-treated group in reassuring since it suggests that TCI does not markedly affect exposure of other organs to doxorubicin. While this is not surprising, it will be important in designing human trials.

The main aim of the current work was to investigate the mechanism by which TCI exerts a beneficial effect on testicular histology and fertility in doxorubicin-treated animals. Since no anthracycline was discovered in TCI-treated testicles (while levels of Doxorubicin in the controlateral testicles were comparable to levels in controls), the mechanism of protection appears to relate to the vascular isolation, as expected. These data are almost certain to be specific for the species employed, the conditions of TCI, and the drug utilized. Similar work will need to be done before the value of TCI can be demonstrated for other known testicular toxins.

References

1. Lui RC, LaRegina MC, Herbold DR et al (1987) Regional doxorubicin delivery reduces testicular toxicity. J Surg Res 43 : 286-295
2. Liebscher GJ, Janney CG, LaRegina MC et al (1990) Preservation of fertility after doxorubicin administration. Surgical Forum 41 : 680-682
3. Stern JA, Lui RC, LaRegina MC et al (1990) Long-term outcome following testicular ischemia in the rat. J Androl 11 : 390-395
4. Van Lancker MA, Bellemans LA, DeLeenheer AP (1986) Quantitative determination of low concentrations of adriamycin in plasma and cell cultures, using a volatile extraction buffer. J Chromatogr 374 : 415-420
5. Formelli F, Carsana R, Pollini C (1987) Pharmacokinetics of 4'-deoxy-4'-iodo-doxorubicin in plasma and tissue of tumor-bearing mice compared with doxorubicin. Cancer Res 47 : 5401-5406
6. Calabresi P, Chabner BA (1990) Antineoplastic agents. In : Gilman AG, Rall TW, Nies AS, Taylor P (eds) The pharmacological basis of therapeutics. Pergamon Press, Elmsford, NY, pp 1241-1244

Abstract. Temporary testicular circulatory isolation (TCI), a regional drug delivery approach to avoid drug-related infertility, decreases Doxorubicin-induced testicular injury in the rat and provides partial protection from Doxorubicin-related infertility. We evaluated the distribution of Doxorubicin in rats trea-

ted with TCI and controls (treated identically but without TCI). Drug levels in all organs were comparable in the 2 groups, except that no Doxorubicin was detected at any time in the left testis of the TCI group. This work indicates that TCI completely protects the testis from Doxorubicin exposure in this model and does not affect distribution of Doxorubicin in other organs.

Early postoperative intraperitoneal Adriamycin. Pharmacologic studies and a preliminary clinical report

PH Sugarbaker*, TW Sweatman**, T Graves***, W Cunliffe****, M Isreal*****

Glen and coll established the frequency with which locoregional treatment failure occurs following complete surgical removal of the primary cancer in 43 retroperitoneal sarcomas. Two thirds of the patients who recurred had peritoneal sarcomatosis. This was the most common site for disease recurrence. The patients reported by Glen et al had maximal treatment with abdominal radiotherapy and maximal systemic chemotherapy. Aggressive systemic chemotherapy was not thought to improve survival in this prospective and randomized clinical trial [1].

The present pharmacological and clinical studies with early postoperative intraperitoneal Adriamycin had limited goals. They were to determine a dose and schedule of intraperitoneal Adriamycin that could be used in an attempt to prevent local (resection site) and regional (peritoneal surface) recurrence. Systemic treatment failures, in these authors' opinion, must be addressed by further studies with systemic chemotherapy. Optimal adjuvant chemotherapy will, most likely, represent combinations of regional and systemic treatments.

Results

Pharmacokinetics study of early postoperative vs. delayed intraperitoneal Adriamycin

Two complete pharmacokinetics studies were performed to compare the concentrations of intraperitoneal Adriamycin early postoperatively with an identical study in the same patient 8 weeks later. This experiment would determine the regional nature of intraperitoneal drug administration in patients with heavily traumatized peritoneal surfaces. Figure 1 presents Adriamycin concentration over time on the first postoperative day and at 8 weeks postoperatively. The dose of Adriamycin was 2.5 mg in 2 liters of fluid with peritoneal fluid sampled as indicated. In the early and delayed intraperitoneal instillations a prolonged exposure of peritoneal surfaces to drug was recorded. Nearly identical results were obtained in a second study.

* The Cancer Institute, Washington Hospital Center, Washington, DC ; **,***** Department of Pharmacology, College of Medicine and the Cancer Center, University of Tennessee, Memphis, TN ; *** Emory University Hospital Pharmacy, Atlanta, GA., USA. **** Consulting Surgeon, Queen Elizabeth Hospital, Gateshead, U.K

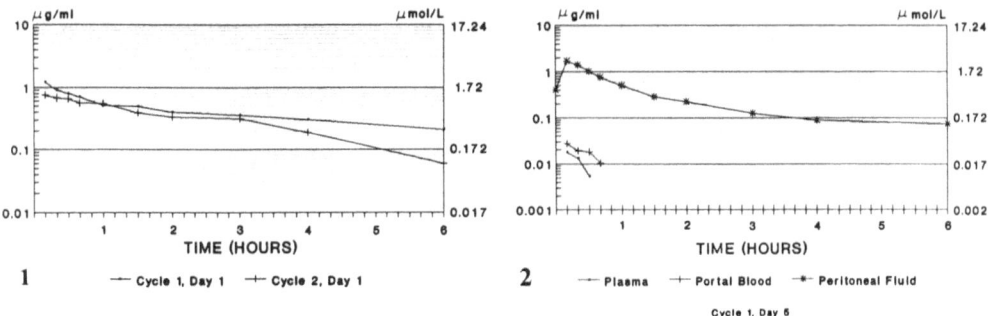

Fig. 1. Pharmacokinetics of early postoperative and delayed postoperative intraperitoneal Adriamycin. A dose of 2.5 mg in 2 l of fluid was instilled into the abdomen. Early treatments were on the first postoperative day. The delayed intraperitoneal Adriamycin was given in a similar fashion 2 months postoperatively

Fig. 2. Pharmacokinetics of intraperitoneal Adriamycin. Intraperitoneal, systemic plasma, and portal plasma Anthracycline following the instillation of Adriamycin (2.5 mg in 2 l)

Intraperitoneal, systemic plasma and portal plasma concentrations

On 2 patients, a portal venous catheter was positioned within this vessel at the level of the porta hepatitis. In the early postoperative period plasma, systemic plasma and peritoneal fluid were assayed for Adriamycin concentration. Figure 2 presents these data.

Discussion

The ratio of intraperitoneal versus systemic area under the curve from concentration-versus time curves showed a medial of 230 : 1 (range 48 : 1 to undetectable). It is clear that there is a marked treatment advantage within the abdominal cavity if Adriamycin is given through the intraperitoneal route. It should also be noted that increased portal blood levels of Adriamycin are present with intraperitoneal administration. Whether this increase in hepatic drug exposure represents a clinically important effect has yet to be determined. This elevation of portal chemotherapy after intraperitoneal instillation is seen with other drugs that show a « single pass effect » through the liver. The phenomenon has been studied by Speyer and colleagues with 5-FU [2].

Conclusion

Even limited effects of intraperitoneal chemotherapy may have profound quality of life benefits in patients with intra-abdominal sarcoma. Sarcomatosis is heretofore a deadly incurable pattern of disease recurrence associated with a long term morbidity. Chemotherapy that is instilled into the peritoneal cavity prior to the formation of scar tissue may be completely effective in preventing the diffuse implantation of malignant cells.

References

1. Glenn J, Kinsella TJ, Glatstein E, Tepper JE, Baker AR, Sugarbaker PH, Sindelar WF, Roth JA, Brennan MF, Costa J, Seipp CA, Wesley RA, Young RC, Rosenberg SA (1985) A randomized prospective trial of adjuvant chemotherapy in adults with soft tissue sarcomas of the head and neck, breast, and trunk. Cancer 55 : 1206-1214
2. Speyer JL, Sugarbaker PH, Collins JM, Dedrick RL, Klecker RW Jr, Meyers CE (1981) Portal levels and hepatic clearance of 5-Fluorouracil after intraperitoneal administration in humans. Cancer Research 41 : 1916-1922

Abstract. To date, no effective adjuvant therapies for retroperitoneal or visceral sarcoma have been reported. Following complete surgical excision of the intra-abdominal neoplasm, peritoneal sarcomatosis is the most common site for disease recurrence. These studies were designed to test intraperitoneal treatments with Adriamycin given early postoperatively in a large volume of dialysis fluid. The goal of this approach was to eradicate minimal residual disease present at the margins of surgical excision and to prevent the implantation of tumor cells disseminated by the trauma of surgery onto free peritoneal surfaces. The early postoperative period was selected so that chemotherapy was present in the abdomen before tumor cells were entrapped by adhesions and scar tissue. Pharmacological studies showed median area under the curve ratios of 230 : 1 for intraperitoneal verses intravenous exposure. Drug concentrations comparable to those maintained in vivo would produce complete destruction of sarcoma cells in vitro. Seventeen patients were treated without mortality. The major adverse side effect was pyrexia seen in 3 of 17 patients. One patient who received 2 cycles developed peritoneal sclerosis requiring prolonged parenteral feeding. Currently the treatment regimen employed is Adriamycin 0.1 mg/kg in 1 liter 1.5 % dextrose dialysis solution given on postoperative days 1 through 5. Our conclusion is that early postoperative intraperitoneal Adriamycin has the potential to develop into a useful surgical adjuvant treatment.

Surgical treatment of pseudomyxoma peritonei

PH Sugarbaker

The surgical treatment of cancer is dictated by the anatomic location of the tumor and its histologic grade of malignancy. In lesions of low-grade malignancy such as mucinous adenocarcinoma which may appear in the colon or appendix, resection including minimal margins (less than 1 mm) of healthy tissue has resulted in cure. Unfortunately, when the primary tumor extends through peritoneal cavity. The resulting clinical entry is commonly referred to as cystadenocarcinoma, malignant pseudomyxoma peritonei or mucinous peritoneal carcinomatosis. In the past, it was considered impossible to render patients, who had peritoneal carcinomatosis, clinically free of tumor.

Surgical technique for cytoreduction

With sufficient courage, knowledge of anatomy, patience and persistence, the surgeon can dissect all peritoneal surfaces within the abdomen free of tumor using ball-tipped electrocautery on pure cut at a high voltage. Dissection with the ball tip just beneath the tumor leaves visceral structures intact removing only the lesion and involved peritoneal surfaces. An important aspect of this technique is strong traction and countertraction between tumor and normal tissue. This will expose vascular and ductal structures and avoid damage to them as a dissection proceeds. Technique for immediate postoperative intraperitoneal lavage when the dissection is completed a Tenckhoff catheter is placed through the abdominal wall at a convenient location lateral to the rectus muscles and anchored at the peritoneal level by a purse string suture.

Postoperatively, the abdominal cavity is lavaged for 24 hours with a dialysis solution containing antibiotics. This will remove blood and tissue debris which may plug the catheter and will help prevent infection and the formation of adhesions.

Early postoperative intraperitoneal chemotherapy

Intraperitoneal chemotherapy has been used to combat the regrowth of cancer within the fibrous adhesions that form after cancer surgery. Optimally, the drugs should be instilled in a large volume of fluid to distend the abdomen and reach all exposed surfaces. The chemotherapy does not penetrate tumor masses of appreciable size but should destroy all small-volume disease. It is best utilized in the first 5 postoperative days when drug distribution to all intra-abdominal surfaces is complete.

The Cancer Institute, Washington Hospital Center, Washington D.C., USA

Delayed postoperative intraperitoneal chemotherapy

It is designed to augment the effects of the surgery and the early postoperative intraperitoneal chemotherapy. Drug distribution is less uniform after abdominal adhesions have formed and retroperitoneal fibrous reaction has occurred.

The current plan for early and late intraperitoneal chemotherapy for large bowel tumors is shown in Table 1.

Table 1. Early and delayed post-operative intraperitoneal chemotherapy for peritoneal carcinomatosis from large-bowel cancer

	Cycle			
Time	1	2*	3*	4*
Day of surgery Postop day 1	Abdominal lavage only			
	Mit C 10 mg/m² in 1 L 1.5% dextrose dialysate solution. Infuse as rapidly as possible; 23-hour dwell time. Maximum dose 20 mg. Drain abdomen completely before next instillation	5-FU 900 mg/m² plus 50 mmol sodium bicarbonate in 2 L 1.5% dextrose dialysate solution. Infuse as rapidly as possible; 24-hour dwell time and no drainage	Mit C 12 mg/m² in 2 L	5-FU 900 mg/m² plus 50 mmol sodium bicarbonate in 2 L
Postop day 2 to 5	5-FU 800 mg/m² plus 50 mmol sodium bicarbonate in 1 L 1.5% dextrose dialysate solution. Infuse as rapidly as possible; 23-hour dwell time. Maximum dose 1600 mg. Drain abdomen completely before next instillation	Same dose of 5-FU in 1 L solution. The soft tube used for peritoneal access is removed after instillation on day 5	5-FU 900 mg/m² plus 50 mmol sodium bicarbonate in 1 L	Same dose of 5-FU in 1 L
Postop day 6	Drain abdominal cavity as completely as possible and remove Tenckhoff catheter			

* Approximately 4 weeks separate cycles of intraperitoneal chemotherapy; drugs are instilled through a soft catheter positioned by paracentesis. Mit C = mitomycin C, 5-FU = 5-fluorouracil

Results

Patients who seemed to profit most over the long term had 3 clinical features in common. First, and most important, they did not have distant lymphatic or hematogenous spread of disease. Second, patients who were made clinically disease free by cytoreductive surgery seemed to be in a favorable group even though some required several staged surgical procedures to reach this status. Only patients who had intraperitoneal chemotherapy in addition to surgery remained well for long periods. Over 3/4 of the patients with peritoneal carcinomatosis from mucinous adenocarcinoma may be expected to have prolonged disease free survival. They represent the first report of cure after treatment for peritoneal carcinomatosis.

Abstract. Tumor spread onto peritoneal surfaces is frequent in patients who have recurrent gastrointestinal cancer. In this study the author describes (a) a cytoreductive surgical technique of ball-tipped electrocautery dissection which can rapidly and definitively remove large volumes of intra-abdominal tumor, (b) a procedure for immediate postoperative lavage of the abdominal cavity to remove blood and tissue debris, and (c) a regimen of early and delayed intraperitoneal chemotherapy to destroy small quantities of residual cancer cells on intra-abdominal surfaces. Seventy-seven patients underwent cytoreductive surgery to remove large volumes of adenocarcinoma widely disseminated through the abdomen. Patients had intraperitoneal chemotherapy to destroy small volumes of cancer remaining within the abdomen. Long term disease-free survival correlated with low tumor aggressiveness, adequate cytoreductive surgery and the use of intraperitoneal chemotherapy.

Rationale for integrating early postoperative intraperitoneal chemotherapy into the surgical treatment of gastrointestinal cancer

PH Sugarbaker*, WJ Cunliffe**, J Belliveau***, EA deBruijn****,
T Graves*****, RE Mullins******, P Schlag*******

Despite potentially curative surgical removal of gastrointestinal (GI) cancers, over 50 % of patients eventually die of their disease. The mechanisms behind GI cancer recurrence have not been convincingly described. The resection site and peritoneal surfaces are extremely common sites of GI cancer recurrence. It seems unlikely that disease spread to the tumor bed and to peritoneal surfaces occurs preoperatively. No cancer can be appreciated by direct visualization of these anatomic sites at the time of surgery. The most common locations for GI cancer recurrence, the resection site and peritoneal surfaces, are involved not by preoperative but by intraoperative and perioperative tumor dissemination.

Our goal in this report is to present a new concept regarding the mechanisms by which the spread of surgically treated GI cancer can be better understood. Also, we present a rationale for treating some (but perhaps not all) of the anatomic sites of surgical treatment failure using intraperitoneal (IP) chemotherapy in the early postoperative period. Our hypothesis suggests that adjuvant chemotherapy that exerts an effect on the surgical procedure can have a favorable impact on the survival of patients with GI cancer.

Tumor cell entrapment hypothesis

Surgical treatment failures at the resection site or on peritoneal surfaces may be caused by a different mechanism than cancer recurrence at other anatomic sites. Hematogenous or lymphatic and peritoneal-surface disease. A new hypothesis was created to explain the most prominent sites of GI cancer recurrence ; these are within the resection site and on peritoneal surfaces (Fig. 1). The tumor cell entrapment hypothesis suggests that spread of disease to these sites is related to implantation of cancer cells traumatically disseminated at the time of surgical removal of the primary tumor.

As the surgeon dissects close to the lateral margins of the specimen, tumor cells may be disrupted and spilled into the operative field. Probably more important, lymphatic channels that must be transsected leak tumor cells from their cut surface. It is naive to think that tumor emboli exist only within lymph

* The Washington Hospital Center, Washington, DC ; ** St. Mark's Hospital, London ; *** The Laboratory of Cancer Research and Clinical Oncology, University of Antwerp, Belgium ; ****, *****, ****** Providence College, Providence, Rhode Island ; ******* Chirurgische Klinik, Heidelberg, Germany

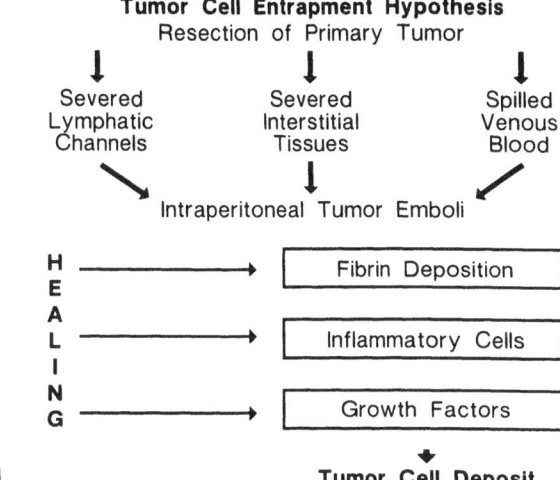

Fig. 1.

nodes. Free tumor cells are common place within lymph channels. With the surgical trauma of excising the primary tumor, release of tumor emboli from lymphatic channels and interstitial tissue spaces into the free peritoneal space is common, especially with advanced cancers. Also, venous blood allowed into the operative field will contain tumor cells. Cancer emboli are released into the peritoneal cavity and readily implanted on the raw tissue surface from which the primary tumor was removed. Also, scuffed peritoneal surfaces are a site on which free-floating tumor cells may stick. Both the resection site and abraded peritoneal surfaces become layered in the immediate postoperative period with fibrinous exudate. This fibrin layer implants the tumor cells and protects them from host defenses.

Early postoperative IP chemotherapy to control IP spread of tumor cells

Tumor cells traumatically dispersed into the peritoneal space by surgical dissection cannot be treated using conventional routines. Intraoperative saline irrigation will remove some spillage, but adequate irrigation of a body cavity with many crevices and an extensive surface area is not possible.

Intraoperative instillations of chemotherapy (mitomycin C may be the drug of choice) into the abdominal cavity at the time of surgery will reduce the quantity of spilled cells, but exposure time and drug distribution will be inadequate. Also, there are hazards to operating room personnel. The effect of a chemotherapeutic agent depends on drug concentration and time for drug contact with the malignant cells (area under the curve [AUC]). Exposure time is of necessity, greatly limited with intraoperative irrigation. Also, with this treatment only, some peritoneal surfaces will have little or no exposure. For example, the parietal peritoneum beneath the anterior abdominal wall cannot be adequately treated by intraoperative chemotherapy irrigations.

To optimally destroy free IP tumor cells we have used early postoperative IP chemotherapy (EPIC) treatments, which continue five to seven days postoperatively. During this time period there is no healing within the abdomen so drug distribution to all abdominal surfaces is expected. The chemotherapy is given in a large volume (usually 1 L) of fluid. This ensures wide drug distribution and provides sufficient dilution. The sclerotic effects of vesicant drugs such as Mitomycin C and Doxorubicin, are less prominent. These treatments are given through a large-bore Silastic catheter that penetrates the anterior abdominal wall. A Tenckhoff catheter is usually used but a closed suction drain is adequate.

Early postoperative IP 5-FU

Figure 2 shows the concentration versus time curves for early postoperative IP 5-FU. A remarkably similar concentration advantage for IP 5-FU is seen in patients with normal mesothelial-lined peritoneal surfaces. Approximately 100 times the AUC exists within peritoneal fluid as compared with the plasma. In our studies, escalating doses of 5-FU have been used in the early postoperative period. 5-FU 15 mg/kg was used as a once daily IP instillation for 5 consecutive postoperative days. At this dosage, prolonged ileus was observed in some patients undergoing extensive surgical procedures.

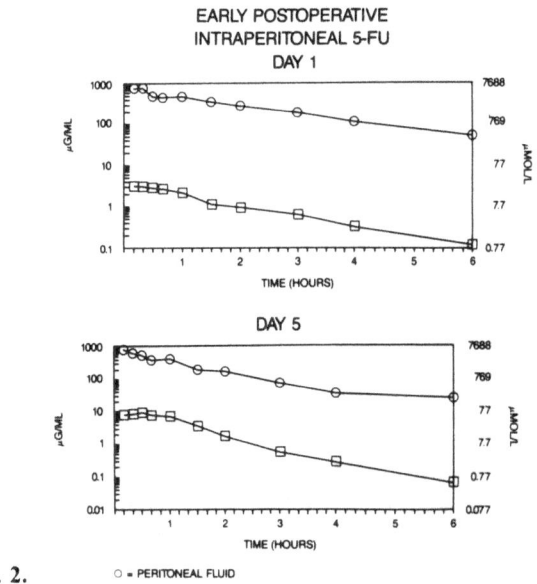

Fig. 2.

Fig. 2.

○ = PERITONEAL FLUID
□ = PLASMA

Abstract. A new concept in the natural history of gastrointestinal (GI) cancer suggests that recurrence of this malignancy can be separated into two types. Hematogenous and lymphatic metastases occur before surgical removal of the primary cancer. The spread of cancer to the resection site and to peritoneal surfaces occurs at the time of surgical removal of the primary tumor. Surgical trauma leads to a dispersal of malignant tumor emboli which then implant within the raw tissue surfaces of the resection site and abraded peritoneal surfaces. Instillation of chemotherapy directly into the peritoneal cavity, as part of GI surgery, provides cytotoxic levels of drug that may change the natural history of GI cancer. The most common sites of disease recurrence have been in the past at the resection site and on peritoneal surfaces. With the optimal use of intraperitoneal chemotherapy these sites of surgical treatment failure should now suggest that an effective dose and schedule have been achieved, that toxicity is at reasonable levels, and that responses with small volumes of intra-abdominal cancer are exceptionally high. Chemotherapy that has its impact by decreasing cancer spread to the resection site and to peritoneal surfaces may significantly improve survival and quality of life in patients with GI cancer.

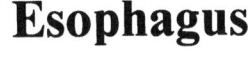

Esophagus

Neo-Adjuvant therapy for esophagus cancer : a coming of age

L Leichman

The experimental introduction of systemic chemotherapy into the initial therapeutic regimen of esophageal cancer had sound rationale. Clinical and autopsy series have demonstrated that even when local treatment with radiation or surgery has been effective most patients with esophageal cancer develop distant metastatic cancer [1]. This suggests that the metastatic process occurs early in the course of esophageal cancer. Over the past decade neo-adjuvant chemotherapy alone or with concomitant radiation has been investigated as a strategy to improve the outcome of patients with esophageal cancer. This approach imitated the effective neo-adjuvant therapy developed for tumors of the anal canal [2].

Clinically evident tumor remissions of short duration for patients with incurable or disseminated esophageal cancers may be achieved using standard chemotherapeutic agents. By combining these relatively active drugs to treat the primary tumor and disseminated disease while still occult, investigators have aimed at increasing the overall survival and cure rate for patients with localregional esophageal cancer. A series of clinical trials have treated patients with local-regional esophageal cancers with Cisplatin-based chemotherapy combinations. The results of these studies have established that approximately 50 percent of the primary tumors have a meaningful clinical responses to chemotherapy alone [3-5]. Approximately 10 percent of patients treated with combination chemotherapy have no cancer in the resected esophagus [6].

When radiation and chemotherapy are combined prior to surgery, symptoms of dysphagia almost always improve and esophagoscopy frequently reveals the absence of lesions within the esophageal mucosa [7]. When the modalities of radiation and chemotherapy are combined before surgery, the resected esophageal tissue is free of tumor in 18 percent to 30 percent of patients [8-10]. Current reports of trials using combined Cisplatin-5-FU or Mitomycin-5-FU, radiation and surgery indicate that 25 to 40 percent of the patients are alive without cancer at 2 and 3 years [11]. Tumors recurrence (as late as 4 to 6 years after cessation of treatment) in distant metastatic sites is still far more common than cure for most patients [12].

Earlem and Cunho-melo reviewed the results of thousands of patients treated for esophageal cancer with either radiation or surgery. The median survival at 2 years for patients treated with either of these local modalities was less than ten percent [13, 14]. Although the results of the combined modality treatments have apparently improved survival over that achieved with surgery or radiation alone, strong arguments have been made that patient selection may have biased these outcomes.

Two recently reported trials scientifically tested the premise that chemotherapy influences the survival of patients with local-regional esophageal cancer. The Eastern Cooperative Oncology Group prospectively randomized esophageal cancer patients across two arms : radiation (4,000 cGy) followed by surgery, and radiation (4,000 cGy) plus 5-FU infusion and Mitomycin-c followed by surgery. The median survival for patients with clinical stage II esophageal tumors treated with chemotherapy and radiation is 14.8 months versus 9.3 months for those treated with radiation alone (p = .02) [15]. A National Cancer Institute Intergroup Trial randomized patients with local-regional esophageal cancer to receive either radiation alone or Cisplatin-5-FU and radiation. Forty-two percent of those who received 5-FU and Cisplatin are alive (and without cancer) at two years whereas ten percent of those who received radiation alone are alive at two years (p = 0.0017) [16]. Treatment for cancer of the esophagus remains inadequate. But, these results indicate that the addition of systemic chemotherapy to local therapy prolongs survival for those with local-regional esophageal cancer.

References

1. Mandard AM, Chasle J, Marnay J et al (1981) Autopsy findings in 111 cases of esophageal cancer. Cancer 48 : 329-335
2. Leichman L, Nigro N, Vaitkevicius VK, Considine B, Buroker T, Bradley G, Seydel HG, Olchowski S, Cummings G, Leichman CG, Baker LH (1985) Cancer of the anal canal : a model for pre-operative adjuvant combined modality therapy. Am J Med 78 : 211-215
3. Kelsen DP, Bains MS, Hilaris B et al (1984) Chemotherapy of esophageal cancer. Sem Oncol 11 : 159-168
4. Carey R, Hilgenberg AD, Wilkens AW et al (1986) Preoperative chemotherapy followed by surgery with possible postoperative radiotherapy in squamous cell carcinoma of the esophagus : evaluation of the chemotherapy component. J Clin Oncol 4 : 697-701
5. Forastiere A, Gennis MK, Orringer M et al (1987) Cisplatin vinblastine and mitoguazone chemotherapy for epidermoid and adenocarcinoma of the esophagus. J Clin Oncol 5 : 1143-1149
6. Hilgenberg AD, Carey RW, Wilkens EW et al (1988) Preoperative chemotherapy, surgical resection and selective postoperative therapy for squamous cell carcinoma of the esophagus. Ann Thoracic Surg 45 : 357-363
7. Franklin R, Steiger Z, Vaishanplayan G et al (1983) Combined modality therapy for esophageal squamous cell carcinoma. Cancer 51 : 1062-1071
8. Leichman L, Steiger Z, Seydel HG et al (1984) Combined preoperative chemotherapy and radiation therapy for cancer of the esophagus : the Wayne State University, Southwest Oncology Group and the Radiation Therapy Oncology Group Experience. Sem Oncol 11 : 178-185
9. Poplin E, Fleming T, Leichman L et al (1987) Combined therapies of squamous cell carcinoma of the esophagus : a Southwest Oncology Group Study (SWOG 8037). J Clin Oncol 5 : 622-628
10. Seydel HG, Leichman L, Byhardt R et al (1988) Preoperative radiation and chemotherapy for localized squamous cell carcinoma of the esophagus : an RTOG study. Int J Rad Oncol Biol Phys 14 : 33-35
11. Forastiere AA, Orringer MB, Perez-Tamayo C et al (1990) Concurrent chemotherapy and radiation therapy followed by transhiatal esophagectomy for local-regional cancer of the esophagus. J Clin Oncol 8 : 119-127

12. Leichman L, Herskovic A, Leichman CG, et al (1987) Non-operative therapy for squamous cell cancer of the esophagus. J Clin Oncol 5 : 356-360
13. Earlem R and Cunha-melo JR (1980) Oesophageal squamous cell carcinoma I : a critical review of surgery. British J Surg 67 : 381-390
14. Earlem R, Cunha-melo JR (1980) Oesophageal squamous cell carcinoma II : critical review of radiotherapy. British J Surg 67 : 457-461
15. Sischy B, Ryan L, Haller D et al (1990) Interim report of EST 1282 phase II protocol for the evaluation of combined modalities in the treatment of patients with carcinoma of the esophagus, stage I & II (abstr). Proc Am Soc Clin Oncol 9 : 105
16. Herskovic A, Martz K, Al Sarraf M et al (Submitted for publication) Results of the intergroup randomized trial of combine modality treatment versus radiation alone for esophageal cancer

Symptomatic improvement and esophagoscopic response after Neo-Adjuvant chemotherapy with Cisplatin, Vindesine and Bleomycin in patients with esophageal cancer (EC)

JJ Illarramendi, A Guerra, M Aizcorbe, F Arias, MA Dominguez, E Martinez, JJ Valerdi

Long-term survival is short in patients with EC, and neo-adjuvant chemotherapy (N-CT) programs have been developed with the aim of improving long-term control of this neoplasm [1]. Besides this potentially curative approach, the early use of chemotherapy in these patients allows a better assessment of the N-CT impact on dysphagia and endoscopic tumor features in patients without previous therapy.

Material and methods

Forty-three patients (41 male, 2 female) with previously untreated EC. Median age : 62 years (35-79). All the group had a pathologic diagnosis of epidermoid carcinoma. Location : upper third 12/43, middle third 25/43, lower third 6/43. Clinical stage (AJCC) : I 1/43, II 14/43, III 28/43. Staging procedures included endoscopy and esophagogram in all the patients, and thoracoabdominal CT scan in 33/43.

Therapeutic schedule comprised two cycles of Cisplatin, Vindesine and Bleomycin [2], followed by megavoltage radiation therapy (60 Gy/6w). Endoscopy was repeated after completion of the two N-CT cycles, and following the end of radiotherapy.

Response criteria (endoscopy) was as follows : a) complete response (CR) status needed a total disappearance of the previous tumor image plus a negative biopsy and cytology. b) partial response (PR) is defined as an « inequivocal » improvement or total dissapearance of endoscopic image, with positive biopsy and/or cytology.

Symptomatic improvement was measured through the use of a four grade dysphagia scale (passage-score PASS), with the following described grades : 3 able to use solide food, 2 semisolid food, 1 liquid food, 0 no possible passage at all.

Results

After N-CT the endoscopic response rate was 49.9 % in 30 evaluable patients (16.6 % CR, 33.3 % PR). Symptomatic improvement was found in 68 % of the patients. Response rates improved after completion of the treatment (55.2 %

Hematology, Oncology and Surgery. Hospital Virgen del Camino. Servs. of Radiation Oncology and Gastroenterology. Hospital de Navarra. Navarre Health Service-Osasunbidea, Pamplona, Spain

CR, 26.3 % PR). Only 7/22 patients are alive after more than 20 months follow up. Local relapse rates in these patients (22 %) scores similar to systemic failure (27 %). Three years overall survival was 17 %. Toxicity was moderate, but 4/43 patients experienced life-threatening sepsis, with 2 neutropenic deaths. Radiotherapy delay was only needed in 9/43 patients previously treated with N-CT.

Discussion and conclusion

Our patient population displayed a rate of endoscopic responses comparable to other radiologically evaluated series treated with N-CT [3]. CRs were found in a significant percentage of our group. Symptomatic improvement rates are even higher, probably reflecting the palliative impact of minor responses. These results are comparable to published studies on symptom improvement after therapy with standard radiotherapy [4]. In fact, a recent randomized study has disclosed similar response rates after radiotherapy or chemotherapy in EC [5].

CRs were common after completion of the N-CT plus radiation program. These results are comparable to other series that use concomitant chemotherapy and radiotherapy [6], and seem largely better than radiation alone. Nevertheless, long term survival and local control score less than in series with surgically proved responses. We conclude that esophagoscopy is not an appropiate predictor of durable local control and survival.

The long-term results of chemotherapy in EC are doubtful. Short and mainly outpatient programs of chemotherapy are able to display a significant palliative effect in locally advanced esophageal cancer.

References

1. Kelsen DP (1989) Neo-adjuvant therapy of esophageal cancer. Can J Surg 32 : 410-414
2. Kelsen DP, Bains M, Chapman R, Golbey R (1981) Cisplatin, vindesine and bleomycin combination for esophageal carcinoma. Cancer Treat Rep 65 : 781-785
3. Kelsen DP, Hilaris B, Coonley C, et al (1986) Cisplatin, vindesine, and bleomycin chemotherapy of local-regional and advanced esophageal carcinoma. Am J Med 75 : 645-652
4. Caspers RJL, Welvaart K, Verkes RJ et al (1988) The effect of radiotherapy on dysphagia and survival in patients with esophageal cancer. Radiother Oncol 12 : 15-23
5. Forastiere AA, Orringer MB, Perez-Tamayo C, et al (1990) Concurrent chemotherapy and radiation therapy followed by transhiatal esophagectomy for local-regional cancer of the esophagus. J Clin Oncol 8 : 119-127
6. Kelsen DP, Minsky B, Smith M, et al (1990) Preoperative therapy for esophageal cancer : a randomized comparison of chemotherapy versus radiation therapy. J Clin Oncol 8 : 1352-1361

Non surgical multimodality treatment of squamous cell cancer of the esophagus

T Zenone, R Lambert, P Romestaing, JP Gerard

Combined modality treatment for inoperable or unresected cancer of the eso-phagus can be used in a curative approach with encouraging results [1, 2, 4, 5]. In this perspective, this paper describe our experience in Lyon with eso-phagus cancer using a radical non surgical treatment.

Materials and methods

Between April 1982 and June 1989, 65 patients (63M/2F, mean age 64 years, WHO performance status 0-1 50, 2-3 15) with biopsy-proven squamous cell carcinoma of the esophagus were treated in a curative intent with multimoda-lity combined treatment (laser or photodynamic therapy, chemotherapy, radiotherapy + /- brachytherapy). Staging was done according to the criteria of TNM-classification UICC 1987 (15 T1, 13 T2, 32 T3, 5 T4 and 34 N0, 8 N1, 23 Nx). The mean tumor size was 4.6 cm. The site distribution was : cervi-cal 2, upper thoracic 17, mid 39, lower 7.

Chemotherapy was administered as follows [3] :
— 5-Fluorouracil 1,000 mg/m^2/d as continuous infusion on days 1-4 ;
— Cisplatin as bolus 80-100 mg/m^2 day 2 or 25 mg/m^2/d on days 2-5.

The standard treatment was to give a first course of chemotherapy during the work up period especially if a laser therapy was used (first part of treat-ment : chemotherapy + /- laser). NdYAG laser was used for rapid improvement of dysphagia and in order to reduce tumor volume before radiation therapy. Photodynamic therapy (hematoporphyrin derivative laser treatment) has been used in 5 cases of early superficial esophageal cancer.

Two courses of concomitant chemotherapy were given during the radiation therapy (second part of treatment). In fact, only 55 patients received conco-mitant radiation-chemotherapy. In 10 cases, chemotherapy was administered only before radiotherapy because of poor general conditions. Irradiation was initiated 4 weeks after induction chemotherapy and concomitant chemotherapy was started usually at the first day of radiotherapy during the first week of treatment. The second course of chemotherapy was given on week 4 or during the second cycle if a split course radiation therapy schedule was used. In case of side effect, the second course of chemotherapy has been given in a few cases with half dose or omitted.

As far as the radiation therapy parameters are concerned, a dose of 50 Gy in 5 weeks was given with a four fields technique (18 MV X rays) ; then a

Service de radiothérapie, Centre Hospitalier Lyon Sud, 69310 Pierre Bénite ; Service d'hépato-gastro-entérologie, Hopital Edouard Herriot, 5 place d'Arsonval, 69003 Lyon, France

dose of 10 to 20 Gy was added with a rotational Cobalt technique. Median total dose was 64 Gy. In 18 cases, a split course schedule has been used. Brachytherapy (Low Dose Rate with Iridium-192) was used in 5 cases as a booster dose (18-20 Gy at the mucosal surface of esophagus) following external irradiation.

Results

By August the first 1990, 45 patients were dead (25 of malignant disease, 2 of secondary malignancy, 7 of associated chronic disease but NED for esophageal cancer and 11 of unknown causes). Nineteen patients are alive and well (mean survival 44 months, range 15-94). Only, one patient was lost to follow-up.

Probability of survival according to Kaplan-Meier method was 79.6 % at 1 year, 40.5 % at 2 years, 36.7 % at 3 years and 26.7 % at 5 years. The median survival was 18 months. The 5 years survival rate was 56.3 % for T1, 29.8 % for T2, 12.9 % for T3. All T4 died within 16 months and all N1 within 17 months.

After first part of treatment (chemotherapy + /- laser), objective response superior to 50 % (CR + PR) was observed in 70 %. An improvement of dysphagia was observed in 80 %. At the end of the treatment, complete initial disease response was achieved in 76 %.

Treatment tolerance was good. Four patients developed neutropenia less than 1 Giga/l (degree 4). One patient had severe myelodepression with fever and systemic candidiasis. Three patients developed angina pectoris with 5-Fluorouracil and one polyneuritis after two courses of CDDP. Seven patients had severe radiation esophagitis with dehydratation and weight loss requiring hospitalisation for symptomatic treatment. Four patients had cutaneous reaction especially after photodynamic therapy (photosensitization). Four patients developed bronchial or tracheal esophageal fistula but it was probably related to progression of their persistent malignancy and not a consequence of the therapy. Six patients required dilatations later to maintain their nutritional status.

Among 6 patients with a survival of more than 5 years, 4 of them have developed a second cancer (3 head and neck, 1 cardia).

Conclusion

Our results demonstrate that patients with squamous cell carcinoma of the esophagus can have a long term survival and may be cured with combined modality treatment without surgery. When patient's general condition is medically inadequate to tolerate an esophagectomy, this treatment is safe and has low morbidity. Twenty six % 5 year survival in this large serie (65 patients) and with a long follow up can be considered as a very encouraging result. The multimodality treatment with induction chemotherapy can be proposed in a curative intent and may be as an alternative to radical surgery at least when there is some risk of operative mortality.

References

1. Coia LR, Engstrom PF, Paul A (1987) Non surgical management of esophageal cancer : report of a study of combined radiotherapy and chemotherapy. J Clin Oncol 5 : 1783-1790
2. Herskovic A, Leichman L, Lattin P et al (1988) Chemo/radiation with and without surgery in the thoracic esophagus : the Wayne State Experience. Int J Rad Oncol Biol Phys 15 : 655-662
3. Kies MS, Rosen ST, Tsang TK et al (1987) Cisplatin and 5-Fluorouracil in the primary management of squamous esophageal cancer. Cancer 60 : 2156-2160
4. Leichman L, Herskovic A, Leichman CG et al (1987) Non operative therapy for squamous cell cancer of the esophagus. J Clin Oncol 5 : 365-370
5. Richmond J, Seydel HG, Bae Y et al (1986) Comparison of three treatment strategies for esophageal cancer within a single institution. Int J Rad Oncol Biol Phys 12 : 118 Abstract

Role of pathologic response after primary chemoradiotherapy and esophagectomy for predicted T3-4 N0-1 M0 squamous carcinoma of the thoracic esophagus

M Valente, M Alloisio, P Bidoli, U Pastorino, A Santoro,
L Tavecchio, S Spinazze, G Muscolino, R Zucali, G Ravasi

A large number of pilot studies [1-4] have investigated primary chemoradiotherapy and esophagectomy in esophageal cancer both for resectable and unresectable tumours.

The regimens used are based on the use of infusional 5-FU combined with mitomycin or cisplatin.

These studies clearly show that concomitant chemoradiotherapy is feasible without any difference between mitomycin or cisplatin regimens, but conflicting conclusions regard the impact on survival, the role of esophagectomy after chemoradiotherapy and the prognostic factors are reported.

The survival of partial responders after esophagectomy is the most conflicting point, as no survival after partial response, reported in the oldest studies [1, 2] is a compelling argument for excluding surgery and treating patients with combined modality therapy consisting solely of chemotherapy plus radiotherapy.

Studies on higher dose of radiotherapy and chemotherapy without surgery showed unsatisfactory local control except for T1 tumours (X-rays staging) [5-7] but unfortunately the majority of patients present with more advanced disease.

The accuracy of pretreatment staging of esophageal cancer is low either for TNM classification and for resectability, but CT or MR imaging providing information about wall penetration and nodal status, overcomes X-rays imaging regard resectability.

Except for tumour located in the cervical esophagus and in the gastroesophageal junction, CT is able to separate patients in two different group respectively with high and low probability of complete resection [8, 9].

In 1985 we start a prospective study on primary concurrent chemoradiotherapy and esophagectomy for esophageal cancer and in this paper we report the data regarding the role of pathologic response in patients with CT predicted T3T4 squamous carcinoma of thoracic esophagus.

Methods

Starting with May, 15th of 1985, patients with predicted T3-4 N0-1 MO squamous carcinoma of the thoracic esophagus and adequate renal and hematological functions have been treated by primary chemoradiotherapy followed, whenever possible, by esophagectomy or higher dose of radiochemiotherapy according to the reclassification of tumour extent and the risk of the resection.

Istituto Nazionale per lo Studio e la Cura per dei Tumori, Milan, Italy

Preoperative evaluation of the tumour extent was performed by barium swallow, endoscopy and computed tomography or magnetic resonance imaging of thorax and upper abdomen and lymphnodes sized > 1 cm were considered positive.

Two cycles of 5-FU 1,000 mg/sqm for 4 days infusion and CDDP 100 mg/sqm, the first day every 29 days, synchronous with radiotherapy (30 Gy days 1 to 19) were given.

After 29 days from the beginning of the second cycle, according to clinical tumour response and medical operability, esophagectomy or supplementary dose of chemoradiotherapy, therapy was given.

Esophagectomy by transthoracic approach for upper and mid-located tumours and by transhyatal approach for lower located tumours was scheduled.

Two to three cycles of 5-FU 1,000 mg/m^2 in 4 days infusion and CDDP 100 mg/m^2, day 1 every 29 days, synchronous with radiotherapy (20 Gy days 1 to 12) was scheduled as supplementary dose of chemoradiotherapy.

Results

Up to November the 6th of 1990, 52 consecutive patients with predicted T3-4 N0 or N1 underwent primary induction radiochemiotherapy followed whenever possible by standard esophagectomy or higher dose of chemoradiotherapy.

Compliance rate of planned treatment was (38/52), 32 patients underwent esophagectomy (22 % operative mortality and 72 % complete resection rate) and 6 patients higher dose of radiochemiotherapy.

Responders were considered 18 (56 %) patients, 8 (25 %) without tumour in the esophageal wall (complete response) and 10 (31 %) without tumour in the esophageal mucosa (partial response) and non responders 14 (44 %) patients with evidence of the tumour in all the layers of the esophageal wall.

Complete resection rate was 89 % in the responders and 43 % in the non responders but the percentage of pathologic nodal diffusion was the same in the two groups (31 % VS 35 %).

After a median follow-up of 40 months, the median survival time (MTS) of the 52 patients was 10 months and 27 % three years survival rate ; without survival for patients who do not underwent esophagectomy.

Regarding the prognostic factors valuable before treatment, tumours location in the upper esophagus showed a significant negative correlation with survival (Table 1) whereas predicted cN1 and predicted cT4 showed non significant lower survival.

For patients who underwent esophagectomy, MST of non responders was 10 months and not reached for responders without any difference between partial and complete responders (Table 1).

For patients who underwent complete resection MST was not reached and there was no difference between responders and non responders.

Table 1. Survival

	N	Median	36 Mo
T3-T4	52	10 mo	27%
Upper	25	8 mo	12%
Lower-Mid	27	15 mo	42%
Partial Response	10	NR	51%
Complete Response	8	NR	58%
No Response	14	10 mo	21%
Complete Resection	23	NR	51%
Incomplete Resection	9	10 mo	10%
CR + RT only	6	12 mo	0%

NR, median not reached

Conclusion

The data regarding the pathologic response indicates that chemoradiotherapy can be more effective for small tumours located only in the mucosa rather than for large tumours or with nodal diffusion.

For predicted T3T4 tumours the expected complete response rate is low and there is little difference in survival between partial and complete response as reported by recent studies [3, 4], and this is a compelling argument to include esophagectomy after induction chemoradiotherapy for esophageal cancer.

References

1. Steiger Z, Franklin R, Wilson RF et al (1981) Eradication and palliation of squamous cell carcinoma of the esophagus with chemotcrapy, radiotcrapy and surgical therapy. J Thorac Cardiovasc Surg 82 : 713-719
2. Poplin E, Fleming T, Leichman L et al (1987) Combined therapies for squamous cell carcinoma of the esophagus, a Southwestern oncology group study (SWOG 8037). J Clin Oncol 5 : 622
3. Forastiere AA, Orringer MB, Perez-Tamayio C, Urba SG, Husted S, Takasugi BJ and Zahurak M (1990) Concurrent chemotherapy and radiation therapy followed by transhiatal esophagectomy for local-regional cancer of the esophagus. J Clin Oncol 5 : 1783-1790
4. Lackey VL, Reagan MT, Smith A and W Anderson (1989) Neo-adjuvant therapy of squamous cell carcinoma of the esophagus : role of resection and benefit of partial responders. Ann Thorc Surg 48 : 218-21
5. Leichman L, Steiger Z, Seydel HG, et al (1984) Preoperative chemotherapy and radiation therapy for patients with cancer of the esophagus a potentially curative approach. J Clin Oncol 2 : 75
6. Leichman L, Herskovic A, Leichman CG (1987) Non operative therapy for squamous cell cancer of the esophagus. J Clin Oncol 5 : 365
7. Coia LR, Engstrom PF, A Paul (1988) Non Surgical management of esophageal cancer. J Clin Oncol 5 : 1783-90

8. Skinner DB, Ferguson MK, Soriano A, Little A and Staszak VM (1986) Selection of operation for esophageal cancer based on staging. Ann Surg 204 : 391-401
9. Halvorsen RA and Thompson WM (1989) CT of Esophageal Neoplasms. Radiologic Clinics of North America 27 : 667-85

Abstract. Fifty-two consecutive patients with predicted T3-4 NO N1 MO squamous carcinoma of the thoracic esophagus and adequate renal and hematological functions underwent induction chemotherapy (5-FU 1,000 mg/sqm 24 hours infusion, days 1 to 4 and CDDP 100 mg/sqm, day 1 (2 courses)), 30 Gy, days 1 to 19, followed, whenever possible, by esophagectomy or radiochemiotherapy. Compliance rate of planned treatment was 73 %, 32 patients underwent esophagectomy and 6 higher dose of radiochemiotherapy. At pathologic evaluation 25 % complete response (CR), 31 % partial response (tumour clearance in the esophageal wall) were observed. At a median follow-up of 40 months, the median survival time (MST) was 10 months for all patients, 20 months for esophagectomy and 12 months for radiochemiotherapy completion and not reached for patients who underwent complete resection. For patients who underwent esophagectomy, MST of non responders was 10 months and not reached for responders without any difference between partial and total responders. For patients who underwent complete resection MST was not reached and there was no difference between responders and non responders. This data confirm a potentially curative role of surgery in partial responders after induction chemoradiotherapy for predicted T3T4 squamous carcinoma of thoracic esophagus.

Gynecology

Neo-Adjuvant chemotherapy in cervical cancer stage IIB ; PEC + RT vs RT. Preliminary results

J Cardenas, A Olguin, F Figueroa, F Becerra, J Pesa, R Huizar

In Mexico, Latin America, and in general in the third world countries, cervical cancer constitutes a real health problem. One out of five malignant tumors in general is a cervical cancer, and almost one out of three women tumors are of this kind. On the other hand, due to the lack of health education, generally associated to the people with less economical resources, the number of patients who are at advanced stages at the moment of diagnosis is too high. In the General Occident Hospital where people of few resources are mainly assisted, the 23 % of the 384 cases were disgnosed in the stage II, the 10 % in the III stage, and the 5 % in stage IV.

The progress on patients in the advanced stages has been very poor. Since many decades ago the radiotherapy has proportioned a consistent, but limited, curative range. It is known that the recovering opportunities particularly in stage II cases, are of about 50 %, which means that a high number of women in productive age, and most of the time with large families, will die for this reason. That is why we believe that it is necessary to investigate new methods to improve the healing perspectives of this kind of tumors in advanced stages, while we cannot reach a complete coverage of the early detection methods.

As a general idea, it is accepted that the actual chemotherapy could offer very few perspectives to the recurrent patient after radiotherapy. All drugs individually and many combination schemes, have been used, but only a 20 % of objective response has been obtained, rarely complete, and with a 4 to 6 months median duration. The drugs' little effectiveness has been related with a poor drug diffusion, in the previously radiated zones, in a low marrow and renal reserve, and a poor general state after the primary treatment.

The neo-adjuvant or initial therapy before the radiated treatment has just begun being used a few years ago. The first trials demonstrated that the cervical epidermoid cancer, was much more sensible to chemotherapy than it was thought. Objective responses above the 50 % or 60 % were observed with schemes such as MOB-P (Mitomycin C (M), Vincristin (O), Bleomycin (B), and Platinum (P)), and others, obtaining very important tumor reductions, that were after followed by conventional treatment. However, even when results were very promising, it could not be demonstrated that this treatment meant an increase of the free progression time and the overall survival.

Based on pilot studies made in Mexico and in other countries, it was decided to start a prospective randomized trial, to investigate the neo-adjuvant chemotherapy impact in a group of patients with porgression risk or known recurrence.

Chimalpopoca, 314 Guadalajara Jalisco, Mexico

Material and methods

Since 1987, in the « Hospital General de Occidente » and in the « Centro Medico de Occidente » in Guadalajara, Mexico, a comparative prospective randomized trial was begun, comparing neo-adjuvant chemotherapy + conventional radiotherapy vs. radiotherapy alone. The inclusion criteria were as follows : patients with cervical epidermoid cancer histologically proven stage II B ; within normal limits of haematologic, renal and liver functions ; younger than 65 ; without any previous treatment ; PS 0-1 ; socially and geographically controllable for follow-up. The IIB stage classification was made according to the FIGO (Obstetrics and Gynaecology International Federation), corroborated by at least 2 oncologists. Later on extension assays were made, thorax X-rays, and excretory urography, also rectosigmoidoscopy and cytoscopy to reject possible invasion of rectum or bladder. All these assays should have been negative or normal, in order to accept the patient for the trial.

Patients were allocated into two groups. The first group consisted of induction chemotherapy with the PEC scheme for 4 cycles according to the following dosage : P = Platinum 50 mg/m^2, E = Epirubicin 75 mg/m^2, C = Cyclophosphamide 500 mg/m^2.

Cycles were repeated every 3 weeks, with previous assays of haematic biometry, platelets, urea, creatinine, hepatic function tests. On the twelfth day of each cycle a biometry, platelet acccount, urea, and creatinine were recorded.

Previously to each treatment all patients were assessed for response, by two doctors of the Oncology Service. By the end of the fourth cycle, patients began receiving external radiotherapy, based on Cobalt 60, 5,000 cGy and later on intracavitary 3,320 cGy. The other group was treated with normal radiotherapy, according to conventional doses, and in exactly equal fields than the ones in the group of induction chemotherapy. These doses and fields are the same as those used as a standard in our radiotherapy department.

Results

Up to now 28 patients have been included, from which 4 are not evaluable, 2 because they did not receive complete treatment ; one loss at the beginning of the trial, and one more still in treatment.

CT + RT group

Eleven patients are evaluable for response to the induction CT, obtaining the following results :

CR, 1 (9 %) ; PR, 7 (64 %) ; C, 1 (9 %) ; PD, 2 (18 %) ; CR + PR 8/11 (73 %).

After the RT, 7/10 (70 %) reached CR, and others one PR. PEC toxicity after 42 CT cycles is summarized in the following chart according to the WHO.

Table 1. Survival

	Grade 1-2	Grade 3
N & V	100%	0%
Alopecia	39%	61%
Diarrhoea	11%	0%
Anorexia	91%	0%
Anaemia	27%	0%
Leucopenia	7%	0%
Leucopenia (nadir)	62%	14%
Plaquetopenia	0%	0%
Renal	8%	0%

RT alone group

Fourteen patients in the RT alone arm, are evaluable. Thirteen reached CR (93 %) and other one PR.

Nowadays, with a media follow-up of 19 months (2-34), 6 out of 10 patients treated with the combined scheme, and 8 of 14 patients with RT alone, are free of tumor.

Discussion and conclusion

Neo-adjuvant CT is being used more frequently in different kinds of tumors. In the case of cervical carcinoma, preliminary trials show that this tumor, traditionally considered little sensible to antineoplasic drugs, can really respond when they are used early. Objective responses above 50 or 60 % have been reported, when using combined schemes that generally include platinum. Nevertheless, the true impact of this kind of treatment has not been adequately evaluated. Well designed, controlled studies, that compare the conventional RT versus induction CT previous to the conventional treatment are necessary.

This trial pretends to evaluate in a homogeneous group of patients, the importance of the PEC scheme as neo-adjuvant therapy. At the present time, with the few number of entered patients in both groups, it is not possible to conclude yet that the addition of the induction CT, with 4 cycles of PEC, means any advantage for patients with cervical cancer stage IIB. Even though, we believe that the inclusion of a major group of patients will help us to elucidate if neo-adjuvant CT could have any future for this kind of tumors.

References

1. De Vita V (1984) Cancer. Principios y practica de oncologia. Salvat, p 760
2. Edmonson JH (1986) Comparison of bleomycin, cyclophosphamide and cisplatin (BCAP) vs bleomycin and cisplatin (BP) in advanced cervical carcinoma. Proceedings of ASCO, abstract C-474

3. Young J (1986) Combination cisplatin and mitomycin-C in patients with advanced or recurrent cervical cancer. Proceedings of ASCO, abstract C-471

4. Kavanagh J (1986) Fluorouracil, doxorubicin and cisplatin (FAP) for the treatment of recurrent or metastatic adenocarcinomas of cervix. Proceedings of ASCO, abstract C-445

5. Baker L (1985) Combination chemotherapy for patients with disseminated carcinoma of the uterine cervix. Proceedings of ASCO, abstract C-465

6. Hakes T (1984) Adjuvant chemotherapy for poor risk stage Ib-IIa cervix carcinoma patients. A pilot study with cisplatin-bleomycin. Proceedings of ASCO, abstract C-669

7. Thomas GA (1984) A phase II study of mitomycin-C, fluorouracil and radiation therapy (rt) in poor prognosis carcinoma of cervix. Proceedings of ASCO, abstract C-648

8. Bauer K (1984) Cis-DDP, bleomicyn, MTX-LCV chemotherapy in advanced previously untreated carcinoma of cervix. Proceedings of ASCO, abstract C-659

9. Jobson V (1984) Cisplatin chemotherapy (CT) followed by radiotherapy (RT) in patients with advanced cervical carcinoma. Proceedings of ASCO, abstract C-665

10. De la Garza J (1987) Cisplatin (P), Epirubicin (E) and Cyclophosphamide (C) + radiotherapy (RT) in stage IIb-IIIb cervix carcinoma. Proceedings of ASCO, abstract C-441

11. Tattersall M (1986) Epirubicin in cervical carcinoma

Abstract. Twenty-eight patients with Cervical Epidermoid Cancer Stage IIB, were randomized to receive whether 4 cycles of Neo-Adjuvant Chemotherapy (CT) of PEC (platinum 50 mg/m² (P), Epirubicin 75 mg/m² (E) and Cyclophosphamide 500 mg/m² (C)) + conventional radiotherapy (RT) vs. radiotherapy alone. At present 24 patients are evaluable. The results for the induction CT were : CR 1/11, PR 7/11, CR + PR 73 % (8/11). After RT 7/10 reached the CR and 1/10 PR. In the group of RT alone, 13 out of 14 patients reached CR (93 %). Nowadays, with a follow-up median of 19 months (2-34), 6/10 treated with CT (60 %), and 8/14 treated with RT alone (57 %) are free of tumor. The CT has been well tolerated, excepting alopecia, no other toxicity was observed grade 3-4. Until now, with this number of patients, it is not possible to demonstrate any advantage with the adding of the neo-adjuvant chemotherapy based on PEC.

Follow-up of treated gynecologic cancer : CT and MRI contribution

D Buthiau*, D Khayat**, D Nizri***, J Chantelard***, M Weil**, JP Lefranc****, Cl Jacquillat**

We present the result of a study on the interest of CT and MRI for the following of gynecologic cancer after treatment, compared with clinical, surgical and histological data.

Materials and methods

One hundred and forty-two women underwent pelvic MRI between january 1984 and september 1990. The patients were aged 21-74 years (mean age : 48 years). The MR imaging findings were correlated with the findings at physical pelvic examination and at surgery and biopsy. For these women with previous pelvic malignancy, histologic proof of the MRI findings was achieved with laparotomy (82 patients) or transvaginal biopsy (60 patients). MRI imaging observations were correlated with those of axial CT in 87 % of cases.

Imaging was performed on CGR CE 12,000, Elscint 2,400 for CT scanner and 1.5 T Signa General Electric, 1 T Siemens, 0.5 T Philips and General Electric for MR imaging. Section thickness in most images was 8 or 10 mm for CT and 5 mm with 2.5 mm intervals for MRI. CT scans with contrast media were always attempted as well as spin-echo pulse sequences for MRI.

Seventeen breast neoplasms were studied by MRI with and without DOTA Gadolinium (paramagnetic contrast media).

Results

Radiation-induced uterine changes

— On CT, there is a decrease in uterine size, 3 months after therapy ended and a thin endo-uterine lumen.
— On MRI, we noted a decrease in thickness and signal intensity of the endometrium on T2, 6 months after therapy, a decrease in signal intensity of the myometrium on T2 early after therapy, loss of uterine zonal anatomy (low intensity band) after 3 months. Post-irradiation changes increase significantly with the dose. The post-irradiation MR changes appear similar to those usually seen on non irradiated post-menopausal uterus.

* Centre RMX, Paris XVᵉ ; ** Service d'Oncologie Médicale, Hopital de la Salpétrière ; *** Service de Radiothérapie, Hopital de la Salpétrière ; **** Service de Gynécologie, Hopital de la Salpétrière, 47 boulevard de l'Hopital, 75013 Paris, France

After surgery

— On CT, the surgical zone appears normaly symetrical, with variable local pelvic fat inflation and thickening of pelvic fascias.
— On MRI, the surgical zone is normaly dark, with low signal intensity on T2, and with same other changes than CT.

CT and MRI evaluation of therapeutic response after pelvic malignancies treatments

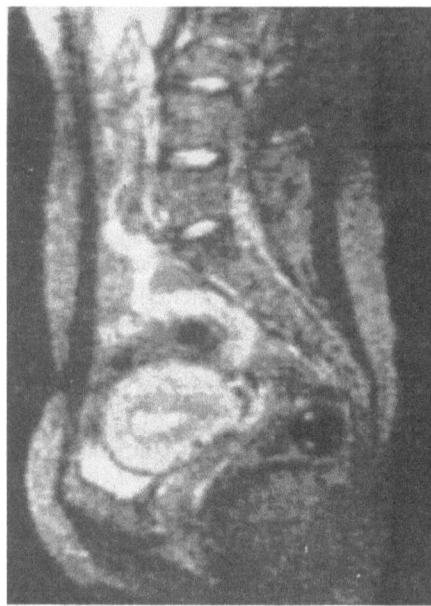

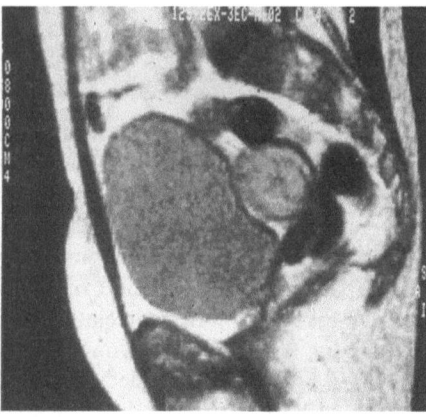

2

1

Fig. 1. Normal uterus on MRI (T2) : note the normal endometrium, with high signal, the myometrium with intermediate to high signal, and the zonal anatomy with hyposignal band (within the myometrium)

Fig. 2. Normal cervix on MRI (T2) with dark signal intensity due to high connective tissue content

— After radiotherapic treatment, CT can evaluate the local responses, particularly the decrease in tumor size ;
— MRI can demonstrate the decrease or loss of abnormal high signal intensity of tumor on T2 and evaluate the local spread ;
— These techniques can appreciate the local response and help future treatments.

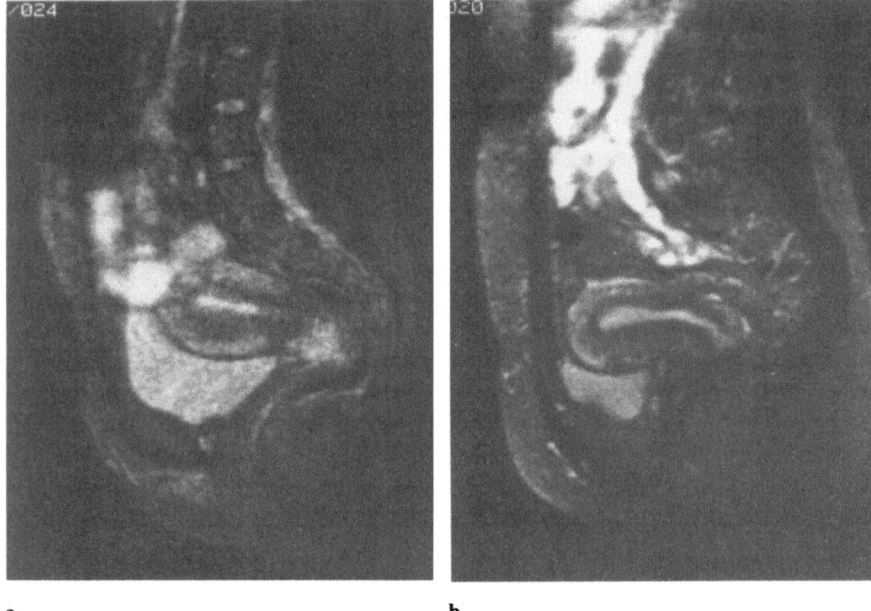

a   b

Fig. 3 a, b. Cervical carcinoma on MRI (sagittal plane, T2) : following of post-irradiation and chemotherapic response : 3 months after therapy, there is a decrease of tumor size and signal *a* and a recovering of normal aspect of cervix, *b* MRI can evaluate the persistance of this aspect with time.

Tumor recurrence versus fibrosis

— This characterisation is not well allowed by CT, because both densities are similar, even after contrast media injection. The only way that can help this differenciation is to compare with previous CT exam and appreciate the local evolution. This is to remain the great interest to realise initial CT scan, 4 to 6 months after any therapy, representing a referency cartography.

— On MRI, post-therapeutic early fibrosis (1-6 months after first treatment) has a low intensity on T1 and high on T2. After one year, the fibrosis has low local signal intensity on T1 and T2. MR imaging demonstrated in 88 % of cases the recurrent tumor as an aera of increased signal intensity on T2. MRI can help to differenciate tumor recurrence versus fibrosis not on T1, but on the contrary on heavy T2, only after 6 months and better one year after first treatment. There is no specificity before 6 months.

— When tumor recurrence is more evident, CT and MRI can demonstrate centropelvic mass, parametrial or parietal spread, bladder of rectum changes, extensive venous thrombosis, important and asymetric hydronephrosis...

— Such a difference on signal intensity between recurrence and fibrosis can be observed on residual lymph nodes, with quite high sensitivity (87 %), but without specificity (inflammatory lymph nodes can appear with high intensity on T2).

Problem of ovarian carcinoma recurrence

Both CT and MRI are limited in this indication, by their difficulties to detect peritoneal implants.

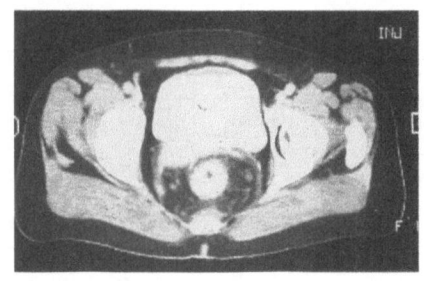
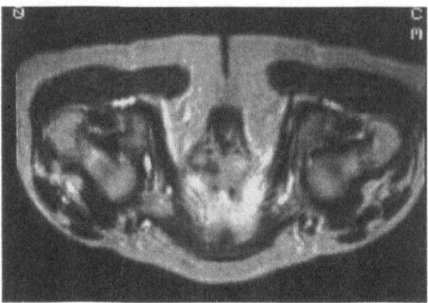

4

5

Fig. 4. Local tumor recurrence on CT, after injection : non symmetrical aspect of the right part of surgical area, with tissular densities

Fig. 5. Vaginal recurrence on MRI (axial plane, T2) : there is a high signal intensity at the basis of centro-pelvic area, correlated, at surgery, with tumor recurrence (22 months after any treatment ended)

Problem of breast cancer recurrence

MR can show significant enhancement on recurrent carcinoma tissue, after Gadolinium injection, with good histological correlation (sensitivity : 92 %).

Nevertheless, such enhancement are encoutered in others breast diseases such as fibroadenomas, proliferative dysplasia, inflammatory disease... When limitations of this technique were considered, MRI can be sometimes beneficial as a supplement in selected difficult cases.

Conclusion

We tried, with this study, to remind of the interest of MRI for the differentiation tumor recurrence versus fibrosis, for the evaluation of chemo- and radiotherapic treatment ; also to remind of the interest of CT for the general spread evaluation, the preradiotherapic dosimetry and for the following after therapy (except for breast disease), providing that a reference CT examen has been done 4 to 6 months after any treatment.

References

1. Arrivé L, Chang YCF, Hricak H et al (1989) Radiation-induced uterine change. MR imaging. Radiology 170 : 55-58
2. Buthiau D, Dargent D, Nizri D et al (1991) TDM et IRM en gynécologie. In : Buthiau D (ed) TDM et IRM cliniques. Frison Roche, Paris (in press)
3. Ebner FE, Kressel HY, Mintz MC et al (1988) Tumor recurrence versus fibrosis in the female pelvis : differentiation with MR imaging at 1.5 T. Radiology 166 : 333-340

Intra-arterial chemotherapy in uterine cancer

P Manivit, R Polo, M Nabet, M Polo, B Rubini, JM Fromaget

We performed intra-arterial chemotherapy in few cases of uterine cancer :
— as a salvage procedure in recurrences after primary treatment ;
— as a complementary procedure after partial surgery ;
— as a neo-adjuvant chemotherapy in bulky tumors before radiobrachy-therapy and surgery.
The method, the material, the follow-up and the discussion are presented.
The number of patients is not sufficient to come to a conclusion, but the fast decrease of tumor volumes and sterilization — from the pathological point of view — are obvious in some of theses observations, and finally the decrease of the tumor volume is constant.
The help of this method, in conjunction with others therapies is to be discussed.

Methods

A catheter is put in each internal iliac artery by Seldinger way. Serum, drugs and heparin are pushed by two arterial infusion pumps (IVAC 531), one on each side ; the sequence is extended during 48 hours. I.V continuous infusion, antiemetics, diuresis control, diet without residuum.

Drugs

Dose per day via I.A route :
— squamous epithelioma of the cervix : MTC 6 to 8 mg/m^2 ; BLM 25 mg/m^2 ; 5-FU 1,000 mg/m^2 with I.V CVF ; CDDP 30 to 50 mg/m^2. Systemic VCR 1 mg/m^2 or VDS 2 to 4 mg/m^2 are sometimes associated.
— adenocarcinoma : the same schedule, or ADR instead of MTC.
— uterine sarcoma : the same schedule without 5-FU.
Number of cycles : 2 to 4.
Interval : 4 to 5 weeks according to clinical and haematological status.

Material

Only 11 patients. Age 28 to 67 : 3 kinds of indications :
1) Four, as recurrences after a primary complete treatment (brachy with or without external radiotherapy and surgery) : 2 cervix (T2b and T2a) and

Hopital Claude Bernard, 57070 Metz, France

2 corpus (T2). Delay of relapse after the initial treatment : 9 to 23 months, a laparotomy and biopsy asserted the pathological malignancy, but the surgeon could not excise the recurrence. 2 to 3 I.A chemo courses were performed.

2) Two after partial surgery, age 44 and 49 ; one leiomyosarcoma, one T2a cervix cancer and bladder — vaginal fistula ; 2 to 4 I.A chemo before iterated laparotomy, excision or biopsies.

3) Four patients had locally advanced tumors : I.A chemotherapy performed as neo-adjuvant method ; age 33 to 64 ; T2 en barillet, T2b, T3b, T3c : 2 to 3 I.A cycles before external irradiation, brachytherapy 3 times and surgery (Wertheim) ; the fifth patient PS 3 had a contra-indication to surgery because of heart and pulmonary insufficiency : 4 I.A sequences, then 10 Gy external radiotherapy and she died.

Follow-up and results

1) Four recurrences after primary treatment : I.A chemo gave PR or CR clinical response and then, all but one are pathologically NED at the microscopic examination of the excised tumor :

2 cervix : 1 local and iliac *lymph node* evolution at 8 months, death at 11, 1 relapse at 49 months as a small mass in the bladder wall : cyctectomy, DFS at 66 months.

2 corpus : 1 iliac and lumbar *lymph node* evolution at 12 months, death at 19, 1 NED at 22 months.

2) Two partial surgery : after I.A chemotherapy, laparotomy and microscopically examination : NED :

1 sarcoma : at 22 months bronchial unique metastase = left inferior lobectomy ; DFS at 60 months.

1 cervix : at 47 months inguinal then lombo aortic *lymph node* and death at 52 months.

3) Five neo-adjuvant I.A chemotherapy had all a good clinical response (2 CR 2 PR and the T3b have a good mobilization from the pelvic wall) after I.A chemotherapy.

After surgery, 4 were NED at pathological examination ; 1 T3c dead at 16 months after local and *lymph node* relapse at 8. Three others are DFS at 35, 60 and 78 months.

The last one T2b with cardiopulmonary insufficiency had 4 I.A chemo courses, 10 Gy external RX well tolerated and she died : at autopsy, uterus and parameters were NED and one iliac lymph node was positive.

Discussion

1) I.A CT alone is able to obtain pathological sterilization of cancer masses : 3 to 4 cases of recurrences, 1 neo-adjuvant I.A chemo and 10 Gy. But it is not an isolated, for itself procedure.

2) I.A chemo appears to be faster and more effective than the systemic route.

3) Before radiotherapy and surgery, I.A chemotherapy needs an intact arterial bed and gives a higher drug concentration than the IV route.

3) Before radiotherapy and surgery, I.A chemotherapy needs an intact arterial bed and gives a higher drug concentration than the IV route.

4) The decrease of tumor mass was constant and sometimes impressive ; this decrease of volume gives a good geometry before brachytherapy.

5) I.A chemotherapy appears to be feasible.

6) Side effects :

— twice, sciatica after one cycle, one had complete regression, one with some sequellae ;

— 1 peripheral neuropathy ;

— 1 thrombosis of the external iliac artery with moderate discomfort.

7) To be discussed :

— number of I.A sequences ;

— other associated drugs ;

— going I.V chemotherapy after surgical treatment.

8) Nevertheless I.A chemotherapy is limited :

— time limited, 2 to 4 cycles ;

— locally limited to the pelvis : 5 of our 11 observations had lymph node evolution.

9) This recording is in the same way as some actual recommandations to perform iliac and lomboaortic surgical curage in stages IIb and III.

10) Four indications can be discussed :

— salvage therapy (alone or preceding brachytherapy) in cases of pelvic recurrence after treatment run normally, when iterative radiotherapy is discussed and at risk because of small intensive complications and skeletal necrosis.

— After partial surgery as overall cleaning method, before radiotherapy and/or iterative surgery.

— As a neo-adjuvant chemotherapy in locally advanced stage III, bulky cervix en barillet stage II, and in stage IIb, to bring out :

• a considerable reducing of tumor burden ;

• a mobilization from the pelvic wall in stage IIIb.

— Occasionally as an antalgic procedure, as observed in 2 of our observations.

Conclusion

We have not enough observations to talk about results. We only can say that :

— the method is feasible ;

— it contributes to a fast decrease of tumor masses ;

— it has been able to sterilize some lesions ;

— it may be used as a salvage therapy after complete use of the classical methods ;

— other experiments and trials are necessary to know if I.A chemotherapy before radiotherapy and surgery had better results than the two usual methods, in locally advanced uterine tumors.

Concomitant chemotherapy and radiotherapy in the treatment of advanced cervix carcinomas

M Resbeut, M Noirclerc, G Houvenaeghel, P Viens

Although early stage cervix carcinoma can be controlled successfully by radiotherapy alone or surgery and radiotherapy with high 5 years survival rate, more than 90 % in stage (St) IB and than 80 % in St IIA [6, 7, 10], the influence of the tumor volume is well documented and advanced lesions carry a bad prognosis. The break seems to appear with St IIB. Most of the studies show a similar actuarial 5 years survival rate in St IIb : [1, 9] 60 % up to 70 % but bulky diseases St IIB have a substiantially worse 5 years survival rate : less than 50 % [1, 14]. In St IIIB, these rates range from 25 % to 50 % with markedly worse results when disease is fixed to both pelvic side walls [2, 4, 14]. Long-term survivors are less than 20 % in St IV [8, 15]. Lymph node involvement implies a poor prognosis specially, in some series [1, 5] if there are 3 or more positive nodes. This paper analyses 22 patients with such advanced cervix carcinomas treated with concomitant chemotherapy and radiotherapy (CCR). The aim of this study is to examine the frequency of local control and side-effects of treatment.

Patients and methods

Between April 1989 and June 1990, 7 patients with bulky (> 6 cm) St IIB and 8 with St IVA carcinoma of the cervix were treated with CCR as a first treatment (group A). Seven patients with more than 3 positive nodes (or capsular effraction) on a previous lymphadenectomy underwent CCR after surgery (group B). All patients were under 60 years old. Staging was checked by examination under anaesthetic with an intracavitary ultrasonography. CCR was a radiotherapy on the whole pelvis (18 MeV X-ray) delivering 45 Gy/25 F/33 days with a chemotherapy on days 1 and 21 which delivered CDDP 60 mg/m^2 followed by 5-FU 600 mg/m^2 for 4 days. In the group A patients, a brachytherapy (15 Gy) was performed after CCR and finally a parametrial boost up was done to 55-60 Gy on the involved side. Four to 6 weeks after brachytherapy these 15 patients underwent surgery (colpohysterectomy with lymphadenectomy or anterior pelvectomy). In the group B, all patients were St IB. Node involvement was demonstrated on lymphadenectomy which was done with a colpohysterectomy after a brachytherapy. CCR was delivered 4 weeks after this surgery and then, a 9 Gy boost was delivered on the positive areas.

232, bd de Sainte Marguerite, 13273 Marseille Cedex 9, France

Results

Tolerance is evaluable in the 22 patients. Mild hemaetologic side effects were observed in only 2. A diarrhea led to a break in the treatment (8 to 15 days) in 4 of them. Serious small bowel troubles required special medical care in 3 patients, with 2 parenteral nutritions before surgery in group A patients and a postoperative fistula. A bladder necrosis was noted in 1 after pelvectomy, an other one died 1 month after the 2nd chemotherapy course with an infectious syndrom (candida albicans) without aplasia. Histological response rates were : 7 CR in the 7 St IIB patients, and in the 8 stage IVA patients : 2 CR, 4 PR and 2 NC. With 1 years median follow-up, 2 CR St IIB patients are alive with evolution, others are NED. 2 PR and the 2 NC St IVA patients are dead (3, 6, 6, 11 months), others are NED.

Discussion

Cure rates for patients with advanced solid tumors remain low as well for those with advanced cervix carcinoma.

In these uterine lesions, loco-regional evolution is the critical point. In order to improve the loco-regional control, several therapeutic modalities can be considered. Few neo-adjuvant chemotherapy studies are available and despite high response rates in some studies [3, 11] long terms results must be confirmed. Hypoxia is one among other radio resistance factors, and sensitizers such as misonidazole [13] or more recently etanidazole could provide some benefit.

The use of combined chemotherapy and radiation therapy could lead to a « spatial cooperation » and the drugs could be a « potentiator » of radiation as formulated by Steel and Peekham [13].

Theoretical mechanisms between chemotherapy and radiation are not yet well known, as well as the best timing, but an additive effect could be expected [16]. This enhancement could be higher since cervix carcinoma cells can be sensitive both to CDDP and 5-FU. Unfortunately « toxicity independence » is not achieved with this CCR. Bladder carcinoma combined treatments point out that even in this case where small bowel is present in the radiation fields, such positive interactions can be available.

In our study we must also consider the role of surgery since we noted 2 major complications after surgery.

Thus, the optimal doses have to be defined before a comparative study and long-term complications have to be studied.

References

1. Ashby MA, Sarales E (1987) Invasive carcinoma of the cervix in young women : clinical data and prognostic features. Radiotherapy and Oncology 10 : 167-174
2. Benstead K, Cowies UJ, Blair V, Hunter RD (1986) Stage III carcinoma of the cer-

vix. The importance of increasing age and extent to parametrial infiltration. Radiotherapy and Oncology 5 : 271-276

3. Buston EJ, Meanwell EA et al (1989) Bleomycine : Fosfamide and Cisplatin chemotherapy in cervix cancer : a highly active regimen that may improve survival. ASCO proceed 585

4. Hanks GE, Herring DF, and Kramer S (1983) Patterns of care outcome studies. Results of the National Practice in Cancer of the Cervix. Cancer 51 : 959-967

5. Inone T, Morita K (1990) The prognostic significance of number of positive nodes in cervical carcinoma. Cancer 65 : 1923-1927

6. Jampolis S, Andras J, Fletcher GH (1985) Analysis of sites and causes of failure of irradiation in invasive squamous cell carcinoma of the intact uterine cervix. Radiology 115 : 681

7. Mendenhall WM, Thar TL, Bova FG, Marcus RB, Jr, Morgan LS and Million RR (1984) Prognostic and treatment factors affecting pelvic control of stage IB and IIa carcinoma of the intact uterine cervix treated with radiotherapy alone. Cancer 53 : 2649-2654

8. Million RR, Rutlege F, Fletcher GH (1972) Stage IV carcinoma of the cervix with bladder invasion. Am 3. Obstet Gynecol 113 (2) : 239-246

9. Montana GS, Fowler WC, Varia MA, Walton LA, Mack Y (1985) Analysis of results of radiation therapy for Stage II carcinoma of the cervix. Cancer 55 : 956-962

10. Perez CA, Breaux S, Askin F et al (1979) Irradiation alone or in combination with surgery in stage IB and IIA carcinoma of the uterine cervix : a non-randomized comparison. Cancer 43 : 1062

11. Roger KM, McKay LE et al (1989) Continuous infusion 5-FU and Cisplatin for advanced squamous cell carcinoma of the cervix. ASCO proceed 613

12. Steel GG, Peckham MJ (1979) Exploitable mechanisms in combined radiotherapy-chemotherapy : the concept of additivity. Int J Radiat Oncol Biol Phys 5 : 85-91

13. Stehman FB, Bundy BN, Keys H et al (1988) A randomized trial of hydroxyurea versus misonidazole adjunct to radiation therapy in carcinoma of the cervix. Am J Obstet. Gynecol 159 : 87-94

14. Sinistrero G, Sismondi P, Zola P (1988) Results of treatment of uterine cervix cancer by radiotherapy. Radiotherapy and Oncology 13 : 257-265

15. Upadhyay SK, Symonds RP, Haeterman M, Watston ER (1988) The treatment of stage IV carcinoma of cervix by radical dose radiotherapy. Radiotherapy and Oncology 11 : 15619

16. Vokes EE, Weichselbaum RR (1990) Concomitant chemotherapy : rationale and clinical experience in patients with solid tumors. J Clin Oncol 8 : 911-934

High-dose chemotherapy

High-dose chemotherapy with hematologic rescue for high-risk non-seminomatous germ cell tumors

JL Pico, JP Droz, E Zambon, M Montastruc, A Gouyette, PY Dietrich, M Hayat

Despite progress in the treatment of disseminated non-seminomatous germ cell tumors (NSGCT), 20-30 % of patients do not achieve CR or relapse [1]. We evaluated high-dose chemotherapy (HDC) followed by autologous bone-marrow transplantation (ABMT) in selected poor-prognosis NSGCT patients. These patients were young, had a chemosensitive tumor with a well-established dose-response relationship [7-10] and rare bone marrow involvement [2]. The HDC associated Cisplatin, Etoposide and Cyclophosphamide (PEC protocol) were used ; Carboplatin recently replaced Cisplatin in a pilot study.

Patients and methods

From April 1984 to July 1990, 65 patients (mean age 26 yrs, range 13-50 ; 6 women) underwent 71 courses of HDC + ABMT. The primary tumor was testicular in 47 cases, ovarian in 6 and extragonadal in 12 (7 abdominal, 5 mediastinal). All had received Cisplatin-containing chemotherapy (CT). Group I consisted of 18 heavily-pretreated patients with progressive disease despite multiple standard drugs. Group II consisted of 14 patients who had relapsed after achieving remission with Cisplatin-based CT but who responded to second-line therapy. Group III consisted of 33 patients in first CR or PR after two courses of conventional CT and who received the PEC protocol as consolidation. They were selected, after multivariate analysis, on the basis of poor prognostic factors [3]. PEC consists of Cisplatin, 40 mg/m^2 days 1-5 ; Etoposide, 350 mg/m^2 D1-D5 ; and Cyclophosphamide, 1,600 mg/m^2 D2-D5 followed by ABMT on day 8. In 7 cases, Cisplatin was replaced by Carboplatin (800-1,600 mg/m^2 total dose). Surgery for residual disease was considered shortly after ABMT.

Results

Group I (refractory disease)

The 18 patients underwent a total of 22 courses of HDC + ABMT. There were two iatrogenic deaths. In the 19 evaluable procedures, there were 15 responses (5 CR, 10 PR) and 4 failures. Only 1 patient is in continuous complete remis-

Institut Gustave Roussy, Villejuif, France

sion (CCR) at 13 months ; the remaining 15 patients died of tumor progression after of 9 months average (2-18 months).

Group II (non-resistant relapse, n = 14)

Four patients were in CR after conventional salvage therapy. Among the 10 evaluable patients, there were 6 CR and 3 PR ; one patient failed to respond. Four patients died of tumor progression at 9, 11, 15 and 24 months. Three are alive with disease at 6, 22 and 26 months. The other 7 patients are alive in unmaintained CR at 4, 13, 18, 62, 70, 72 and 76 months.

Group III (consolidation of first PR-CR, n = 33)

A total of 35 courses of HDC + ABMT were administered. Ten courses were not evaluable, either because of existing CR (n = 8) or iatrogenic death (n = 2). In the 25 evaluable procedures, there were 4 PR and 21 CR on the basis of histology following surgery (n = 21) and/or CT scan. Twenty patients are alive in unmaintained CR after a median of 40.5 months (range 11-63) and one patient is alive with disease at 30 months. Eight patients died, 5 of tumor progression after 11 months (range 7-30) and 3 of other causes.

Two patients are lost to follow-up.

Hematologic toxicity

HDC induced profound myelosuppression. The median duration of granulocytopenia ($0.5 \times 10^9/1$) was 17 days (range 6-180) and that of thrombocytopenia ($0 \times 10^9/1$) was 18 days (range 6-210).

Non-hematologic toxicity

There were moderate or severe nausea and vomiting in 63 procedures, diarrhea in 31, mucositis in 60 and œsophagitis in 13. Nineteen patients developed a peripheral neuropathy. Other adverse effects included transient liver malfunction (n = 12), transient kidney malfunction (n = 6), skin rash (n = 11), inappropriate secretion of antidiuretic hormone (n = 4) and hemorrhagic cystitis (n = 1). One patient with extragonadal NSGCT and a gastric mass died at day 14 post-ABMT of a massive GI hemorrhage due to tumor lysis.

Discussion

Our use of high-dose chemotherapy is based on the dose-response relationship and synergism of Cisplatin, Etoposide and Cyclophosphamide [3-5]. The overall response rate was high, with 49 responses in 54 evaluable procedures (90.7 %), including 32 CR (59.2 %). The 18 heavily-pretreated patients with refractory disease (group I) showed a high response rate but a short survival. The results for the 14 patients with non-resistant relapse (group II) were good, since seven are in CCR ; 4 have a long period of disease-free survival (62-70 months) and are probably cured. Similarly, the results for the 33 patients receiving HDC + ABMT as consolidation of a first remission were encouraging, with 20 patients (60 %) in CCR with a median follow-up of 40.5 months (range 11-63). The incidence of hematologic toxicity and documented infections was similar to that in other comparable studies. Other adverse effects were gastro-intestinal tract toxicity and peripheral neuropathies. Four treatment-related deaths occurred during the 71 HDC courses, a low rate (5.6 %) compared to other studies involving ABMT. We conclude that the HDC + ABMT protocol we use is effective for the treatment of poor-prognosis NSGCT patients. Tolerance is acceptable. Patients with progressive disease have a disappointingly short response. We recommend this protocol for patients with non-resistant relapse. The results of consolidation in patients with initial poor prognostic features are being compared with a conventional treatment in a prospective trial. Surgery is indicated after HDC for the removal of residual masses and to obtain histologic information. Cisplatin might be favourably replaced by high-dose Carboplatin.

References

1. Bosl GJ, Gluckman R, Geller N, Golbey RB, Whitmore WF, Herr H, Sogani P, Morse M, Martini N, Bains M, McCormac P (1986) VAB-6 : An effective chemotherapy regimen for germ cell tumors. J Clin Oncol 4 : 1493-1499
2. Pico JL, Droz JP, Ostronoff M, Baume D, Gouyette A, Beaujean F, Hayat M (1989) Proceedings of the Fourth International Symposium (ed) The University of Texas MD Anderson Cancer Center : high-dose chemotherapy with autologous bone marrow transplantation for poor prognosis non-seminomatous germ cell tumors
3. Droz JP, Kramar A, Ghosn M, Piot G, Rey A, Theodore C, Wibault P, Court BH, Perrin JL, Travagli JP, Bellet D, Caillaud JM, Pico JL, Hayat M (1988) Prognostic factors in advanced non-seminomatous testicular cancer. Cancer 62 : 564-568
4. Nichols CR, Tricot G, Williams SD, Van Besien K, Loehrerp J, Roth BJ, Akard L, Hoffman R, Goulet R, Wolff SN, Giannone L, Greer J, Einhorn LH, Jansen J (1989) Dose-intensive chemotherapy in refractory germ cell cancer — A phase I/II trial of high-dose carboplatin and etoposide with autologous bone marrow transplantation. J Clin Oncol 7 : 932-939
5. Ozols RF, Ihde DC, Lineman WM, Jacob J, Ostchega Y, Young RC (1988) A randomized trial of standard chemotherapy versus a high-dose chemotherapy regimen in the treatment of poor prognosis non-seminomatous germ cell tumors. J Clin Oncol 6 : 1031-1040

High-dose chemotherapy and autologous bone marrow transplantation

GN Hortobagyi

Chemotherapy is the treatment of choice for most advanced, or metastatic malignancies. The efficacy of chemotherapy varies from tumor type to tumor type, being curative for some (Hodgkin's disease, non-Hodgkin's lymphoma, testicular cancer) but palliative only for most others (bronchogenic carcinoma, colorectal carcinoma, breast carcinoma). The evolution of curative chemotherapy for advanced stages indicates that long lasting complete remissions, some of which turn out to be cures, appear only after a substantial fraction of the treated patients achieves a complete remission. For most malignancies, only complete remissions alter survival, whereas partial remissions or minor responses have no impact. For most human malignancies complete remissions are more frequent after combination cytotoxic therapy than after single agent treatment.

Complete remissions after chemotherapy are dependent on a variety of interacting factors. The extent of tumor involvement, the general condition of the host (performance status), the functional status of major organs, and the extent of prior therapy all influence the frequency and quality of responses. Tumor heterogeneity and dose-intensity are additional factors that have been shown to influence the outcome of treatment [1]. The former can be addressed by the utilization of multiple agents, with minimally overlapping mechanisms of action and patterns of toxicity. Dose-intensity, on the other hand, is highly dependent on the host's tolerance. For most cytotoxic agents the dose-limiting toxicity is myelosuppression. A certain degree of reversible myelosuppression is acceptable during the standard utilization of most antineoplastic agents. However, when infectious complications increase in frequency and severity to the extent that they exceed the potential benefits of treatment, then toxicity is no longer tolerable.

Preclinical experiments have demonstrated in several systems that the higher the dose, or dose intensity, of a cytotoxic regimen, the higher the prolongation of survival or cure rate [2]. Retrospective analyses of dose-intensity in clinical trials have often supported the dose-response correlation in many human malignancies [1-3]. Prospective, randomized trials have been performed in some tumors. In most responsive tumors the dose-response correlation has been quite well established. In the more resistant, common adult malignancies, the data about the importance of dose-intensity have been conflicting.

During the last 15-20 years harvesting and reinfusion of autologous stem cells from the bone marrow, or peripheral blood has become an established technique, that is both safe and effective in restoring progenitor cells, and peripheral blood components [4]. Armed with this support system, many investigators initiated high-dose chemotherapy regimens for many human malignan-

The University of Texas MD Anderson Cancer Center, Department of Medical Oncology, Breast Medical Oncology Service, 1515 Holcombe Boulevard, Houston, Texas 77030, USA

cies. Initially single drugs, mostly alkylating agents were used [5]. More recently, high-dose combination chemotherapy with autologous stem cell support was employed. Tables 1 and 2 show the initial results of this treatment strategy. It is apparent that high-dose chemotherapy, employing doses 2 to 15 times higher than the maximum tolerated dose without autologous stem cell support, resulted in a high overall remission rate, and the appearance of a substantial complete remission rate in many malignancies. For some neoplasms, complete remissions, achieved by this strategy, yielded a cure fraction, even in patients refractory to standard chemotherapy. In some other tumors, responses have been short lasting and relapses, the rule.

Table 1. High-dose chemotherapy plus autologous bone marrow transplantation for solid tumors

Tumor Type	No. of Pts.	% CR	% CR + PR
Melanoma	187	12	49
Colon	100	14	53
Glioma	95	27	32
Breast	71	7	37
SC Lung	57	37	54
Neuroblastoma	39	33	46
Sarcoma	35	28	57
Testis	33	18	49
Ewing	21	33	71

Modified from Cheson BD et al — Ann Int Med 110:51-65, 1989

Table 2. Combination chemotherapy plus autologous bone marrow transplantation for malignant tumors

Tumor Type	No. of Pts.	% CR	% CR + PR
SC Lung	157	54	90
Melanoma	96	10	61
Testis	74	30	81
Breast	67	58	79
Neuroblastoma	45	40	44
Ovary	21	38	57
Sarcoma	17	12	71
Hodgkin's	90	65	87
Non-Hodgkin's	77	69	78
ALL	29	69	69
ANNL	162	62	62
CML	17	65	65

Modified from Cheson BD et al — Ann Int Med 110:51-65, 1989

Initially the morbidity of these regimens was very high, and the mortality rate approached 25 % in most centers [5]. During the last five years, careful modifications of dose and schedule of administration of the cytotoxic agents, as well as optimization of the reinfusion of autologous stem cells, have decreased substantially the serious morbidity and mortality of most high-dose chemotherapy regimens. Still, mortality is observed in 10-12 % of patients in most recently published reports.

This group of clinical trials have demonstrated that an objective response to therapy, even a complete remission does not always have an impact on survival. Furthermore, we have also learned that an objective response is usually but it is not always sufficient for palliation of symptoms. On the other hand, cures have never been achieved without reaching a complete remission first.

The next five presentations will review the state of the art in high-dose chemotherapy regimens with autologous stem cell support in selected human malignancies, where the strategies have been most successful. They will point out the lessons learned thus far, the place these strategies have in the overall management of each tumor, and sketch future trials to optimize the outcome of these therapies.

References

1. Hryniuk WM, Figueredo A, Goodyear M (1987) Applications of dose intensity to problems in chemotherapy of breast and colorectal cancer. Sem Oncol 14 : 3
2. Schabel FM (1975) Animal models as predictive systems. In : cancer chemotherapy-fundamental concepts and recent advances. Year Book Medical Publishers, Inc, Chicago, p 323
3. Frei E, Canellos GP (1980) Dose : a critical factor in cancer chemotherapy. Am J Med 69 : 585
4. Dicke KA, Spitzer G (1986) Evaluation of the use of high-dose cytoreduction with autologous marrow rescue in various malignancies. In : transplantation. The Williams & Wilkins Co, p 4
5. Cheson BD, Lacerna L, Leyland-Jones B, Sarosy G, Wittes RE (1989) Autologous bone marrow transplantation. Current status and future directions. Ann Intern Med 110 : 51

High-dose therapy in breast cancer

G Spitzer

The concept of high-dose intensification and the recent clinical results in metastatic breast cancer, and high-risk early stage breast cancer are discussed. High-dose therapy studies in hormone refractory metastatic breast cancer are discussed.

High-dose therapy studies in hormone refractory metastatic breast cancer

Initial clinical trials with high-dose, single agent chemotherapy have demonstrated that in a patient with metastatic breast cancer refractory to standard chemotherapy, higher objective response rates can be achieved (30-70 %) than with any cytotoxic agent used at « standard doses » [1, 2]. However, complete remissions with single agent high-dose chemotherapy were uncommon (< 10 %), remission durations short (3-4 months), and no detectable impact on survival could be observed. High-dose combination chemotherapy (usually with combinations of alkylating agents) has been more successful in increasing the overall response rate in patients with refractory metastatic breast cancer (60-80 %), and achieving a substantial percentage of complete remissions (20-50 %). Remission durations are short (2-7 months) with minimal or little impact on overall survival. The dose response of metastatic breast cancer is modestly shallow and drug resistance prevalent. The timing of high-dose strategies should be early, at a time of low tumor burden and less drug resistance.

The most recent generation of clinical studies with high-dose chemotherapy have included a « standard dose » combination chemotherapy induction regimen to the point of maximal response, followed by the administration of high-dose chemotherapy in responsive and sometimes stable patients as « consolidation » treatment. Standard dose therapy has included Anthracycline combined with either antimetabolites or alkylating agents and intensification has incorporated combinations of alkylating agents combined with Cisplatin or Carboplatin or the double high-dose CVP (Cyclophosphamide, Etoposide (VP-16) and Cisplatin) combination used by us [3-6].

The controversy relates to the uncertainty of the natural history of the subgroup of patients who entered in these trials and the magnitude of the selection in choosing the patients who have been offered marrow transplantation. The patients who entered in metastatic disease trials had been previously untreated for metastatic disease with chemotherapy and were either estrogen recep-

St. Louis University Medical School, Division of Medical Oncology and Bone Marrow Transplantation, 3635 Vista, PO Box 15250, St. Louis, MO 63110-0250, USA

tor negative (ER-) or hormone refractory. The median survival of patients with ER- tumors approximates at best 15-18 months, with at the most a 10 % three-year progression-free and overall survival [7]. Follow-up of high-dose therapy intensification strategies in metastatic disease is maturing, several studies now having significant median follow-up. The complete response rates achieved with this strategy (47-70 %) are higher than those achieved with any other treatment approach to metastatic breast cancer. Approximately 50 % of patients with residual measurable disease following induction therapy are converted to CR, and an approximate 20-30 % of patients in several trials remain in complete remission for periods exceeding 24 months [3-6]. The controversy centers around the probability that selection of patients alone could account for the probable 15 % increment in long-term survival. Our own studies demonstrate that patients with lesser volume of disease (1 or 2 metastatic sites only), and without liver involvement are the patients with prolonged disease-free survival [4, 8]. These patients, analyzed separately, have a projected 40 % disease-free survival. Patients with more extensive disease will require different strategies of high-dose therapy.

Studies in stage III and stage II breast cancer

The studies in stage IV breast cancer would seem to suggest that high-dose intensification has improved by some 10-15 % the proportion of long-term disease free survivors. This effect is however, only, in patients with lesser volume of disease.

Obviously, the introduction of these approaches into still earlier stages of breast cancer in subgroups associated with poor long-term outlook may show more dramatic results. To comprehend the potential impact of high-dose therapy in these patients the natural history of these patients with the use of conventional therapy must be understood.

The groups proposed, and in whom studies have already been initiated, are stage II and stage III disease patients with greater than 10 positive lymph nodes. Eight to 10 year follow-up reports with adjuvant combination chemotherapy suggest a superior outcome to that previously expected [9]. There is an approximate a 30-45 % DFS. At shorter periods of follow up DFS ranges from 50 % to almost 80 % at 2 years and is 35-65 % at 3 years.

Peters [10] in 53 patients (43 Stage II with more than 10 nodes and 10 stage III) used 4 cycles of the equivalent to FAC followed by a single cycle of high dose chemotherapy consolidation with Cyclophosphamide 5,600 mg/m^2, Cisplatin 165 mg/m^2 and BCNU 600 mg/m^2 and subsequent autologous bone marrow infusion. With a median follow up of 14 months and a lead time of 40 months there have been 6 relapses, 3 local relapses in 6 patients who did not receive local irradiation. The estimated 3 year DFS is 80 %. Studies from Japan in a small group of women with greater than 10 nodes show an impressive estimate of 80 % DFS at 5 years (30). These outcomes with high-dose therapy suggest a superior outcome than conventional therapy but disease-free outcomes are estimates derived from short follow-up. Proponents of conservative therapy suggest that these results cannot yet be interpreted as positive without longer follow-up.

Conclusion

There has been a recent rapid expansion of the application of high-dose chemotherapy and autologous stem-cell transfusion in the treatment of subgroups of breast cancer with probable small increments in survival in selected patients. Further studies and follow-up should resolve more accurately the impact of this aproach. Innovations to enhance the quality of the infused product should reduce toxicity.

References

1. Antman K, Bearman SI, Davidson N, de Vries E, Gianna AM, Giesselbrecht C, Kaiser H, Lazarus H, Livingston RB, Maraninchi D, McElwain TJ, Ogawa M, Peters W, Rosti G, Slease RB, Spitzer G, Tajima T, Vaughan WP, Williams S (1990) Dose intensive therapy in breast cancer : current status. In : RE Champlin and RP Gale (ed) New Strategies in bone marrow transplantation. Alan R Liss Inc, New York, p. 423
2. Antman K, Gale R (1988) Advanced breast cancer : high-dose chemotherapy and bone marrow autotransplants. Ann Intern Med 108 : 570-574
3. Antman K, Eder J, Elias A, Ayash L, Wheeler C, Schnipper L, and Frei III E (1990) High-dose cyclophosphamide, thiotepa & carboplatin intensification with autologous bone marrow support in patients with breast cancer responding to standard dose induction therapy. Proc ASCO 9 : 10, 33
4. Dunphy F R, Spitzer G, Buzdar AU, Hortobagyi GN, Horwitz LJ, Yau JC, Spinolo JA, Holmes F, Jagannath S, Bohannan PA, Dicke KA (1990) Treatment of estrogen receptor-negative or hormonally refractory breast cancer with double high-dose chemotherapy intensification and bone marrow support. J Clin Oncol 8 : 1207-1216
5. Peters WP, Eder JP, Henner WD, Schryber S, Wilmore D, Finberg R, Schoenfeld D, Bast R, Gargone B, Antman K, Anderson J, Anderson K, Krusall M S, Schnipper L, Frei E III (1986) High-dose combination alkylating agent chemotherapy with autologous bone marrow support for metastatic breast cancer. J Clin Oncol 4 : 646-654
6. Williams SF, Mick R, Desser R, Golick J, Beschorner J, Bitran JD (1989) High dose consolidation therapy with autologous stem cell rescue in stage IV breast cancer. J Clin Oncol 7 : 1824-1830
7. Livingston R, Schulman S (1987) Combination chemotherapy and systemic irradiation consolidation for poor prognosis breast cancer. Cancer 59 : 1249-1254
8. S Huan, J Yau, R Wallerstein, F Dunphy, V Spencer, D Williams, C LeMaistre, A Deisseroth, G Hortobagyi, A Buzdar, R Thierault, J Spinolo, K Dicke and G Spitzer (1991) Characteristics of long-term progression free survivors after tandem high-dose cyclophosphamide, etoposide and cisplatin (hdcvp) for breast cancer patients. Proc ASCO 10 : in press

9. Kau SW, Buzdar A, Fraschini G, Hug V, Holmes F, Hortobagyi G (1989) Impact of adjuvant chemotherapy with FAC in patients with ten or more positive nodes in operable breast cancer. Proceedings of the American Society Clinical Oncology 8 : 30
10. Peters WP, Davis R, Shpall EJ, Jones R, Ross M, Marks L, Norton L, Hurd D, Durham NC (1990) Adjuvant chemotherapy involving high-dose combination cyclophosphamide, cisplatin and carmustine and autologous bone marrow support for stage II/III breast cancer involving ten or more lymph nodes (CALGB 8782) : a Preliminary report Proc ASCO 9 : 10

Radio-chemotherapy

Differential expression of P-glycoprotein and certain other multidrug resistance characteristics in tumour cells pre-exposed in vitro either to antitumour drugs or to fractionated radiation

BT Hill, WCM Dempke, LK Hosking, S McClean, RDH Whelan

Clinical resistance to antitumour drugs is noted in patients previously treated not only with chemotherapy, but also with radiotherapy. We have proposed that although radiation-induced vascular fibrosis may limit drug delivery to the tumour, exposure to radiation may « induce » or « select » for drug resistance [1, 2]. We have examined this hypothesis using an *in vitro* model system and shown that exposure of mammalian tumour cells to fractionated X-irradiation results in the expression of resistance to a range of antitumour drugs. We have also selected for drug resistance by in vitro drug exposure and then examined the drug resistance phenotype of these various independently-derived sublines

Materials and methods

The AuxB1 Chinese hamster ovary cell line received ten 9 Gy fractions of X-rays (a dose reducing their cell survival fraction to 0.01) as detailed earlier [1]. The human tumour cell lines received 8 to 11 X-ray fractions at a dose which reduced the cell survival fraction to 0.1, to a total dose approximating to that used clinically for each tumour type [2]. Sublines were derived from cancers of the tongue (HN-1), breast (MCF-7), testis (SuSa), bladder (RT112) and ovary (SK-OV-3 and JA-T). Drug and X-ray cytotoxicities were evaluated by colony-forming assay [1-3]. Published methods were used to monitor drug uptake, assess glutathione S-transferase (GST) activities and for Western, Southern and Northern blot analyse [1-2].

Results

Studies with Chinese hamster ovary cell lines

The irradiated sublines designated DXR-10I and DXR-10II proved resistant to vincristine (VCR) and etoposide (VP16). Levels of resistance were relatively modest (i.e. 2- to 8-fold), but highly significant and considered clinically relevant. These sublines exhibited certain characteristics of the classic multidrug

Imperial Cancer Research Fund Laboratories, London WC2A 3PX, UK resistance phenotype, showing cross resistance to Vinblastine, Colchicine and Actinomycin D, elevated activity (2-fold) of GST, modified VCR accumulation, partial reversal of VCR resistance by Verapamil and overexpression of P-glycoprotein (Pgp) [1].

However, in these X-ray-pretreated cells, in which resistance proved co-dominant, Pgp overexpression occurred despite a lack of gene amplification or any significant alteration in Pgp messenger RNA levels. Furthermore, these DXR sublines showed no cross resistance to the anthracyclines.

Studies with human tumour cell lines

Data shown in Table 1 illustrate that this range of human tumour X-ray-pretreated sublines also proved consistently resistant to VCR and VP16, but not to Adriamycin (ADR). A comparison of VCR — and X-ray-selected MCF-7 sublines indicated that only the drug-selected sublines showed cross resistance to ADR and had elevated GST activity [4]. In addition, whilst the drug-selected VCR resistant sublines failed to express detectable œstrogen or progesterone receptors, X-ray-selected VCR resistant cells retained parental cell values of both steroid receptors [5]. Furthermore, quantitation of epidermal growth factor receptors revealed comparable levels in the parental and X-ray-pretreated cells, contrasting with an approximate 10-fold elevation in the drug-selected VCR resistant sublines [5].

Table 1. Summary of human tumour subline drug responses*

Cell Line	VP16	VCR	ADR
HN-1/DXR-11	R+	R+	S
MCF-7/DXR-10	R+	R++	S
SuSa/DXR-10	R+	R+	S
RT112/DXR-8	R+	R++	S
SK-OV-3/DXR-10	R+	R++	S
JA-T/DXR-10	R++	R++	S

* Ratio of IC_{50} values for a 24-h drug exposure of each subline compared with the parental line: R++ = 3-6; R+ = 1.8-2.9

Discussion and conclusion

Identification of these differential characteristics expressed by independently-derived drug — or X-ray-selected VCR resistant cell lines lends support to our contention that different resistance mechanisms may operate depending on the agent(s) to which tumour cells may have been previously exposed.

These data suggest a biological basis for the clinical problem of drug resistance that can occur in previously irradiated tumours. These observations have clinical implications for the combined modality approach and need to be considered when attempting to identify resistant tumour cells in clinical specimens with the aim of monitoring or identifying effective drug regimens.

References

1. Hill BT, Deuchars K, Hosking LK et al (1990) Overexpression of P-glycoprotein in mammalian tumour cell lines after fractionated X-irradiation *in vitro*. J Natl Cancer Inst 82 : 607-612
2. Hill BT, Whelan RDH, Hosking LK et al (1988) Interactions between antitumor drugs and radiation in mammalian tumour cell lines : differential drug responses and mechanisms of resistance following fractionated X-irradiation or continuous drug exposure *in vitro*. NCI Monogr 6 : 177-181
3. Hill BT, Whelan RDH, Gibby EM et al (1987) Establishment and characterisation of three new human ovarian carcinoma cell lines and initial evaluation of their potential in experimental chemotherapy studies. Int J Cancer 39 : 219-225
4. Whelan RDH, Hosking LK, Townsend AJ et al (1989) Differential increases in glutathione S-transferase activities in a range of multidrug-resistant human tumour cell lines. Cancer Commun 1 : 359-365
5. Hill BT, McClean S, Whelan RDH (1991) Human breast cancer cells exposed *in vitro* to fractionated X-irradiation express drug resistance yet retain functional hormone receptors and unaltered levels of epidermal growth factor receptors. Proc Am Soc Clin Oncol 10 (in press)

Abstract. Drug resistance can be expressed by tumour cells following in vitro *exposure to fractionated X-irradiation, as well as to antitumour drugs. Our results suggest that different mechanisms may operate or predominate depending on the agent to which tumour cells may have been previously exposed. These observations have potential clinical significance.*

Simultaneous chemo-radiotherapy in advanced head and neck cancer

TG Wendt, TPU Wustrow, A Schalhorn

In patients suffering from locally advanced squamous cell carcinoma of the head and neck conventionally fractionated radiotherapy results in five-years-survival probability of less than 30 % mainly due to loco-regional failure. In controlled studies chemotherapy preceding radical radiotherapy produced high response rates but failed to influence the long term results consistently. Another approach to overcome the radioresistance of large squamous cell carcinomas adopts accelerated fractionation. In this prospective single arm study a twice daily fractionated split-course radiotherapy is combined with simultaneous administration of Cisplatin (DDP) and 5-Fluorouracil (FUra) with Leucovorin (LV) enhancement.

Patients and methods

Patients are eligible for this protocol if they have a previously untreated, biopsy proven, squamous cell carcinoma of the tonsils, or the base of the tongue, the floor of the mouth, the mobile part of the tongue, the hypopharynx or the supraglottic larynx, which were considered inoperable because of local extension. This surgical decision is made by inspection, palpation and endoscopy under general anaesthesia and is also based on radiographic findings in computer tomography scans. Patients are excluded if aggressive chemotherapy is limited by severe concomitant diseases such as decompensated liver cirrhosis (pseudocholinesterase < 3,000 U/1), damage of renal function (131-iodohippurate clearance < 300 ml/min/1.73 m^2) or cardiac diseases, that do not allow hydration.

Chemotherapy was started after hydration (day 1) and consists of DDP i.v. 60 mg/m^2, 5-FUra i.v. bolus 350 mg/m^2 and LV i.v. bolus 50 mg/m^2 on day 2. On the same day, a continuous i.v. infusion over 96 hours of 5-FUra 350 mg/m^2/24 hrs and LV 100 mg/m^2/24 hrs (day 2-5) is started. This regimen is repeated on day 22 and 44.

Radiotherapy encompassed the primary and neck node metastases and was started on day 3, 24 and 46. During one cycle 13 fractions (two per day of 1.8 Gy each) are administered from day 3 to 11 (Fig. 1), up to a total tumor dose of 70.2 Gy through 3 cycles in 51 days. Shrinking field technique is applied after 60 Gy when possible. In case of severe mucositis the rest periods from day 12 to 21 and from day 34 to 43 are prolonged by one additional week.

Mucositis showed a typical triphasic pattern with its maximum during the rest intervals. Hematologic toxicity observed in a subset of the cohort has been

Klinikum Grosshadern Univ. of Munich, Marchioninistr. 15, 8000 Munich 70, Germany

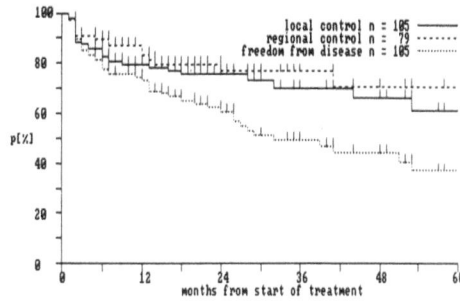

Fig. 1. Local control, regional control and disease free survival probability in 105 patients with advanced head and neck carcinoma after simultaneous radio-chemotherapy

reported earlier [1]. Tumor response was assessed clinically, biopsy was not performed routinely but was carried out during follow-up in patients showing some suspicious residum or regrowth of tumor.

From 1984 to 1989 a total of 109 patients were entered. Four patients died during treatment, 3 of them from carotid hemorrhage, one from uncontrolled infection. One hundred and five patients (11 women, 94 men) were eligible for evaluation. Distribution of TNM-stages is show in Table 1. The site of primary was the floor of mouth in 16, the supraglottic larynx in 19, the oropharynx in 44 and the hypopharynx in 26 patients.

Table 1. Distribution of tumor and nodal status according to UICC

	N0	N1	N2A	N2B	N2C	N3	total
T1	-	-	-	-	-	-	-
T2	-	-	1	1	-	2	4
T3	10	10	5	2	3	4	34
T4	16	13	12	2	15	9	67

Stage III: 20 stage IV: 85

Results

The local tumor control rate (Kaplan-Meier) amounts to 66 %, the node control rate in 79 nodal positive patients to 70 % at 4 years (N1, N2a-c : 74 %, N3 : 55 %, log-rank-test : $p < 0.02$). The 4 year's disease free survival rate is 44 % (Fig. 1).

Thirty-two out of 105 patients failed at the primary, 16/79 nodal positive necks were not controlled (N1 : 1/23, N2a-c : 9/41, N3 : 6/15). Twelve distant metastases were observed during follow-up. Neither site of primary for T-stage influenced the local tumor control probability.

Despite these promising results the value of concomitantly administered chemotherapy in these tumors is not established. In an ongoing randomized study this protocol is compared to radiotherapy alone.

Reference

1. Wendt TG, Hartenstein RC, Wustrow TPU, Lissner J (1989) Cis-platinum, 5-FU with folinic acid enhancement and synchronous accelerated radiotherapy in the management of locally advanced head and neck cancer : a phase II study. J Clin Oncol 7 : 471-476

Pediatric tumors

Two different regimens with ifosfamide as preoperative chemotherapy in children with unresectable rhabdomyosarcoma. A report from the German soft tissue sarcoma study CWS-86 and the Italian rhabdomyosarcoma study ICG-88

E Koscielniak*, M Carli**, L Andrello**, J Treuner*

The degree of the initial tumour regression produced by chemotherapy was shown in the German Soft Tissue Sarcoma Study CWS-81 to correlate with improved survival [1]. Patients with primary unresectable RMS, who achieved complete remission after 7 weeks of chemotherapy with VCR, CYC, ADR and AMD (VACA), as well as patients with primary, completely resected tumors (post-surgical stage I) had a similar DFS-rate. Therefore, it was the aim of the subsequent study, CWS-86, to increase the rate of complete responders by replacing CYC in the VACA combination through ifosfamide (IFO). IFO has been shown to be highly effective alone or in combination in the treatment of RMS [2]. Since there was no optimal dosage schedule established, we decided together with the ICG-88 to compare two different dosages and the mode of application of IFO. The study designs of the two groups were planned to allow a comparison between them.

Study design and methods

In both studies, the preoperative chemotherapy for primary non-resectable RMS (post-surgical Stage III) consisted of VCR (1.5 mg/m^2/day at wk 1, 2, 3, and 4), AMD (0.5 mg/m^2/day × 3 at wk 1, 7), ADR (40 mg/m^2/day × 2 at wk 4) and IFO at wk 1, 4 and 7. The Italian group decided to give an IFO dose of 2 g/m^2/day × 5, in contrast to the German study, in which the dose was 3 g/m^2/day × 2. IFO was given in both studies as a 24 h continuous infusion with Mesna uroprotection. The tumor response to this combination was evaluated according to the degree of tumour volume regression at week 7-9. The volume was measured before each course of chemotherapy by CT scanning [1]. The patients were divided into 4 groups according to the degree of the tumor volume regression : 1. complete regression, 2. good response : tumor regression of > 2/3 of the original tumor volume, 3. poor response : regression between 2/3 and 1/3, 4. no response : < 1/3 regression.

---

* Dep. Ped. Oncology/Hematology, Olga Hospital, Stuttgart, Germany ; ** Dep. Ped. Oncology/Hematology, University of Padova, Italy

Patients' characteristics

There were 72 children under 18 years of age with unresectable RMS registered in the CWS-86 Study and 41 in the ICG-88 Study who were evaluable for this analysis. None of them had received prior treatment with chemotherapeutic agents. The pretreatment tumor characteristics of these two groups is shown in Table 1.

Table 1. Distribution of patients' characteristics according to primary site, histology and size

Category	CWS-86 n (%)		ICG-88 n (%)
Site*			
Orbit	13 (18)		6 (15)
H/N	3 (4)		9 (22)
PM	34 (47)		9 (22)
BP	8 (11)	$p < 0.05$	6 (15)
GU-non-BP	2 (3)		1 (2)
EXT	2 (3)		2 (5)
OTH	10 (14)		8 (19)
Pathology			
embryonal	58 (80)		28 (68)
alveolar	11 (15)	$p > 0.05$	13 (32)
other	3 (4)		0
Size			
< 5cm	33 (46)	$p > 0.7$	20 (49)
> 5cm	39 (54)		21 (51)

* H/N: head/neck non-parameningeal, PM: head/neck parameningeal, BP: bladder/prostate, GU-non-BP: genitourinary non-bladder/prostate, EXT: extremity, OTH: other

Results

The regression of the tumor volume after 7-9 weeks of chemotherapy in the analyzed groups is shown in Table 2. There were no major differences between the distribution of the patients with complete response (18 % vs 15 %)

Table 2. Tumor regression in patients with primary unresectable RMS after 7 weeks of chemotherapy (VAIA)

Response	CWS 81 n (%)		ICG 88 n (%)
Complete	13 (18)		6 (15)
Good	36 (50)	$p < 0.05$	28 (68)
Poor	14 (19)		3 (7)
No	9 (12)		4 (10)

and no response (12 % vs 10 %). However, a trend towards a higher percentage of good responders in the ICG-88 was seen in comparison to the CWS-86 (68 % vs 50 %, p = 0.04).

Discussion and conclusions

In several studies testing IFO in pediatric tumors [2, 3], a 5-day schedule and a 2-day schedule with different doses was used. No definitive conclusion, however, could be drawn concerning the optimal therapeutic schedule i.e. one having the best anti-tumor efficacy and less toxicity.

Since we have shown previously, that the replacement of CYC through IFO in the four-drug combination of the preoperative chemotherapy given to RMS patients resulted in a better response rate [4], our nex step was to compare the different schedules of IFO for their anti-tumor efficacy. This was one of the objectives of the cooperation between the German CWS-86 and Italian ICG-88 studies. We did not observe any difference in the rates of complete and non responders between the studies. It is, however, worth mentioning that a statistically significant shift from the poor responder group towards the good responder group was found (ICG-88 : 7 % vs 68 %, CWS-86 : 19 % vs 50 %).

Since, on the basis of the CWS-81 data, a clear advantage in survival could be seen only in the group of complete responders after 7-9 weeks of chemotherapy, the question arises, as to whether the higher rate of good responders will influence the prognosis. The preliminary analysis of prognosis for the stage III RMS patients in the CWS 86 revealed that the DFS rate for good responders was 75 % in comparison to 55 % in the CWS- 81 Study (data not shown). One can speculate that the « quality » of partial remission was changed due to the replacement of CYC through IFO. Would the same be the case if the 2-day schedule with IFO at 6 g/m^2 would be compared with the 5-day schedule with IFO at 10 g/m^2 ? It is too early to draw definitive conclusion whether the higher rate of good reponders for the 5 day schedule would affect the long term survival. One has also to take the psychological and financial problems associated with the longer hospitalization into account if the 5-day cycle is given.

It was not the main objective of this study to compare the toxicity of the different IFO schedules. The preliminary analysis, however, revealed no major differences (data not shown).

Future analyses of the survival of different response groups will probably show whether there is any prognostic significance of the differences in distribution of good and poor responders in the German and Italian studies.

References

1. Treuner J, Suder J, Keim M, Kaatsch P, Niethammer D (1989) The predicitive value of initial cytostatic response in primary unresectable rhabdomyosarcoma in children. Acta Oncol 28 : 67-72

2. Pratt CB (1990) Ifosfamide studies for primary or recurrent malignant solid tumors and leukemia. Sem Oncol 17 : 31-40
3. Juergens H, Treuner J, Winkler K, Gœbel U (1989) Ifosfamide in pediatric malignancies. Sem Oncol 16 : 46-50
4. Treuner J, Koscielniak E, Keim M (1989) Comparison of the rates of response to ifosfamide and cyclophosphamide in primary unresectable rhabdomyosarcomas. Cancer Chemother Pharmacol 24 : 48-49

Abstract. One of the objectives of the cooperation between the German (CWS-86) and Italian (ICG-88) Rhabdomyosarcoma (RMS) Studies was the comparison of the response to preoperative chemotherapy in children with RMS. In both studies the same chemotherapy cycle comprising Vincristine (VCR), Ifosfamide (IFO), Dactinomycin (AMD) and Doxorubicin (ADR) was used, with differences in dosage and in he mode of IFO administration. In the German protocol, the IFO dose of 3 g/m²/day was given for two consecutive days. The Italian study used the dose of 2 g/m²/day × 5. There were 72 RMS patients in the CWS-86 and 41 in the ICG-88 who were evaluable for this analysis. No difference in the rates of complete responders and non-responders was observed. There was, however, a significant difference in the distribution of good responders (> 2/3 tumor volume regression) and poor responders (< 2/3 tumor volume regression) between the studies (p = 0.04). We conclude that the IFO dose of 2 g/m²/day × 5 seems to be more effective than the 3 g/m²/day × 2 dose in terms of the degree of tumor volume regression.

Limb sparing treatment in osteosarcoma with Neo-Adjuvant chemotherapy and intraoperative radiotherapy in pediatric patients. Analysis of local control

F Antillón, L Sierrasesúmaga, I Villa, F Calvo*, I Bilbao**,
S Amillo***, Canadell***

Until scarcely a decade ago no one challenged the principle that conventional treatment for osteosarcoma (OS) required a radical surgical approach (amputation and/or desarticulation). The survival rate of patients who underwent this treatment was 20 % five years from diagnosis [1].

From 1970 onwards the introduction of guidelines for neo-adjuvant, chemotherapy to complement surgery, improved these results significantly, the relevant literature reports survival figures ranging from 40 % to 70 % five years from diagnosis [2, 3].

In an attempt to improve the effects of neo-adjuvant chemotherapy, several groups have used intra-arterial therapy [5].

Intraoperative radiotherapy (IOR), is a treatment technique with the aim to sterilize surgically non-resected microscopic disease, by releasing a high dose of radiation into the tumor bed area. Some normal structures, organs and tissues can be shielded or kept out of the irradiation field [4].

Our experience using neo-adjuvant chemotherapy (i.a. + i.v.) and IOR in pediatric patients affected by OS is reported.

Material and methods

From August 1985 to November 1990, pediatric patients with proven pathology, previously untreated OS, entered into a prospective treatment protocol consisting of : neo-adjuvant chemotherapy with 3 cycles of i.a. Cisplatin and systemic Adriamycin, repeated every 3 weeks and followed by conservative limb sparing surgery (the methodology included a wide « en bloc » tumor resection, by removing all the involved bone and a macroscopic margin of normal surrounding tissues), and a IOR boost to the tumor bed.

Patients were included in the study independently of the grade of local extension, with or without pathological fracture.

IOR was carried out using a linear accelerator (Mevatron 77). Single or multiple fields were used depending on anatomic location and size of tumor bed area. Cone size ranged from 5 to 12 cm in diameter. The electron beam energy ranged from 10 to 20 Gy and it was selected depending on the tumor burden after surgery and normal tissues included in the field. The planning of each treatment program was performed by computer using a dosimetric system, able

* Departments of Pediatrics, Radiotherapy, ** Radiology, and *** Orthopedic Surgery. Clínica Universitaria Fac. Med. Univ. Navarra. Av. Pio XII s/n. 31080, Pamplona, Spain

to handle data and results from radiation beam calibration and also from the CT scan images.

Three weeks after surgery, adjuvant chemotherapy was given using 2 alternating regimens :

a) HDMTX + Cisplatin + Adriamycin and

b) HDMTX + Bleomycin + Cyclophosphamide + VCR + Act D., maintained for 48 weeks [3].

Results

A total of 28 patients have been treated. There were 17 females and 11 males, mean age 14 years (limits 7-16). Twenty six had localized disease and 2 had lung metastases at diagnosis. Two patients had pathologic bone fractures. Tumor location femur 19, tibia 7, and humerus 2, being the Enneking surgical staging 23 stage IIB, and 2 stage III. Histologic sub-type was osteoblastic 20, chondroblastic 6, and fibroblastic 2.

At the time of this report 26 patients remain alive (92.8 %). Mean follow-up has been 25 months (limits 3-63). According to the Kaplan-Meier method the actuarial survival was of 90 % at 63 months of follow-up.

All patients attained complete remission ; 3 patients had disease progression, 1 had local relapse, 1 had local and lung relapse, and 1 had lung progression. The 2 patients with lung disease died of progression. The actuarial survival rate free of disease has been of 82 % at 63 months.

The pathological study of necrosis in the tumoral piece, after resection, was for osteoblastic OS 14 cases with > 90 % and 6 with < 90 % ; chondroblastic OS 6 cases with < 90 % and for fibroblastic OS sub-histology 1 with < 90 % and 1 non evaluable.

All patients were treated with limb sparing techniques, 22 had allograft bone implantation and 6 had custom endoprostheses implanted. The two local relapses were at 12 and 20 months from diagnosis. The former had a wide amputation above the knee, and the later had a second limb salvage procedure with allograft implantation. The event-free local control was of 26/28 (92.8 %), and the global final local control has been 27/28 (96 %). In this series there is no correlation between grade of necrosis and histologic subtype with the rate of local control.

Eighteen patients had no complications, 4 had deep infections, 3 had loosening of fixation of the endoprostheses or the allograft, 2 had transitorial peripheric neuropathy, and 1 had allograft fracture.

Dicussion and conclusion

The multidisciplinary approach, that includes i.v. neo-adjuvant chemotherapy brought significant advances in the local control of OS, which allows more conservative attitudes in surgery, without detriment to the long term survival rates. Some authors have reported rates between 70 % to 90 % of local control [1-3].

The analysis of local recurrences shows that this is a consequence of microscopical residual disease, which remains behind at the time of maximal surgical debulking, and these residual cells are highly resistant to complementary conventional chemotherapy. For this reason, some investigators postulate local intensification of treatment by means of intra-arterial neo-adjuvant administration of drugs (CDDP, ADR) [5]. Although there isn't evidence about efficacy of radiotherapy in OS, by translation of previous experiences [6], IOR is emerging as an interesting alternative in the attempt to sterilize the tumor beds from possible minimal residual disease.

The high local control observed in our study (96 %), is attributed to an intensive therapeutic local approach, without jeopardazing long term survival (92.8 %). Local toxicity is acceptable, and functional results are comparable to other series. At the moment, our data suggest efficacy, but this is not enough to support definitively the application of IOR in the local control of OS, until the realization of a comparative trial.

References

1. Goorin Am, Abelson HT, Frei M (1985) Osteosarcoma : fifteen years later. N Engl J Med 313 : 1637-1643
2. Link MP, Goorin AM, Miser AW et al (1986) The effect of adjuvant chemotherapy and relapse free survival in patients with osteosarcoma of the extremity. N Engl J Med 314 : 1600-6
3. Rosen G, Caparros B, Huvos AG et al (1982) Preoperative chemotherapy. Cancer 49 : 1221-30
4. Abe M (1984) Intraoperative radiotherapy : past, present and future. Int J Radiat Oncol Biol Phys 10 : 1987-90
5. Jaffe N, Kevin A, Ayala A et al (1989) Analysis of the efficacy of intra-arterial cis-diamminedichloroplatinum-II and high dose methotrexate with citrovorum factor rescue in the treatment of primary osteosarcoma. Reg Cancer Treat 2 : 157-63
6. Calvo F, Sierrasesumaga L, Martin I et al (1989) Intraoperative radiotherapy in the multidisciplinary treatment of pediatric tumors. Preliminary report of initial results. Acta Oncol 28 : 257-260

Bone and soft tissue sarcomas

The combination of Etoposide and Cyclophosphamide as Neo-Adjuvant chemotherapy for osteosarcoma

WF Cassano, J Graham-Pole, N Dickson

The ability of adjuvant chemotherapy to improve survival in patients with non-metastatic osteosarcoma of the extremity has been proven by randomized, clinical trials comparing surgery alone to surgery followed by combination chemotherapy [1, 2]. The study by Link et al reported an actuarial, relapse-free survival (RFS) rate of 17 % at 2 years in the surgery alone group and 66 % in the surgery plus adjuvant chemotherapy group (p < 0.001). Eilber et al reported similar results of 20 % RFS at 2 years in a control group receiving no chemotherapy while those who received adjuvant chemotherapy achieved a 55 % RFS rate (p < 0.01). These results agree with historical data prior to 1970 when patients with osteogenic sarcoma, treated by surgery alone, had 5 year RFS rates less than 20 % [3].

Many single and multi-agent chemotherapy trials demonstrated the effectiveness of Methotrexate, Doxorubicin, Cisplatin, and Cyclophosphamide in the treatment of osteosarcoma [4, 5]. Several non-randomized studies of multi-agent adjuvant chemotherapy, some including preoperative (neo-adjuvant) chemotherapy, have reported actuarial survival rates for non metastatic disease from 38 to 93 % [6-9]. Neo-adjuvant chemotherapy administered prior to definitive surgery to treat both the primary tumor and any micro-metastases present at diagnosis has been advocated by Rosen [10], Winkler [11], and Jaffe [12], but no randomized trials comparing neo-adjuvant to adjuvant chemotherapy have been completed to determine whether there is an advantage for this approach.

Recent phase 2 trials using VP-16 in children with recurrent malignant solid tumors including osteosarcoma have shown a high proportion of complete and partial responses [13]. Our phase 2 data for the combination of VP-16 and Cyclophosphamide in 40 patients with a variety of recurrent solid tumors demonstrated a 58 % response rate [14]. These encouraging data prompted our evaluation of this drug combination as neo-adjuvant therapy for osteosarcoma. Data from the first 17 osteosarcoma patients treated with Etoposide and Cyclophosphamide showed an 88 % overall response rate [15]. We hypothesized that this high initial response rate might also translate into an improved relapse free survival. We now report follow-up data on 37 consecutive osteosarcoma patients treated with this combination, including the original 17 patients whose initial neo-adjuvant response was previously reported.

Department of Pediatric Hematology-Oncology, University of Florida, College of Medicine Gainesville, Florida 32610, USA

Materials and methods

Study population

All patients less than 25 years of age with a histologic diagnosis of osteosarcoma, spindle cell sarcoma of bone or malignant fibrous histiocytoma (MFH)
of bone were referred to the Pediatric Oncology Service at the University of
Florida between October 1987 and April 1990 were entered on this study. There
were no other entry exclusions and no selection or referral biases identified
during this study. All patients were evaluated for metastatic disease by computed tomography of the chest and radionuclide bone scan. Primary lesions
were evaluated with computed tomography and magnetic resonance imaging.

Chemotherapy

All patients received their first course of chemotherapy within two weeks of
registration on this study. As outlined in Figure 1, chemotherapy consisted of
two courses each of Etoposide/Cyclophosphamide (VP/CY) and Cispla-
tin/Doxorubicin (CIS/DOX) prior to definitive surgery followed by alternating courses of VP/CY and CIS/DOX for a total of 8 postoperative chemotherapy courses. Drug doses were as follows : Etoposide 200 mg/m^2/day by
continuous infusion for 72 hours (600 mg/m^2/course) ; Cyclophosphamide
300 mg/m^2/dose every 12 hours for 6 doses (1,800 mg/m^2/course) ; Cisplatin
100 mg/m^2 as a single dose per course ; Doxorubicin 40 mg/m^2 as a single
dose per course.

week :	0	3	6	8	10	13	16	19	22	25	28	31	34
	VP	VP	P	P	S	VP	P	VP	P	VP	P	VP	P
	CY	CY	A	A	U	CY	A	CY	A	CY	A	CY	A
					R								
					G								
					E								
					R								
					Y								

VP = etoposide 200 mg/m^2/day continuous infusion × 72 hr (600 mg/m^2/course)
CY = cyclophosphamide 300 mg/m^2/dose q12h × 6 doses (1800 mg/m^2/course)
P = cisplatin 100 mg/m^2
A = doxorubicin 40 mg/m^2

Fig. 1.

Surgery

All patients with extremity lesions had wide local excisions of the primary
tumor and limb salvage procedures chosen by the patient in consultation with
his orthopedic surgeon.

Patient registration

At the time of initial diagnosis of osteosarcoma, MFH or spindle cell sarcoma of bone by either needle aspirate or open surgical biopsy, patients were entered on study by registration with our data manager.

Statistical analysis

Log rank analysis was performed with the LIFETEST procedure from the SAS PC statistical software [16].

Results

Thirty-seven consecutive patients were entered on this study between October 1987 and April 1990. Patient characteristics are detailed in Table 1. None of the patients had previous neoplasms, and none had prior radiation therapy.

Table 1. Patient characteristics

Age (years)			Primary site		
mean	14.3		extremity	34	
median	15		distal femur		21
range	4-24		proximal tibia		6
Sex			proximal humerus		2
male	23		proximal femur		1
female	14		proximal fibula		1
Race			distal fibula		1
white	31		calcaneus		1
black	6		distal radius		1
Mctastatic discasc at diagnosis			axial	3	
present	6		vertebral body		2
absent	31		ilium		1
			Histology		
			osteosarcoma		34
			MFH		2
			spindle cell		1

Median follow-up of these patients is 2 years with a range of 5 months to 2.8 years. Six patients (16 %) had pulmonary metastases at diagnosis, 3 (8 %) had primary axial skeletal lesions. Three patients had primary bone tumors with histologies other than classical osteosarcoma, 2 MFH and 1 an unspecified, spindle cell sarcoma of bone. These 3 patients had nonmetastatic, extremity lesions.

Overall, 11 of the 37 patients have relapsed. All tumor recurrences were at distant pulmonary or bone sites. There were no failures at the primary site. Log rank analysis revealed a significant difference in RFS probability between patients with metastases at diagnosis (0 %) and those without metastases at diagnosis (78 ± 9 %) (p < 0.0001) (Fig. 2). Black race was significantly associated with an earlier time to relapse although RFS probability was the same. A serum alkaline phosphatase higher than 300 IU at diagnosis was associated with a significantly poorer RFS probability (p < 0.04) (Table 2). Age, sex, and site were not significant prognostic variables in this group of patients.

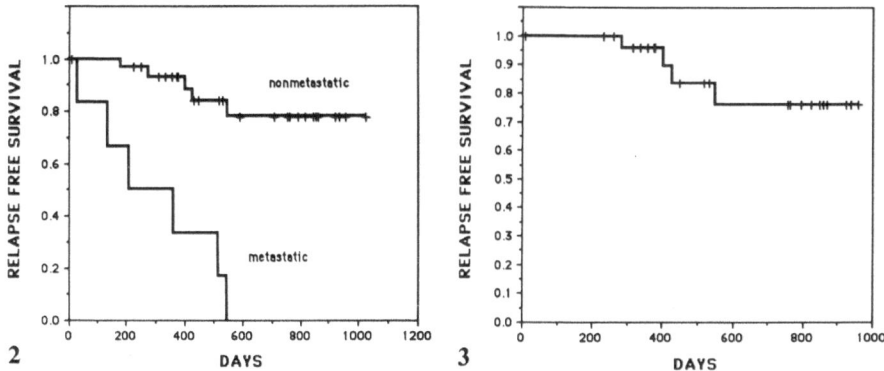

Fig. 2. Actuarial relapse free survival rates for patients with metastases at diagnosis compred to those without metastase at diagnosis

Fig. 3. Actuarial relapse free survival rates for patients with nonmetastatic, extremity osteosarcoma

Table 2. Stratified survival data for all patients entered on study

	STRATUM	N	%RFS ± SE	P value
Age	< 12 yr	9	59 ± 18	
	> 12	28	63 ± 11	NS
Sex	male	23	64 ± 13	
	female	14	58 ± 15	NS
Race	white	31	63 ± 10	
	black	6	67 ± 19	.04
Site	axial	3	50 ± 35	
	extremity	34	62 ± 10	NS
Metastatic at diagnosis				
	yes	6	0	
	no	31	78 ± 9	.0001
Alkaline phosphatase :				
	< 300	19	80 ± 11	
	> 300	18	43 ± 14	.04

To compare our results with most other published studies which exclude metastatic and axial skeleton tumors, we created a subgroup of 26 patients by excluding patients with metastases at diagnosis, axial skeleton primary lesions, and histologies other than classical osteosarcoma. Five of these 26 patients recurred for an overall, actuarial RFS of 78 % ± 9 % (Fig. 3). Log rank analysis of this patient group failed to identify any significant differences in relapse free survival when stratified by age, sex, race, and serum alkaline phosphatase (Table 3).

Table 3. Stratified survival data for patients with nonmetastatic, extremity osteosarcoma only

	STRATUM	N	%RFS ± SE	P value
Age	< 12 yr	7	80 ± 18	
	> 12	19	73 ± 14	NS
Sex	male	18	68 ± 16	
	female	8	88 ± 12	NS
Race	white	23	75 ± 11	
	black	3	100 ± 0	NS
Alkaline phosphatase:				
	< 300	13	88 ± 12	
	> 300	13	66 ± 16	NS
	< 400	17	86 ± 10	
	> 400	9	60 ± 22	NS
	< 500	21	78 ± 12	
	> 500	5	67 ± 27	NS

Transient, severe myelosuppression was the only major toxicity of the Etoposide-Cyclophosphamide courses. No irreversible organ damage or toxic deaths were observed in patients enrolled in this study.

Discussion and conclusion

The proven benefit of adjuvant chemotherapy for osteosarcoma has stimulated further investigation to identify more effective drug combinations. The standard approach of comparing two treatment regimens in a randomized study requires large numbers of patients and several years of follow-up observation. To evaluate new drug combinations, the initial response rates in previously untreated patients can be examined requiring fewer patients and shorter observation times. We found that the combination of Etoposide and Cyclophosphamide in the initial therapy of osteosarcoma produced an 88 % response rate for the primary tumor and metastases. Further observation of outcome in these patients indicate that their actuarial RFS rates are equivalent to those achieved with the best adjuvant results previously reported.

We conclude that the combination of Etoposide and Cyclophosphamide is an effective treatment for osteosarcoma, and when combined with Cisplatin and Doxorubicin, is as effective as any previously reported adjuvant chemotherapy for osteosarcoma. Although patients with metastatic disease at diagnosis have achieved complete remissions with this therapy, all of them eventually developed recurrent disease. Therefore, new therapeutic approaches are needed for these patients with metastases at diagnosis.

References

1. Link MP, Goorin AM, Miser AW et al (1986) The effect of adjuvant chemotherapy on relapse-free survival in patients with osteosarcoma of the extremity. New Engl J Med 314 : 1600-1606
2. Eilber F, Giuliano A, Eckardt J et al (1987) Adjuvant chemotherapy for osteosarcoma : a randomized prospective trial. J Clin Oncol 5 (1) : 21-26
3. Friedman MA, Carter SK (1972) The therapy of osteogenic sarcoma— current status and thoughts for the future. J Surg Oncol 4 : 482-510
4. Weichselbaum RR, Cassady JR, Jaffe N et al (1977) Preliminary result of aggressive multimodality therapy for metastatic osteosarcoma. Cancer 40 : 78-93
5. Rosen G, Huvos AG, Mosende C et al (1978) Chemotherapy and thoracotomy for metastatic osteogenic sarcoma : a model for adjuvant chemotherapy and the rationale for the timing of thoracic surgery. Cancer 41 : 841-849
6. Eilber FR, Rosen G (1989) Adjuvant chemotherapy for osteosarcoma. Sem in Oncology 16 (4) : 312-323
7. Sutow WW, Sullivan MP, Fernbach DJ et al (1975) Adjuvant chemotherapy in primary treatment of osteogenic sarcoma. Cancer 36 : 1598-1602
8. Pratt S, Shanks E, Hustu O et al (1977) Adjuvant multiple drug chemotherapy for osteosarcoma of the extremity. Cancer 39 : 51-57
9. Bacci G, Picci P, Ruggieri P et al (1990) Primary chemotherapy and delayed surgery (neo-adjuvant chemotherapy) for osteosarcoma of the extremities. Cancer 65 : 2539-2553
10. Rosen G, Caparros B, Huvos A et al (1982) Preoperative chemotherapy for osteogenic sarcoma : selection of postoperative adjuvant chemotherapy based on the response of the primary tumor to preoperative chemotherapy. Cancer 49 : 1221-1230
11. Winkler K, Beron G, Kotz R et al (1984) neo-adjuvant chemotherapy for osteosarcoma : results of a cooperative German/Austrian study. J Clin Oncol 2 : 617-624
12. Jaffe N, Robertson R, Ayala A et al (1985) Comparison of intra-arterial cis-diamminedichloroplatinum II with high dose methotrexate in the treatment of primary osteosarcoma. J Clin Oncol 3 : 1101-1104
13. King F, Hayes A, Krischer J (1985) VP-16 in children with recurrent malignant solid tumors. A phase II study. ASCO Proc 4 : 235
14. Grana N, Graham-Pole J, Cassano WF et al (1989) Etoposide (VP-16) infusion plus cyclophosphamide (CY) pulses : an effective combination for refractory cancer (Abstr). Proc Am Soc Clin Oncol 8 : 300
15. Saleh RA, Graham-Pole J, Cassano WF et al (1990) Response of osteogenic sarcoma to the combination of Etoposide and Cyclophosphamide as neo-adjuvant chemotherapy. Cancer 65 : 861-865
16. SAS Institute Inc., Cary, NC

Abstract. We have evaluated the combination of etoposide and cyclophosphamide as initial, presurgical therapy for patients with osteosarcoma and found an 88 % response rate for the primary tumor and any metastases. After definitive, limb salvage surgery and adjuvant chemotherapy with etoposide, cyclophosphamide, cisplatin and doxorubicin, patients without metastases at diagnosis, followed for a median of 2 years from diagnosis, achieved an actuarial, relapse free survival (RFS) rate of 78 ± 9 %. This result is equivalent to what has been achieved with the best adjuvant chemotherapy results reported to date. Patients without metastases at diagnosis had significantly better RFS probability (78 ± 9 %) than those with metastases at diagnosis (0 %). Transient, severe myelosuppression has been the only major toxicity of the Etoposide-Cyclophosphamide courses. No irreversible organ damage or toxic deaths have been observed in patients enrolled in this study. We conclude that the combination of Etoposide and Cyclophosphamide is effective treatment for osteosarcoma, and when combined with Cisplatin and Doxorubicin, is as effective as any previously reported chemotherapy for osteosarcoma.

Dose response relationship in adult osteosarcoma patients treated with Neo-Adjuvant high dose Methotrexate, surgery and adjuvant chemotherapy

B Brun, JF Gimonet, F Feuilhade, G Delepine, P Feuilhade, N Delepine, MC Voisin, JP Le Bourgeois

It is commonly admitted that neo-adjuvant or adjuvant chemotherapy is the main factor responsible for the improvement of prognosis in osteogenic osteo-sarcoma [1, 2]. Surgical treatment may be conservative (with the reserve of needed monobloc surgery) or radical without influence upon general prognosis [3]. We describe here our series of adult patients treated according to a cooperative protocol (GETO SO5 87), which overall analysis is not yet available. This separate report is made in order to analyse the role of neo-adjuvant Methotrexate included in this protocol.

Patients

Ten adult patients with a median age of 40 [19-62] were included, all with an histologically demonstrated high grade osteosarcoma. One patient had a Paget disease. Localizations were : mandibula : 1 ; rib : 1 ; upper femoral extremity : 3 ; upper tibial extremity : 2 ; scapula : 3.

Protocol design

Initial evaluation included radiograph, tomodensitometry, magnetic resonance, angiography of the lesion, and general staging. This evaluation was repeated after the first month just prior to intervention.

Initial part of the treatment was one month of neo-adjuvant weekly high dose Methotrexate. The timing had to be strictly observed. The Methotrexate infusion was given in 6 h, after alcalinisation ; folinic rescue was begun at 14th h after the end of infusion ; it was folinic acid 15 mg/m2/6 hr until Methotrexate serum level was < 0,5 μM/l. At the first cycle the dosage given was 8 g/m^2, but at further cycles the dosage was systematically increased with the aim to achieve a serum peak level above 1,000 μM/l, and even when correct elimination was achieved at previous cycle.

At the end of the first month immediately after response evaluation, the patient was deferred to surgeon and had to received a monobloc surgery with plastic surgery.

CHU Henri Mondor, 51 av. du Maréchal de Lattre de Tassigny, 94000 Créteil, France

The response to neo-adjuvant chemotherapy was judged upon *a)* clinical response *b)* imaging response *c)* necrosis rate on histological examination of resection specimen. In this study we classified a patient as a good responder when at least 2 or 3 of the above criterias were met.

After surgery, the patients received a complex program of perioperative and maintenance chemotherapy administered at maximally tolerated dose during 8 months. Drugs used were THP, Adriamycin, Bleomycin, Actinomycin D, Cyclophosphamide, Phosphamide, Cisplatin. We do not describe this complex program, which is out of the scope of our analysis.

Results

All 10 patients received all projected phases of treatment. A monobloc surgery with plastic surgery was performed in all. However in 2 patients, prothesis infection led to secondary amputation. Median follow up is 24 months. One patient (the one with a Paget disease) had pulmonary metastases at 24 months and subsequently died. Actuarial survival is 87,5 %. We cannot comment upon these results since the patient series is small and follow up too short. But we wish to comment upon the data obtained with neo-adjuvant Methotrexate :

1) Despite the very high dosage used, no important toxicity was observed. There was no myelodepression. Increased level of transaminases was seen one time in 2 patients, and many times in 6 others, without any other liver disturbance, and we never modified the treatment with this anomaly. Two patients, however, developed during maintenance therapy an overt hepatopathy with icterus. In these 2 cases a viral hepatitis was demonstrated by histology. One patient complained of disturbed vision during her third neo-adjuvant methotrexate ; the dosage of the fourth infusion was lowered and the troubles disappeared.

Kinetic studies showed to us that there was not any predictable relationship between administered dose and Methotrexate serum peak level. Indeed different patterns were seen in individuals with a need to very high dose in younger patients to achieve a high serum level.

The response was classified as good in 5 patients and poor in 5 others.

We calculated the mean Methotrexate serum peak level achieved during the neo-adjuvant phase ; No demonstrated correlation between mean serum levels and response was evident. However, surprisingly the mean administered dose of Methotrexate given during neo-adjuvant chemotherapy was significantly different in responders (14 g/m²/wk) and non responders (11,5 g/m²/wk) $p < 0.05$ (Fig.1).

Discussion

The notion of a dose-response relationship in Methotrexate treatment of osteosarcoma is highly suggested by classical papers of Jaffe [4]. The better para-

B Brun et al

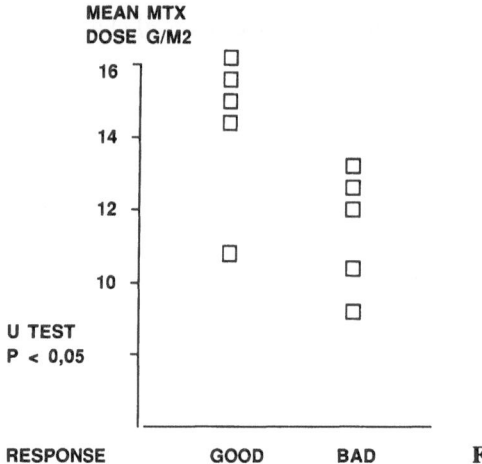

Fig. 1.

meter to deliver the appropriate dosage is perhaps the Methotrexate serum peak level achieved. The correlation may not appear in our very limited series. But perhaps the different kinetic patterns observed do not describe accurately the distribution of methotrexate in the body. Nobody knows if there is, indeed, a correlation between the Methotrexate serum peak level achieved, and the amount of drug entering the tumor cells. This would explain why the dose delivered is not so clearly correlated with the response.

References

1. Link MP, Goorin AM, Miser AW et al (1986) The effect of adjuvant chemotherapy on relapse fee survival in patients with osteosarcoma of the extremity. New Eng J Med 314 : 1600-6
2. Rosen G, Marcove RC, Huvos AC et al (1983) Primary osteogenic sarcoma ; a 8 years experience with adjuvant chemotherapy. J Cancer Res Clin Oncol 106 : 55-67
3. Simon SA, Aschlimna MA, Thomas N et al (1986) Limb salvage versus amputation for osteosarcoma of the distal end of the femur. J Bone Joint Surg 68 : 1331-1337
4. Jaffe N, Frei E, Traggis D (1978) High dose methotrexate in osteogenic sarcoma ; a 5 years experience. Cancer treat Rep 62 : 259-264

Chemotherapy of soft tissue sarcomas with Cyclophosphamid or Ifosfamid, Adriamycin and DTIC (CAD or IAD) preoperatively and in patients with metastatic disease : a non randomized pilot study

HP Honegger, MD Cserhati, A Von Hochstetter, GU Exner

Soft tissue sarcomas are rare tumors, in localized disease most authors report a five year survival between 40 and 60 %. Patients with soft tissue sarcomas mostly present with their primary tumors ; they can be rendered disease free clinically by wide resection. Since local recurrences and metastases, especially in grade II and III soft tissue sarcomas over 5 cm in size are a major therapeutic problem, combined modality treatment with radiotherapy and adjuvant chemotherapy is evaluated in prospective studies. Limb sparing procedures without jeopardizing the result may be used, if they are associated with radiotherapy and chemotherapy (Eilber 1980, Consensus Conference 1985, Eilber 1990). Several chemotherapeutic agents, most recently Ifosfamid was added to the list, are found to be effective ; among the most promising regimes were Cyclophosphamid, Adriamycin, DTIC (CAD, Blum 1980) and in recent years Ifosfamid, Adriamycin, DTIC (IAD, Elias 1989).

Our study was initially designed to examine the effect of intravenous CAD in previously untreated patients with soft tissue sarcomas and was extended after 1985 to IAD in a non randomized fashion as well. In a selected group of patients, mainly with primary tumors > 5 cm in size, we chose to apply chemotherapy preoperatively. The aim was to test its feasability, and to assess its influence on tumor biology and on limb sparing interventions.

Materials and methods

Since 1981, 44 patients with histologically confirmed grade II-III soft tissue sarcomas were treated in our pilot study. There were 22 female and 22 male patients, median age 48 years, mean 43.5 years, range 16-68 y. Patients were ambulatory and had no evidence of heart disease. Diagnostic work up included an abdominal sonography, CT-Scans of lung and bone scans. Twenty-five patients had localized tumors, 19 metastatic disease, mostly multiple in the lung, 1 patient showed a single liver metastasis. Patients with localized disease were selected for the preoperative chemotherapy study if they presented with a big primary tumor (> 5 cm), with invasion of adjacent structures or with a rapidly growing (within 6 months after resection of the primary tumor) locally recurring soft tissue sarcoma. Location of primary tumors were : arms 7, legs 9, trunk 5, inner abdominal/thoracic area : 4. The following histological types

University Hospital Zürich, Section of Oncology, Institute of Pathology, Clinic for Orthopedics and Oncology Institute, Triemli Hospital, Zürich, Switzerland

of grade II and III soft tissue sarcomas were found : leiomyosarcoma 9, MFH8, undifferentiated mesenchymal sarcoma 7, liposarcoma 6, synovialsarcoma 5, neurofibrosarcoma 3, various 6.

Chemotherapy consisted of intravenous Adriamycin 15 mg/m²/day, days 1-4, in continuous infusion ; DTIC 250 mg/m²/day, days 1-4 and Cyclophosphamid 600 mg/m² day 01 or Ifosfamid 2.5 g/m²/day, days 1-3, with mesna uroprotection. Dosage of Adriamycin and Cyclophosphamid/Ifosfamid was increased until a nadir of less than 3,000 white blood cells/mm³ was obtained. The overall response rate was assessed by standard criteria after 3 chemotherapy cycles ; patients who was treated preoperatively and rendered disease free by surgical intervention received radiotherapy (5,500-6,000 rad) and additional 5 chemotherapy cycles. Overall survival was calculated in months begining at definitive evaluation (after 3 chemotherapy cycles) until recurrence or death, or until December 1990. Survival curves were plotted according to Kaplan/Meyer/method ; statistical comparisons were carried out by the log rank test (Peto).

Results

Response to chemotherapy

The overall response rate for all 44 patients after 3 chemotherapy cycles were : CR 2/44 (4 %), PR 17/44 (39 %), NC 13/44 (29 %) and progressive disease 12/44 (28 %). In the 19 patients with metastatic disease no CR was observed, 5 responded partially, 4 NC and 10 (53 %) had progressive disease. Of the 25 patients with localized disease treated preoperatively, 2 had CR (8 %), 12 PR (48 %), 9 NC (36 %) and 2 (8 %) progressive local disease. There was no difference between CAD and IAD in this non randomised study among patients treated preoperatively or with metastatic disease (Table 1).

Surgical intervention after chemotherapy

Twenty-two patients underwent a surgical procedure after 3 chemotherapy cycles. One of 25 patients (5 %) with metastatic disease had a resection of a single liver metastasis. Twenty-one out of 25 patients (84 %) with localized disease had resections, surgery was considered inappropriate in 4, 1 with a primary of lung with mediastinal infiltration without adequate response, 3 with massive pelvic disease that responded only partially to chemotherapy. One patient died 7 days postoperatively with an ARDS syndrom after a chestwall resection. The surgeons obtained a CR in 19/22 patients (86 %) ; in the remaining 3 patients the bulk of tumor was removed, the margins were not completely tumorfree (1 chestwall + vessels ; 1 abdominal wall + inguinal vessels ; 1 inguinal area + vessels). Additional radiotherapy was given to extremity and trunk tumors. None of our patients with extremity tumors were amputated primarily.

Table 1. Soft tissue sarcomas, grade II-III results of chemotherapy, (clinical/radiologic evaluation)

	local		mestastatic		total
	CAD	IAD	CAD	IAD	
CR	1	1	...	...	2
PR	8	4	3	2	17
NL	2	7	4	...	13
P	1	1	4	6	12
N	12	13	11	8	44

Survival data

Median survival time for patients with metastatic disease is 7 months, 2 and 5 years survival 36 % and 21 % respectively. Patients with localized disease had a median survival time of 56 months, survival at 2 and 5 years was 68 % and 44 % respectively. Those 19 patients who were rendered completely disease-free by surgery after preoperative chemotherapy reached a 2 and 5 years survival of 89 % and 58 % respectively (see Fig. 1).

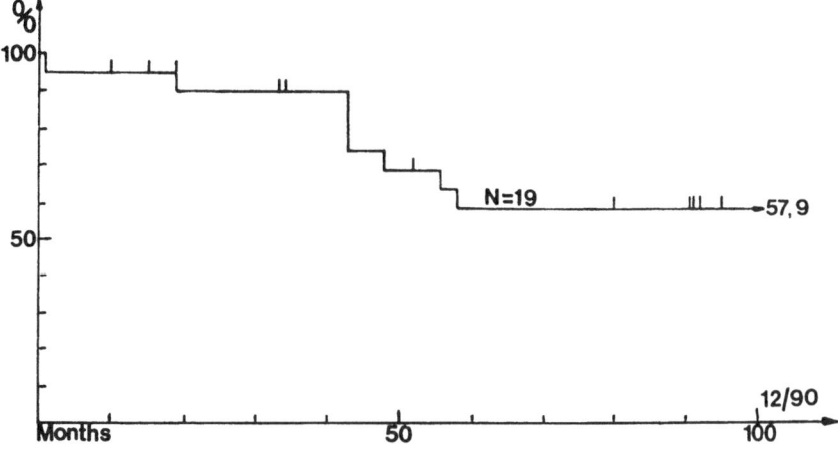

Fig. 1. Soft tissue sarcomas CR after preoperative chemotherapy and surgery

Four out of 16 patients with extremity soft tissue sarcomas and a limb sparing procedure that lead to CR developped a local recurrence after 33 months (range 21-47), 2/16 had then a secondary amputation (13 %). Among the 21 patients with localized disease and preoperative chemotherapy and surgery, 12 obtained a PR, 9 NC after 3 chemotherapy cycles. Survival for those patients was not different whether they obtained PR or NC. Of our whole patient group, 29 are dead by now (29/44 = 66 %) ; death rate for metastatic disease is 79 %, for localized disease 56 %. If only disease-free patients (after preoperative chemotherapy + surgery) are considered, then 7/19 died because of lung metastases, 1 with ARDS, thus 8/19 or 42 % are dead.

Discussion

One of the aims of our pilot study was to assess the effect of chemotherapy in previously untreated grade II-III soft tissue sarcomas. The overall response rate was 43 % (CR + PR), 29 % NC and 28 % progressive disease. Response rates were higher in loco-regional disease (56 %, CR + PR) than in metastatic disease (26 %). Primary progressive disease was seen in 53 % with metastatic and in 8 % with localized disease. We thus confirm our earlier findings (Honegger 1986) and those of others (Blum 1980, Benjamin 1981, Elias 1989). There was no discernable difference between CAD and IAD within this small non randomized study. The desired degree of myelosuppression was reached in 71 % of our patients, all had some degree of nausea and vomiting and alopecia (data not shown).

Chemotherapy treated patients with metastatic disease had a median survival of 7 months ; in those with localized disease, median survival was 56 months (similar data was reported by Elias).

After preoperative chemotherapy, 84 % of patients with loco-regional disease and 5 % of patients with metastatic disease were rendered disease-free by surgery and received additional chemotherapy. No surgical attempt was considered possible in 3 pelvic lesions and a pulmo-mediastinal sarcoma without favourable response to chemotherapy. A CR was obtained in 19/22 (86 %) of patients undergoing surgery, in 3 patients resections were only marginal. A 26 year old female died 7 days after resection of parts of her chestwall of a ARDS syndrom. Among those 19 CR patients, a 2 and 5 year survival of 89 % and 58 % respectively was observed, all 16 patients with extremity soft tissue sarcomas had limb sparing procedures. Four of these 16 patients in CR developed later a local recurrence after a median 33 months, 2/16 then had a secondary amputation (13 %). The extent of response after preoperative chemotherapy was not a significant prognostic factor for survival (PR versus NC).

In summary, we found that preoperative chemotherapy with CAD or IAD resulted in higher response rates than in metastatic disease. As others have seen (Yap 1983, Rouessé 1987) a small group of patients with grade II/III soft tissue sarcomas that reach CR after preoperative chemotherapy plus surgery may have a relatively favourable outcome with 2 and 5 years survival of 89 % and 58 % respectively, some of them may even be cured. Despite promising data, the very limited number of patients with a favourable course asks for cautious interpretation and preclude general application ; preoperative chemotherapy in soft tissue sarcomas should only be used in carefully designed trials in order to clarify the impact of that approach.

References

1. Blum R, Carson J, Wilson R et al (1980) Sucessful treatment of metastatic sarcomas with Cyclophosphamid, Adriamycin and DTIC (CAD). Cancer 46 : 1722-1726
2. Elias A, Ryan L, Sulkes A et al (1989) Response to Mesna, Doxorubicin, Ifosfamid and Dacarbazine in 108 patients with metastatic or unresectable sarcoma and no prior chemotherapy. J Clin Oncol 7 : 1208-1216
3. Consensus Conference (1985) Limb sparing treatment of adult soft tissue sarcomas and osteosarcomas. JAMA 254 : 1791-1796
4. Eilber F, Eckhardt J, Merton D (1984) Advances in the treatment of sarcomas of the extremity. Cancer 54 : 2695-2701
5. Benjamin R, Yap O, Frazier J (1981) Combination chemotherapy for sarcomas with Cyclophosphamid, continuous infusion Adriamycin and Dacarbazine with surgical intensification. Proceedings. Am Soc Clin Onc 22 : 526
6. Honegger HP, Cserhati MD, Von Hochstetter et al (1986) Pilot study of chemotherapy containing Adriamycin by continuous infusion, Cytoxan and DTIC in patients with soft tissue sarcomas, applied preoperatively and in metastatic disease. Neoadjuvant chemotherapy colloque. INSERM/John Libby Eurotex Ltd, Vol 137 : 599-605
7. Yap BS, Sincovics JG, Burgess MA et al (1983) The curability of advanced soft tissue sarcomas in adults with chemotherapy. Prceedings. Am Soc Clin Onc 2 : 239
8. Rouessé JG, Friedman S, Sevin D et al (1987) Preoperative induction chemotherapy in the treatment of locally advanced soft tissue sarcomas. Cancer 60 : 296-300
9. Eilber F, Huth J, Mirra J, Rosen G (1990) Progress in the recognition and treatment of soft tissue sarcomas. Cancer 65 : 660-666

Abstract. From 1981-1990 we treated 44 patients with histologically confirmed grade II-III soft tissue sarcomas, 9 had metastatic disease, 25 a localized primary or recurrent tumor. Response was assessed after 3 chemotherapy cycles. 0/19 patients with metastatic disease had a CR, 5/19 (26 %) PR, 4/19 (21 %) NC, 10/19 (53 %) progressive disease. 14/19 are dead, 5 currently alive, median survival is 7 months, 2 and 5 year survival is 36 % and 21 % respectively. The response rates of 25 patients with localized disease were as follows : 2 (8 %) had a CR, 12/25 (48 %) PR, 9/25 (36 %) NC, 2 (8 %) had a locally progressive disease. 1/19 with metastatic disease (5 %) and 21/25 with localized disease (84 %) underwent then tumor resection. In 4/25patients with localized disease, surgery was considered inappropriate after preoperative chemotherapy because of inadequate response. The 19 patients who were rendered completely disease free by surgery after preoperative chemotherapy had a 2 and 5 y survival of 89 % and 58 % respectively. No significant differences for response rate CR + PR nor for progressive disease for CAD versus IAD was seen in this small none randomized study. In summary : preoperative chemotherapy with CAD or IAD results in higher response rates than in metastatic disease. Patients with CR's, obtained after preoperative chemotherapy and surgery in grade II and III soft tissue sarcomas, have a 2 and 5 y survival of 89 % and 58 % respectively.

Phase II study of THP-Adriamycin (Pirarubicin) and DTIC in advanced soft tissue sarcomas

PA Salem, S Steiger, RS Benjamin

Adriamycin is probably the most effective single agent in the treatment of soft tissue sarcomas with a response rate of approximately 30 % [1]. Reported data strongly suggest a steep dose-response curve [2]. Prior to the emergence of Ifosfamide, the second most important drug in the treatment of sarcomas was Dacarbazine (DTIC) with a response rate of approximately 17 % [3]. The addition of DTIC to Adriamycin increased the remission rate by approximately 10 % [4], and made this combination one of the standard treatments for these diseases.

THP-Adriamycin is a new Adriamycin analog which was synthesized in Japan in 1979 [5] and had undergone extensive phase I and phase II testing by the Japanese. It has been shown to have activity in a wide spectrum of neoplastic diseases [6]. Preclinical studies strongly suggest that it is more active and less cardiotoxic than Adriamycin [7]. Thus, we decided to substitute THP-Adriamycin for adriamycin in the Adriamycin-DTIC combination to study the therapeutic efficacy and toxicity pattern of this new combination and compare it to our own historical control of Adriamycin and DTIC.

Materials and methods

Patients were eligible for this study if they had measurable disease and no prior chemotherapy. Patients with congestive heart failure, cardiomyopathy and unstable angina were excluded. THP-Adriamycin was given in an infusion over half an hour and DTIC was given over a 2 hour infusion. Both drugs were given on the same day. Cycles were repeated every 3 weeks. The starting dose of THP-Adriamycin was 60 mg/m^2 and was increased or decreased depending on the presence or absence of infection, severe stomatitis and/or severe myelosuppression. The dose of DTIC was kept constant at 1,000 mg/m^2.

Results

A total of 17 patients have been treated so far. Sixteen of these patients are evaluable for response and toxicity. Median age was 47 years.

The total response rate was 31 % but no complete remissions were achieved. Time to response was 7 weeks. The median duration of response was 1 year. The median follow-up for live patients was approximately 2 years. Ninety-

The University of Texas, M.D. Anderson Cancer Center, Department of Medical Oncology, 1515 Holcombe Boulevard, Box 77, Houston, Texas 77030, USA

Response

Evaluable patients	16	
Complete response	0	(0%)
Partial response	5	(31%)
Minor response	1	(6%)
No change	4	(25%)
Progressive disease	6	(38%)

four percent of patients who received the first cycle at 60 mg/m^2 were eligible for dose escalation to 75 mg/m^2 in the second cycle. Also 90 % of those who received the second cycle at 75 mg/m^2 were eligible for dose increase in the subsequent cycle to dose level 90 mg/m^2. Accordingly, the starting dose of 60 mg/m^2 was relatively low.

Toxicity

Dose limiting toxicity was neutropenia. Thrombocytopenia was rare.

Hematologic Toxicity

Dose level	Number of cycles	AGC < 0.5	Plt < 50	Hgb < 8
− 2	1	0	0	0
− 1	3	2	1	1
0	42	27	4	2
1	18	12	3	2
2	20	16	1	1

An absolute granulocyte count (AGC) of < 0.5, which lasted for more than 7 days, occurred in 18 % of the cycles. In regard to non-hematologic toxicity, alopecia was observed in all patients but was very mild. No patient developed severe alopecia or severe stomatitis. Grade II stomatitis occurred in 12 out of 80 cycles. Grade III nausea and vomiting occurred in 11 out of 80 cycles.

A total of 5 patients received a cumulative dose of more than 450 mg/m^2 and only in one of these patients the ejection fraction dropped to < 50 %. This patient received a cumulative dose of 1,005 mg/m^2. No endomyocardial biopsy (EMB) was obtained because the patient went off study due to progression of disease. One patient at a cumulative dose of 1,035 mg/m^2 had an EMB of grade 1.5. Another patient had EMB of 2.0 after he received a cumulative dose of 855 mg/m^2 and he subsequently developed congestive heart failure.

Discussion

This study confirms that THP-adriamycin has definite activity in the treatment of soft tissue sarcomas. However, it is impossible to determine the exact magnitude of this activity because of the small number of patients treated and because the overwhelming majority of the patients received a low dose. More than 80 % of the patients who received the starting dose of 60 mg/m² were eligible for escalation to dose level 90 mg/m². This indicates that the starting dose of 60 mg/m² was relatively low and the recommended dose in future studies should be 90 mg/m². In spite of the fact that the overwhelming majority of patients had received a suboptimum dose, the response rate in this preliminary experience was 30 %.

In regard to toxicity, our study confirms the observation that alopecia is much less severe with THP-Adriamycin as compared to Adriamycin. However, from our data, we cannot determine whether THP-Adriamycin is indeed associated with less cardiac toxicity and less mucositis.

In conclusion, our preliminary data strongly suggest that THP-Adriamycin may have comparable efficacy to Adriamycin in soft tissue sarcomas and is less toxic. We recommend that more patients be treated for a total of at least 50. The starting dose we recommend is 90 mg/m².

References

1. Gottlieb JA (1975) Activity in solid tumors. In : Ghione M, Fetzer J, and Maier H (eds) Ergebnisse der Adriamycin-Therapie. Springer-Verlag, Berlin, pp 95-102
2. O'Bryan RM, Baker LH, Gottlieb JA et al (1977) Dose-response evaluation of Adriamycin in human neoplasias. Cancer 39 : 1940-1948
3. Gottlieb JA, Benjamin RS, Baker LH et al (1976) Role of DTIC (NSC 45399) in the chemotherapy of sarcomas. Cancer Treat Rep 60 : 199-203
4. Benjamin RS, Baker LH, Rodriguez V et al (1977) The chemotherapy of soft-tissue sarcomas in adults. In: Proceedings of the 21st Annual Clinical Conference on Cancer, M. D. Anderson Hospital and Tumor Institute, Nov 1976. Current concepts in the management of primary bone and soft-tissue sarcomas. Year Book Med Publ, Chicago, pp 309-315
5. Tsuruo T, Ida H, Tsukagoshi S et al (1982) 4'-0-Tetrahydropyranyladriamycin as a potential new antitumor agent. Cancer Res 42 : 1462-1467
6. Nakada H, Ogawa M, Miyamoto H et al (1984) Phase II study of 4'-0-Tetrahydropyranyladriamycin (THP-ADM). Gan-To-Kagaku-Ryoho 11 : 138-1421
7. Ogawa M, Miyamota H, Inigaki J, Horikashi N, Ezaki K, Inoue K et al (1983) Phase I clinical trial of a new anthracycline : 4'-0-Tetrahydropyranyladriamycin. Invest New Drugs 1 : 169-172

Abstract. The therapeutic efficacy and toxicity pattern of THP-Adriamycin (THP-ADM) were explored in a phase II study using THP-ADM in combination with DTIC in the treatment of previously untreated advanced soft tissue sarcomas. THP-ADM was given in an infusion over half an hour and DTIC was given in a dose of 1,000 mg/m² over a 2 hour infusion. Cycles were repeated every three weeks. The starting dose of THP-ADM was 60 mg/m² and was increased or decreased depending on the presence or absence of infection, severe stomatitis and/or severe myelosuppression. Seventeen patients were entered into the study but 16 were evaluable for response and toxicity. Thirty-one percent had a partial response, 6 % minor response and 25 % stable disease. The median duration of response was one year. Ninety-four percent of patients who received the first cycle were eligible for dose escalation in the second cycle and also 90 % of those who received the second cycle were eligible for dose increase in the subsequent cycle. Accordingly, the starting dose of 60 mg/m² was relatively low. The dose limiting toxicity was neutropenia. Thrombocytopenia was rare. Alopecia was observed in all patients but was very mild. No patient developed severe alopecia or severe stomatitis. Five patients had a cumulative dose > 450 mg/m², and only one of these developed congestive heart failure. This patient had a cardiac biopsy score of 2 after 855 mg/m². Another patient had a score of 1.5 at 1,035 mg/m². A drop in left ventricular ejection fraction to < 50 occurred in 2 patients who received cumulative doses of 855 mg/m² and 1,005 mg/m². In conclusion, although the starting dose of THP-ADM was low, the response rate in this small number of patients was comparable to that of adequate dose Adriamycin + DTIC. THP-ADM is certainly less toxic than Adriamycin in regard to alopecia but whether it is also less toxic in terms of cardiac toxicity and mucositis, more patients should be treated. Our data suggest that this new analog may be as effective as Adriamycin but less toxic.

Combined approach to malignant small round blue cell neoplasms in the adult

P Casali, P Zucchinelli, A Santoro, F Lombardi, L Gandola,
A Azzarelli, U Pastorino, G Bonadonna

Small round blue cell neoplasms are common malignancies in the childhood but are rare in the adults. They include Ewing's sarcoma, peripheral neuro-epithelioma, and rhabdomyosarcoma. *Ewing's sarcoma* and *peripheral neuro-epithelioma* may arise either from bone or soft tissues and share some biological as well as clinical features [1-3] ; *rhabdomyosarcoma* is a soft tissue sarcoma of the same clinical aggressiveness but with a distinct biological pattern [4]. Only a few case series analyses of adult patients with such neoplasms were reported on. They suggested a poorer prognosis than in the childhood [5-7]. Furthermore, in the adults these tumors are sometimes confused with conventional soft tissue sarcomas and treated accordingly. Therefore, to assess prognostic factors of these tumors in the adults and to enlighten their differences from typical soft tissue sarcomas, we decided to prospectively study a consecutive series of such patients at our institution. They were treated with the same integrated approach, on the model of those employed in childhood tumors. The study is ongoing and preliminary results are provided herein.

Patients and methods

Eligible patients had previously untreated Ewing's sarcoma, peripheral neuro-epithelioma, or rhabdomyosarcoma (either embryonal or alveolar). Patients with bone Ewing's sarcoma were enrolled only if they had *bulky* disease, that is a local lesion greater than 8 cm in the maximal diameter.

Twenty-two evaluable patients (M/F = 15/7 ; median age = 24 yrs, range from 17 to 52 ; PS = from 0 to 2) were enrolled : 6 with local disease ; 9 with bulky local and/or regional disease ; 7 with both local and metastatic disease.

Patients were treated with a combined modality approach including chemotherapy, surgery, and radiotherapy. Primary chemotherapy with Epirubicin 90 mg/m² day 1, Ifosfamide 2,500 mg/m² (with hydration and mesna) x 3 days, and Vincristine was repeated every 3 weeks for 4-6 cycles. Patients whose disease was conservatively resectable were operated on. In all cases radiotherapy (45-60 Gy) followed and was delivered with 2 cycles of Cisplatin 30 mg/m² (with hydration) x 3 days and Vincristine. Treatment consolidation with Ifosfamide 2,500 mg/m² (with hydration and mesna) x 3 days, Actinomycin D 0.5 mg/m² x 3 days, and Dacarbazine 300 mg/m² x 3 days, for 4-6 courses, was eventually administered.

Istituto Nazionale Tumori, Milano, Italy

Results

Tumor response after primary chemotherapy was 86 % (CI : 67 % to 95 %). Of 16 patients who completed their treatment program, 4 were in complete remission after primary chemotherapy, 3 were rendered disease-free by surgery, and 3 by radiotherapy.

With a median follow-up of 15 months, the actuarial two-year disease-free survival of patients with only local disease is 36 %, while all patients with metastases at entry relapsed.

Discussion

Our preliminary data confirm that adult small round blue cell neoplasms respond well to polychemotherapy. Their response rate is different from conventional adult soft tissue sarcomas, in which a response rate averaging 85 % is currently unachievable with available regimens. At least for this reason, therefore, they should be clearly distinguished from typical adult soft tissue sarcomas, both in clinical research and in standard practice.

The impact of integrated approaches is left to be determined, since our data should be regarded as preliminary. However, the high rate of relapses within two years, although on a limited number of patients, demonstrates the clinical aggressiveness of these tumors in adults. Relapses occur both at the local level and systemically. Prospective trials are needed to optimize combined modality approaches in adult patients.

References

1. Dehner LP (1986) Peripheral and central primitive neuro-ectodermal tumors. A nosologic concept seeking a consensus. Arch Pathol Lab Med 110 : 997-1005
2. Miser JS, Kinsella TJ, Triche TJ, Stesi R, Tsokos M, Wesley R et al (1987) Treatment of peripheral neuro-epithelioma in children and young adults. J Clin Oncol 5 : 1752-1758
3. Kinsella TJ, Miser JS, Triche TJ, Horvath K, Glatstein E (1988) Treatment of high-risk sarcomas in children and young adults : analysis of local control using intensive combined modality therapy. NCI Monogr 6 : 291-296
4. Donaldson SS (1989) Rhabdomyosarcoma : contemporary status and future directions. Arch Surg 124 : 1015-1020
5. Lloyd RV, Hajdu SI, Knapper WH (1983) Embryonal rhabdomyosarcoma in adults. Cancer 51 : 557-565
6. Miettinen M (1988) Rhabdomyosarcoma in patients older than 40 years of age. Cancer 62 : 2060-2065
7. Siegel RD, Ryan LM, Antman KH (1988) Adults with Ewing's sarcoma. An analysis of 16 patients at the Dana Farber Cancer Institute. Am J Clin Oncol (CCT) 11 : 614-617

Neo-Adjuvant chemotherapy in the management of appendicular soft tissue sarcomas

P Benedetto, W Mnaymneh, L Ghandur-Mnaymneh, M Joppert, D Robinson, G Morillo

Appendicular soft tissue sarcomas (STS) are relatively rare tumors for which standard surgical and radiotherapeutic techniques have provided high levels of local control. Despite such success, distant disease occurs for approximately half of those patients with intermediate or high grade lesions [1]. Strategies utilizing adjuvant chemotherapy to reduce the incidence of post-operative metastatic disease have yielded varying results [2, 3]. Neo-adjuvant chemotherapy (CT) has become a standard principle of treatment for primary bone tumors, with response to pre-operative therapy predictive of overall outcome [4, 5]. Based on these principles, we designed a program to treat STS patients at high risk for occult metastatic disease.

Materials and methods

Patients included those with a diagnosis of primary non-metastatic STS of an extremity (buttock lesions were allowed, as were patients who failed prior local treatment) with American Joint Committee Stage IIB or greater. Pre-treatment workup included CAT scan of the chest, bone scan and CAT or MRI scan or both of the primary tumor. Subsequent to diagnostic biopsy, Cisplatin at a dose of 100 mg/m² in 1 liter of normal saline was infused over 4h through an arterial catheter placed in a feeding vessel, followed by Adriamycin 25 mg/m²/d x 3 consecutive days IVP. This procedure was repeated at day 21. Three to 4 weeks after the second course of intra-arterial therapy, definitive surgical resection was planned.

Pathologic assessment of the extent of viable tumor remaining was made as follows : the resected specimen was grossly measured in perpendicular diameters to estimate tumor volume and breadloafed at 1.5-2 cm intervals along its longest axis and largest diameter. Slices from the slabs with the greatest amount of identifiable tumor were obtained. Two slabs were routinely examined for tumors less than 5 cm. Following fixation the slices were cut into 2.0 x 1.5 cm blocks, embedded and stained. Each slide was then examined for the presence of identifiable tumor « present » or « not present » and replaced by acute necrosis, hemorrhage, fibrin, granulation tissue, or dense fibrous tissue. A ratio of « identifiable tumor » to « replaced tumor » was estimated visually on each slide as a percentage. The percentages from all slides were then averaged resulting in one final percentage figure (= % viable tumor). The final response to neo-adjuvant treatment expressed as a percent tumor volume reduction was defined as follows :

University of Miami Sylvester Comprehensive Cancer Center, PO Box 016960 (D8-4), Miami, Florida 33136, USA

$$\% = \frac{1 - \% \text{ viable tumor x post-Rx tumor size x } 100}{\text{initial tumor volume}}$$

where the initial volume of tumor was calculated as the product of the 3 largest perpendicular diameters obtained from the prebiopsy CT or MRI scan, the post-Rx tumor size was calculated from the gross description of the resection specimen, and the % viable tumor was obtained as described above.

Patients who achieved a final response of > 50 % were considered responders (R) and were to receive further adjuvant CT utilizing the same drugs and dosages pre-op for a total of 6 courses except that the Cisplatin was administered intravenously. All patients undergoing wide local excision received postoperative RT, unless prior RT had been given, within 6 weeks of surgery, or unless delayed by wound healing or toxicity of therapy. The planned dose of RT was 6660-7020cGy in 180cGy fractions.

Results

Eighteen patients have been treated. Median age was 50 (range 20-77). Primary site was upper extremity, 5 ; lower extremity, 10 ; buttock, 3. Final response > 50 % was observed for 2 of 3 AJCC Stage IIB, 5 (2) of 6 (2) IIIA, and 7 (1) of 9 (1) IIIB patients, the numbers in parentheses representing local failures to prior therapy, for an overall rate of response of 79 % (14/18). Concordance between physical examination, radiologic studies and final pathologic assessment was examined. CT or MRI objectively identified tumor response in only 5 of 11 (45 %) responding patients, significantly underestimating the neo-adjuvant chemotherapy effect.

The toxicity of therapy was significant. Only 4 of 14 patients completed the planned 6 cycles of CT. Twenty of 63 courses of chemotherapy were associated with an episode of granulocytopenic fever. Median nadir WBC count was 0.6 ; median nadir platelet count, 62,000. Two-thirds of patients experienced transient elevations of serum creatinine, 3 with persistent values above 2.1 mg/dl. One patient developed cardiomyopathy despite a cumulative adriamycin dose of 386.8 mg/m^2. This patient is alive 38 months after diagnosis without recurrence with well compensated cardiac function.

One of 14 responders (median follow-up 23.5 months) has relapsed in the lung and is at present salvaged by pulmonary resection. This patient had a 65 % final response. The follow-up of the non responders has been considerably shorter at 9 months. One of 4 patients has recurred locally, salvaged by amputation.

Discussion

This study demonstrates a high response rate as defined above for neo-adjuvant CT in patients with STS not previously reported. It underscores the fact that response is considerably underestimated by presurgical evaluation using standard radiologic techniques. At present, the patient population is small, the follow-up short and the number of relapse events data too scarce to comment on the ultimate endpoint of disease-free survival. Three of the patients in the study had previously failed local therapy with surgery and/or RT. Each has achieved local control for extended periods (19 +, 21 +, 38 + mos) with the neo-adjuvant approach ; 2 without definitive post-operative RT. Whether neo-adjuvant therapy will be predictive of the outcome of patients with soft tissue sarcoma as it has been for osteogenic sarcoma will require further follow-up.

References

1. Chang AE, Rosenberg SA, Glatstein EJ, Antman KA (1989) Sarcomas of soft tis- sues. In : DeVita VT Jr (ed) Cancer, principles and Practice of Oncology. JP Lip- pincott Company, Philadelphia, p 1360
2. Rosenberg SA, Chang AE, Glatstein E (1985) Adjuvant chemotherapy for treatment of extremity soft tissue sarcomas : review of the NCI experience. Cancer Treatment Symp 3 : 83-88
3. Lerner HJ, Amato DA, Savlov ED, et al (1987) Eastern Cooperative Oncology Group : a comparison of adjuvant doxorubicin and observation for patients with localized soft tissue sarcoma. J Clin Onc 5 : 613-617
4. Rosen G, Nirenberg A, Caparros B (1981) Osteogenic sarcoma : eighty-percent, three- year, disease-free survival with combination chemotherapy (T-7). Natl Cancer Inst Monogr 56 : 213-220
5. Raymond AK, Chawla SP, Carrasco H (1987) Osteosarcoma chemotherapy effect : a prognostic factor. Seminars in Diagnostic Pathology 4 : 212-236

Hematosarcomas

Neo-Adjuvant treatment in locally advanced thymoma

A Fornasiero, O Daniele, C Ghiotto, D Bernardi, F Rea*,
F Calabro*, MV Fiorentin

Malignant thymomas are relatively rare neoplasms, representing about 0.2 %
to 1.5 % of all malignancies : the main cause of death is due to locoregional
spread and, less frequently, distant metastases [1, 2].

Chemotherapy has usually been administered only after surgical and/or
radiation therapy to patients with unresectable or progressive disease.

The efficacy of the ADOC schedule [3, 4] encouraged us to use it in the
locally advanced disease (as preoperative administration).

Materials and methods

Sixteen patients with locally advanced malignant thymoma (7 males, 9 females)
were treated at our Unit from 1986 to 1990 with ADOC chemotherapy combination, as neo-adjuvant treatment.

All patients were treated with a combination of 50 mg/m² of cisplatin intravenously and 40 mg/m² of doxorubicin on day 1, 0.6 mg/m² of vincristine on
day 3 and 700 mg/m² of cyclophosphamide on day 4 (the cycle was repeated
every 3 weeks).

The stages were classified as suggested by Masaoka [5], and there were
12 patients stage III, 3 patients stage IVa and 1 patient stage IVb.

We administered 4 cycles of ADOC chemotherapy, because our previous
experience [6] demontrated that the maximum response to the treatment occurs
with 4 cycles.

Results

Ten patients obtained a major clinical response to the treatment and underwent an explorative thoracotomy with a radical resection ; a pathologically confirmed complete remission was found in 5. Six patients had non radical surgical approach.

The patients with histologically complete remission were treated with 2 further cycles of ADOC chemotherapy, while the remaining patients were submitted to radiotherapy.

* Divisione di Oncologia Medica, Clinica Chirurgica I, ULSS 21, 35100 Padova, Italy

Toxicity

The treatment was well tolerated. Nausea, vomiting and alopecia occurred at various degrees in all patients. Myelosuppression was the major drug-related toxicity, but never toxic deaths were noted. Renal and cardiac functions ramained normal throughout the study.

Discussion

In 1986 we have designed a pilot study to evaluate a combined modalities program to improve the results in the treatment of invasive thymoma.

Radiation therapy can assure a local control of the disease, especially with a limited extent of the tumor, but its use as adjuvant post-surgical therapy, or in unresectable disease, as a first line treatment, often failed to prevent distant metastases [7].

Moreover, some Centers reported that all objective responses to chemotherapy occurred in non-irradiated patients or in areas of disease not previously irradiated. So, it seems justified to consider radiotherapy as a second line treatment for a large invasive thymomas, while chemotherapy should be given at first.

The rationale for a surgical approach, if possible after chemotherapy, consist in a more appropriate restaging with histologic confirmation and in the resection of a residual tumor (debulking), in order to facilitate further treatments.

References

1. Batata MA, Martini N, Huvos AG (1974) Thymomas-Clinicopathologic features, therapy and prognosis. Cancer 34 : 389-396
2. Verley JM, Hollmann KH (1985) Thymoma : a comparative study of clinical stages, histologic features, and survival in 200 cases. Cancer 55 : 1074-1086
3. Fornasiero A, Daniele O, Sperandio P (1984) Chemotherapy of invasive or metastatic thymoma : report of 11 cases. Cancer Treat Rep 68 : 1205-1210
4. Fornasiero A, Daniele O, Ghiotto C (1990) Chemotherapy of invasive thymoma. J Clin Oncol 8 (8) : 1419-1423
5. Masaoka A, Monden Y, Nakahara K (1981) Follow-up study of thymomas with special references to their clinical stages. Cancer 48 : 2485-2492
6. Fornasiero A, Daniele O, Morandi P (1988) neo-adjuvant chemotherapy in invasive thymoma. Second International Congress on Neo-Adjuvant chemotherapy, Paris 19-21 February
7. Monden Y, Nakahara K, Lioka S (1985) Recurrence of thymoma ; clinicopathological feature, therapy and prognosis. Ann Thorac Surgery 39 : 165-169

Abstract. The efficacy of the ADOC treatment (Adriamycin 40 mg/m² day 1, Cisplatin 50 mg/m² day 1, Oncovin 1 mg day 3 and Cyclophosphamide

750 mg/m² day 4) in metastatic thymoma [3, 4] encouraged us to use it in the locally advanced disease as well. A previous experience of ours (Paris feb. 19-21 1988) demonstrated that the maximum response to the treatment occurs with 4 cycles of chemotherapy. Since 1986 16 patients with locally advanced thymoma (7 males, 9 females ; 12 stage III, 3 stage IVA and 1 IVB according to Masaoka) have been treated with 4 cycles of the ADOC schedule prior to surgery. Ten patients with a clinical response > 70 % underwent radical surgical resection : 5 of them had no hystological residues of neoplasia. Six patients had non-radical surgical therapy. In our opinion, in locally advanced thymoma the first approach is chemotherapy ; in case of a complete clinical response (or higher than 70 %) surgery follows, otherwise radiotherapy consolidates the results obtained with chemotherapy.

Neo-Adjuvant chemotherapy in locally advanced invasive thymomas

AJ Lacave, E Estrada, JA Estrada, C Penin, I Palacio, LMG de Sande, J Cueva, J Rodriguez

Postoperative mediastinal irradiation has been the classical treatment for patients with residual invasive thymomas,but less than 50 % of these patients are free from disease after 5 years [1-2]. In many short reports, chemotherapy has shown activity both in local and metastatic disease [3-5]. Some authors conclude that combination chemotherapy is effective in the first-line post-surgical treatment of incompletely resected thymoma [5]. Considering that Prednisone (P), Adriamycin (A), Iphosphamide (I) and Cisplatin (D) are anticancer drugs proven effective as single agents, we began a study with a combination of these 4 drugs in patients with locally advanced thymomas as neo-adjuvant chemotherapy trying to improve the results.

Material and methods

The pathological classification followed in this study was one that was proposed by Verley and Hollman [6]. All the histologic sections were revised by a pathologist (CP). Immuno-histochemical analysis was performed for this report.

Patients judged to have unresectable tumor by thoracotomy or mediastinoscopy, or patients with partialy resectable tumor with residual disease invading adjacent structures such as pericardium, vessels and pleura, were included in the study. Other selection factors included : no previous treatment with chemotherapy, radiotherapy and adequate cardiac, liver and renal functions.

All patients were treated with a combination of Prednisone 100 mg/m² p.o. daily d1-5, Adriamycin 40-50 mg/m² i.v. d1, Iphosphamide 4 g/m² i.v. d1 and Cisplatin 50 mg/m² i.v. d1 (PAID). Cycles were repeated every 4 weeks. Drug dose was reduced in cases of severe mucositis, renal insufficiency or severe myelosuppresion. The number of cycles was given until maximum response or a maximum of 6. Radiotherapy was proposed to be administered 4-5 weeks after finishing chemotherapy and patients were treated with Co 60 or 18 Mv photons to a tumor-dose of 45-55 Gy (1,8-2 Gy per fraction) 5 fractions weekly, with parallel opposite fields.

Criteria of response and grades of toxicities were used as defined by the WHO [7]. Disease free survival was measured from day 1 of chemotherapy to the first evidence of progression after finishing radiotherapy. Survival time was measured from day 1 of chemotherapy to the day of death. Clinical staging was done according to the criteria of Masaoka et al [8].

Servicio de Oncologia Médica, Hospital General de Asturias, Oviedo, Spain

Results

From October 1986 until February 1991, 4 consecutive patients were treated. In 1 of the patients, previously diagnosed as undifferentiated thymoma, a germ cell tumor was found in the biopsy taken from a vertebral recurrence. When we reviewed the first biopsy we realized that there was not enough material to provide an accurate histological diagnosis. The characteristics of the 3 evaluable patients are described in Table 1.

Table 1. Patients characteristics

Clinical feature	Case 1	Case 2	Case 3
Sex	F	F	F
Age	51	53	19
Stage	IIIa	IIIa	IIIa
Histology	Epithelial	Spindle	Lymphocitic
Resection	Partial	No	Partial
Infiltration	Yes	Yes	Yes
Associate syndrome	No	No	Raynaud and rhinitis

The results in a correlative way (case 1, 2 and 3) were : responses (CR, PR, CR ; number of cycles received (3, 5, 3) ; interval to radiotherapy (4, 8 and 4 weeks) — before receiving radiotherapy case 2 progressed — ; tumor dose administered in Gy (4.6, 5.5, 4.5) ; clinical status after finishing radiotherapy (CR, PR, CR) ; disease free survival in months (33 +, 3,48 +) and overall survival in months (33 +, 19 +, 48 +).

The maximum toxicity per patient was recorded. Vomiting and alopecia grade 3 were present in all 3 cases. Stomatitis grade 3 was developed in case 1 when the dose of Adriamycin was escalated to 50 mg/m^2 in the second cycle. Also case 3 had aplasia after the first cycle with the 50 mg/m^2 of Adriamycin. Case 2 always received 40 mg/m^2 in all 5 cycles and no cases of severe toxicity were present in this patient.

Discussion

The early administration (before radiotherapy) of the PAID combination seems to be effective in the therapeutic management of invasive thymomas. It is not easy to compare our data with other data of the literature due to the small number or patients treated in our study and the relatively recent application of neo-adjuvant chemotherapy in invasive thymomas, resulting in a certain lack of general experience in this subject.

We will continue with this PAID combination considering that these 4 drugs are the most active single agents in the treatment of thymomas. We believe that the appropriate dose of Adriamycin in this combination is 40 mg/m². Only randomized trials could prove whether the disease-free survival and overall survival could be prolonged by neo-adjuvant chemotherapy, but the rarity of this tumor make it difficult to carry out a comparative clinical study.

References

1. Rosenberg JC (1989) Neoplasms of the mediastinum. In : de Vita VT, Hellman S, Rosemberg SA (ed) Philadelphia JB Lippincott Company, p 706-724
2. Curran WJ, Kornstein MJ, Brooks JJ et al (1988) Invasive thymoma : the role of mediastinal irradiation following complete or incomplete surgical resection. J Clin Oncol 6 : 1722-1727
3. Salyer WR, Eggleston JC (1976) thymoma : a clinical and pathological study of 65 cases. Cancer 37 : 229-249
4. Kosmidis PA, Iliopoulos E and Pentea S (1988) Combination chemotherapy with cyclophosphamide, adriamycin, and vincristine in malignant thymoma and myasthemia gravis. Cancer 61 : 1736-1740
5. Göldel N, Böning L, Fredrik A et al (1989) Chemotherapy of invasive thymoma : a retrospective study of 22 cases. Cancer 63 : 1493-1500
6. Verley JM and Hollman AK (1985) Thymoma : a comparative study of clinical stages, istologic features and survival in 200 cases. Cancer 55 : 1074-1086
7. WHO (1979) Handbook for reporting results of cancer treatment. Geneva, World Health Organization
8. Masaoka A, Yasumasa M, Nakahara K et al (1981) Follow-up study of thymomas with special reference to their clinical stages. Cancer 48 : 2485-2492

Neo-Adjuvant chemotherapy for invasive thymoma : an interim analysis

P Macchiarini*, A Chella*, F Ducci**, B Rossi***, G Bevilacqua****, CA Angeletti*

The therapeutic indexes of surgery and/or radiotherapy for invasive thymoma (IT) are often limited by either local involvement of unresectable structure (s) or tumor dissemination outside the radiation fields. An important step forward has been systemic chemotherapy, the efficacy of which has been demonstratedeither as first-line or as adjuvant therapy [1, 2].

This and the provided rationales [3] of neo-adjuvant chemotherapy (NC) stimulated the design of a prospective, single-arm study investigating NC for IT, and preliminary data are presented.

Materials and methods

Eligibility was restricted to previously untreated patients aged less than 75 years with histologically confirmed and clinically staged IIIa IT [4], ECOG PS of 0-3, measurable disease, adequate bone marrow reserve, liver, renal and cardiac function. Initial work-up included a complete history and physical exam, chest X-ray, total-body CT scan and ultrasound, bone [67] Gallium scans. Tumor specimens were pathologically classified according to Rosai and Levine [5]. NC included 3 courses of intravenous cisplatin (75 mg/m^2, day 1), epirubicin (100 mg/m^2, day 1), and etoposide (120 mg/m^2, days 1, 3 and 5), repeated every 3 weeks [6]. After 3 courses, complete or partial responders were submitted to surgery.

Those patients showing either stable or progressive disease were crossed over to radiotherapy (RT). Post-operative RT was given to tumor-bearing areas at doses of 45 Gy (complete resection) or 60 Gy (incomplete resection) over 5 or 6 weeks, respectively.

Results

Between 1/1988 and 6/1990, 7 eligible patients were enrolled ; their demographic data and outcome are shown on Table 1. The total number of courses delivered was 21 ; mean WBC, granulocyte, platelet and hemoglobin nadirs were 1922.2/mm^3, 639.5/mm^3, 115,000/mm^3 and 10.55 g/dl respectively, but a complete recovery by day 21 was obtained in the majority of patients. Non-hematological toxicity included mainly stomatitis, alopecia and nausea and vomiting, usually mild to moderate. The time between start of NC and sur-

Service of Thoracic Surgery* and Radiotherapy**, Institutes of Neurology*** and Pathological Anatomy**** University of Pisa, Pisa, Italy

Table 1. Demographic data of the 7 patients with Invasive Thymoma

Patients No/Sex/Age	ECOG	MG	Clinical Signs	(pre-Surgical Histology)	Extent Tumor	Objective Response	Type of Surgery	Post-Surgical Histology	Radiation Fields: Doses
1/M/51	2	—	SVCS (II)	CT-G needle (E*)	Pleura, pericardium, great vessels	>75%	CR	E*	H:46 Gy
2/F/47	1	—	SVCS (I)	Mediastinotomy (L)	Pleura, Lung great vessels	>50- 75%	PR (R2)	L	H:60 Gy
3/M/26	3	III	—	Echo-guided needle (E*)	Pleura, Lung great vessels	>50 75%	PR (R1)	E*	H:60 Gy
4/M/32	2	—	SVCS (II)	Echo-guided needle (E*)	Pleura, pericardium,	>75%	CR	negative	H:45 Gy
5/M/55	1	—	Chest pain	CT-G needle (E*)	Pleura, pericardium	>75%	CR	E*	H:45 Gy
6/M/62	1	—	Cought	CT-G needle (E)	Pleura, Lung pericardium, great vessels	>50- 75%	PR (R1)	E	H:60 Gy
7/M/42	1	IIa	Chest pain	CT-G needle (L)	Pleura, Lung pericardium	>75%	CR	negative	H:45 Gy

MG: Myasthenia gravis (graded according to Osserman et al., 1971); SVCS: superior vena cava syndrome (graded according to Bariety M and Coury C, 1958); Echo-C: echographic-guided; CT-G: computed-tomography guided; CR: complete resection; PR: incomplete resection; R1: microscopic residual tumor; R2: macroscopic residual tumor; Histology: E: epithelial invasive thymoma ; L: Lymphatic invasive thymoma; *thymic carcinoma; H: involved radiation field

gery ranged from 12 to 15 weeks. There were neither major technical difficulties induced by NC nor operative mortality. Histology of surgical specimens was negative for 2 completely resected patients. Six patients are currently alive and disease-free ; 1 patient died while disease-free from massive pulmonary embolism following craniotomy for a grade IV brain astrocytoma.

Discussion

Preliminary data might provide prima facie evidence that NC is a new therapeutic window and likely to play a major and expanding role in the management of IT. NC was well tolerated and resulted in an acceptable toxicity. More interestingly, it induced a 100 % tumor shrinkage, reversing in all instances an unresectable tumor in a resectable one. This without increasing the surgical-related morbidity and mortality rate. The strict relationship observed among degree of tumor shrinkage, complete resection rate and presence of thymoma cells in post-surgical specimens addresses the issues whether surgical resection should be attempted only after maximum tumor responses to NC (e.g. > 75 %) and/or post-operative RT is worthwhile for completely resected patients displaying features of tumor necrosis. Preliminary data suggest that NC is feasible and might represent a major therapeutic advance for IT ; however, it appears premature to recommend it as a standard therapy until a larger number of patients and longer follow-up are available.

References

1. Uematsu M and Kondo M (1986) A proposal for treatment of invasive thymoma. Cancer 58 : 1979-1984
2. Fornasiero A, Daniele O, Ghiotto C et al (1990) Chemotherapy of invasive thymoma. J Clin Oncol 8 : 1419-1423
3. Frei E III (1988) What's in a name-neo-adjuvant. J Natl Cancer Inst 80 : 1088-1089
4. Verley JM and Hollmann KH (1985) Thymoma : a comparative study of clinical stages, histologic features and survival in 200 cases. Cancer 55 : 1074-1086
5. Rosai J and Levine GD (1976) Tumors of the thymus/ In : atlas of Tumor Pathology, Fascicle 13. Washington, DC : Armed Forces Institutes of Pathology
6. Macchiarini P, Chella A, Riva A et al (1990) Feasibility phase II study of high-dose epirubicin-based regimens for untreated patients with small cell lung cancer. Am J Clin Oncol 13 : 495-500

Involvement of the Interleukin 2/Interleukin 2-receptor system in the proliferation of human immature leukemic T cells

Y Sahraoui, M Allouche, E Spanakis, C Clemenceau, C Jasmin, M Perraki, C Varella-Millot, V Georgoulias

The mechanisms regulating the proliferation of immature T cells are yet elucidated. Previous studies investigating the involvement of IL2/IL2-R system presented evidence that some subsets of human thymocytes (CD2⁻CD8⁻ cells) can express IL2-binding chains and respond to rIL2 [1-2]. More recently, Toribio et al [3] showed that IL2-Rα negative prothymocytes constitutively express IL2-Rβ chains and produce their own IL2 ; the interaction of IL2 with IL2-Rβ induces the expression of IL2-Rα chain and the formation of high affinity IL2-R, thus, suggesting, an IL2-dependent autocrine growth pathway at this stage of T-cell differentiation.

Cells form T-cell Acute Lymphoblastic Leukemias (T-ALL) or T-cell non-Hodgkin's Lymphomas (T-NHL) are often viewed as a clonal expansion of thymocytes « frozen » at different stages of T cell differentiation, and can be used as a model to define the proliferation mechanisms of immature T cells. We have previously reported that clonogenic cells from some T-ALL patients could proliferate spontaneously in semi-solid media ; moreover, in some cases where a low plating efeciency was observed, low concentrations of exogenous recombinant IL2 (rIL2) could enhance colony growth. Both spontaneous and IL2-induced colony growth could be inhibited by monoclonal antibodies (moAb) against IL2-Ra and IL2 [4] suggesting that the IL2/IL2-R system is involved in the proliferation of some T-ALL clonogenic cells.

Materials and methods

Cells

Mononuclear cells were obtained from peripheral blood, bone marrow, pleural effusion or mediastinal tumor from 17 patients with T-ALL or T-NHL by Ficoll-Paque density centrifugation and in all cases blast-enriched cells were used. Phenotypic analysis was performed using appropriate moAbs. Cell proliferation was evaluated by a standard [3H] TdR incorporation assay. Binding of ^{125}I-rIL2 was performed according to Robb et al [5] and the number of binding sites/cell and the dissociation constant (Kd) were evaluated by Scatchard analysis. IL2-Ra mRNA of T-ALL cells was analysed by Northern blot whereas production of IL2 by T-ALL cells was tested in media conditioned by T-ALL cells.

Oncogénèse Appliquée, INSERM U268, Hôpital Paul Brousse, 94800 Villejuif, France and School of Medicine, Department of Clinical Oncology, University of Crete, G-71409, Greece

Results

Leukemic cells did not constituvely express IL2-Ra since only in 2 patients 10 %
and 8 % of the cells could be stained with an anti-IL2-Ra moAb. However,
Tac mRNA trancripts were present in T leukemic cells from all patients tested
(Fig. 1). In addition in 5 out of 12 cases tested, 8-13 % of T-ALL cells could
be stained by the TU-27 moAb. A 24 h cell incubation with culture medium,
without adding mitogens, FCS, or growth factors, induced a substantial Tac
expression in 5 out of 13 patients (11-83 % positive cells ; Table 1).

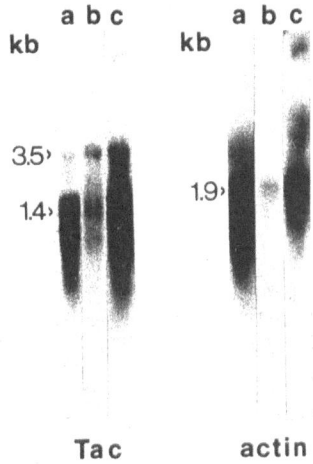

Fig. 1.

Hybridization of mRNA extracted form 2 T-
ALL cells (lanes b and c and norm PHA-blasts
(lane a) with a Tac cDNA probe

Binding experiments with 125 I-rIL2 under high affinity conditions using
fresh leukemic cells from 7 T-ALL patients revealed, in 3 patients, a low number of high affintiy IL2-R(114-200/cell with a Kd ranging between 101 and
181 pM (Table 2).

Aliquots of 1-3 10 fresh cells were incubated for 2 h at 4°C with serial
dilutions of 125 I-rIL2, and the radioactivity of separated supernatants and
precipitated cells was counted. Non-specific binding was estimated by adding
a 500 fold excess cold rIL2.

Cells from patient no 16 were tested both fesh and after a 24 h incubation
in RPMI 1640. Normal peripheral blood MNC were stimulated for 48 h with
PHA-P (0.1 %v/v). Cultured cells were extensively washed, incubated for 1 h
at 37°C, and washed again before performing the binding assay.

Culture supernatants from 10 out of 13 patients' cells were found to contain IL2 activity when tested either in a colorimetric or/and an immuno-
enzymatic assay. IL2-dependent proliferatin of T-ALL cells demonstrated a
dose-dependent rIL2-induced proliferation in 6 out of 15 (40 %) cases. In all
cases proliferating cells displayed a phenotype compatible with stage I or III
but not with stage II of T cell differentiation. IL2-responsivenes was seen with

Table 1. Spontaneous expression of IL2-Ra (Tac) on T-ALL cells incubated with culture medium

Patient	%Tac[+]cells[1]		Detection of Tac mRNA transcripts[2]
	0h	24h	
1	1	0	ND[3]
2	0	16	ND
3	3	69	+
4	0	26	+
5	0	1	+
6	3	3	+
8	0	0	+
9	0	1	+
10	5	3	ND
11	0	1	ND
13	3	11	+
15	0	0	+
16	6	83	+
17	0	0	+

[1] MNC or blast-enriched cell fractions from T-ALL/T-NHL patients were stained with the 10T14 MoAb, immediately after separation (0h), or after a 24h incubation in RPMI 1640, in the absence of FCS (24h).
[2] RNA was extracted from 1-7-108 fresh or cropreserved leukemic cells and was hydribized with a Tac cDNA probe.
[3] Not determined.

Table 2. High affinity binding of 125 I-rIL2 to unstimulated leukemic cells from T-ALL patients

Patients	Cells	Sites/cell	Kd(pM)	%Tac[+]cells
9	Fresh MNC	200	181	0
12	Fresh MNC	114	101	8
16	Fresh MNC	100	115	6
16	24h incubation with culture medium	180	107	55
Normal PHA-blasts	48h stimulation with PHA	3 500	105	85

low concentrations of rIL2 (up 200 pM) and was inhibited by anti-Tac MoAb (Table 3), indicating the specific effect of IL2-induced proliferation on leukemic cells.

Table 3. Inhibition of IL2-induced proliferation of T-ALL cells by anti-Tac MoAb

Patient	3H-TdR incorporation (cpm ± SD)		% of inhibition by anti-Tac mAb		
	$-IL2$	$+IL2$	10^{-3}	10^{-4}	10^{-5}
1	6942 ± 1337	19575 ± 1772	ND[1]	42	27
5	476 ± 122	2285 ± 171	74	52	49
16	355 ± 143	20.16 ± 1445	94	23	17

Blasts from T-ALL patients were pre-incubated with various concentrations of anti-Tac moAb (10^{-6} -10^{-5} v/v of ascites) before being seeded in microtiter plates at 2.10^5 cells/well in the absence or presence of 200 pM (patients n° 1 and 5) or 500 pM (patient n° 16) rIL2. [³H]-TdR incorporation was determined, as described in Materials and Methods. ND[1] (Table 3), not determined (Table 3).

Discussion and conclusion

The results reported here clearly indicate, that immature leukemic cells from some T-ALL patients may respond specifically to rIL2. Indeed, blast cells from 40 % of the studied patients can proliferate in vitro in the presence of a whole range of rIL2 concentrations corresponding, on the basis of binding experiments on normal T cells, to high and intermediate affinity IL2-R [6-11]. In addition, our findings demonstrate that leukemic T cells from the majority of the patients tested release spontaneously an IL2 activity, which was also reactive in an immuno-enzymatic assay using two moAbs recognizing distinct epitopes of IL2 ; thus, these observations strongly suggest that cells release a molecule which is biologically and immunologically very close to IL2. However, in some cases the quantities of secreted IL2 must be very low since its biologic activity could be detected only after concentration of conditioned media. Although immunofluorescence staining of T-ALL cells failed to detect IL2-Rα⁺ cells, Northern analysis of total cellular RNA with a Tac cDNA probe revealed a constitutive presence of specific Tac mRNA transcripts, irrespectively of the in vitro IL2-dependent proliferation of the cells. Therefore, it seems likely that leukemic T-ALL cells display a constitutive expression of IL2-Rα gene and, probably, a very low number of corresponding molecules on the cell surface. This was confirmed by ^{125}I-rIL2 binding experiments, which demonstrated the presence of a low number (less than 200 sites/cell) of high affinity IL2-R in 3 T-ALL cases. Although, the failure to detect IL2-Rα on leukemic T-ALL cells by immunofluorescence could be attributed to the low number of expressed receptors, we cannot, however, completely exclude the possibility that IL2-Rα chains are either down modulated or/and masked by the IL2 activity which was spontaneously secreted by leukemic T cells.

In some patients, high concentrations of rIL2, corrsponding to intermediate affinity IL2-R, could not induce cell proliferation although cells expressed the IL2-Rα chain displayed a constitutive IL2-Rα mRNA expression and could spontaneously release IL2 activity. In addition, the detection of high affinity IL2-binding sites, or the expression of Tac molecules during the culture period were not always correlated with an IL2-induced proliferation. The reasons for these discrepancies are not obvious. Several factors could be responsible for this heterogeneity such as abnormalities of the signal transduction mediated by IL2-Rβ chain in some leukemic T cells, and/or a defect of association of IL2-Rα and IL2-Rβ chains. Moreover, we cannot exclude that some leukemic cells « frozen » at a given differantiation stage require, in addition to IL2, other lymphokines for their in vitro proliferation. It has been reported that Tumor Necrosis Factor (TNF) induces the expression of IL2-Rα chain in normal mature T cells [12] whereas interleukin 4 (IL4) has been, recently, shown to exert an important action on the function and configuration of high affinity IL2-R on anti-m-activated leukemic cells form patients with B-cell Chronic Lymphocytic Leukemia [13].

In conclusion, our findings demonstrated that IL2 could be involved in the proliferation process of some immature T-ALL cells but other leukemic cells have lost, for yet unknown reasons, their sensibility to the IL2/IL2-R system.

References

1. Shimonkevitz R, Husmann L, Bevean M, Crispe T (1987) Transient expression of IL2-receptor precedes the differentiation of immature thymocytes. Nature 329 : 157
2. Reem G, Yeh N, Urdal D, Kilian P, Farrar J (1985) Induction and upregulation by interleukin 2 of high-affinity interleukin 2 receptors on thymocytes and T cells. Proc Natl Acad Sci USA 82 : 8663
3. Toribio M, Gutiérez-Ramos J, Pezzi L, Marcos M, Martinez C (1989) Interleukin 2-depenedent autocrine proliferation in T-cell development. Nature 342 : 82
4. Georgoulias V, Alluche M, Salvatore A, Clemenceau C, Jasmin C (1987) Interleukin 2 responsiveness of immature T-cell colony-forming cells (T-CFC) from patients with Acute T-cell Lymphoblstic Leukemias. Cell Immunol 105 : 317
5. Robb R, Greene W, Rusk C (1984) Low and high affinity cellular receptors for Interleukin 2. Implications for the level of Tac antigen. J Exp Med 160 : 1126
6. Sharon M, Klausner R, Cullen B, Chizzonite R, Leonard W (1986) Novel Interleukin-2 receptor subunit detected by cross-linking under high affinity conditions. Science 234 : 859
7. Tsudo M, Kozak R, Goldman C, Waldmann T (1986) Demonstration of a non-Tac peptide that binds Interleukn 2 : a potential participant in a multichain Interleukin 2 receptor complex. Proc Natl Acad Sci (USA) 83 : 9694
8. Tsudo M, Kozak R, Godman C, Waldmann T (1987) Contribution of a p75 Interleukin 2 binding peptide to a high-affinity Interleukin 2 receptor complex Proc Natl Acad Sci (USA) 84 : 4215
9. Teshigawara K, Wang H, Kato K, Smith K (1987) Interleukin 2 high-affinity receptor expression requires two distinct proteins J Exp Med 165 : 233
10. Robb R, Rusk C, Yodoi J, Greene W (1987) Interleukin 2 binding molecule distinct from the Tac protein : analysis of its role in formation of high affinity receptors. Proc Natl Acad Sci (USA) 84 : 2002

11. Dukowitch M, Wano T, Thûy Ly T, Katz P, Cullen B, Kehrl J, Greene W (1987)
    A second human Interleukin-2 binding protein that may be a component of high
    affinity Interleukin-2 receptors. Nature 327 : 518
12. Lowenthal J, Ballard D, Bogerd H, Böhnlein E, Greene W (1986) Tumor Necrosis
    Factor-activation of the IL2 receptor-a involves the induction of KB-specific DNA
    binding proteins J Immunol 142 : 3121
13. Karran S, Dautry-Varsat A, Tsudo M, Merle-Beral H, Debre P, Galanaud P (1990)
    IL4 inhibits the expression of high affinity IL2 receptors on monoclonal human
    B cells J Immunol 145 : 1152

Abstract. Leukemic cells from 6 out of 17 T-ALL/T-NHL patients with a prothymocyte or mature thymocyte, but not common thymocyte phenotype, could proliferate, in a dose dependent manner, in response to rIL2 and anti-Tac moAb could inhibit this IL2-induced cell proliferation. Both crude or/and Amicon-concentrated media conditioned by T-ALL cells from 10 of 13 patients contained IL2 activity. Although less than 10 % of fresh leukemic cells expressed IL2-Rα chain, a 24 h cell incubation in the absence of any mitogenic stimulation induced IL2-Rα expression in 5 of 13 patients. Tac mRNA transcripts could be detected in fresh cells from all 10 patients tested. Four to 13 % of leukemic cells also expressed IL2-Rβ chain and binding experiments with ^{125}I-rIL2 showed a small number of high affinity IL2-R on fresh cells from 3 T-ALL patients. These observations suggest that an IL2/IL2-R-dependent mechanism could be involved in the proliferation of some T-ALL cells.

Pharmacokinetic

Issues in multidrug resistance

WT Beck, MK Danks, T Funabiki

Tumor cell resistance to multiple « natural product » anticancer drugs, known as multidrug resistance (MDR), is now a well-documented phenomenon, and some excellent reviews have recently summarized its pharmacology and cell and molecular biology [1-5]. Several types of natural product MDR have been described : one is associated with P-glycoprotein overexpression (Pgp-MDR) [1-5], another with alterations in DNA topoisomerase II (at-MDR) [6], and a third with features similar to Pgp-MDR but without Pgp overexpression [7, 8]. Although Pgp-MDR appears to have clinical correlates, we do not yet know about the clinical relevance of other forms of MDR.

Key issues in MDR

Pgp-MDR

While we know much about the expression of Pgp-MDR and are learning more about at-MDR, important questions remain. For example, we need to ask whether Pgp expression correlates with clinical response. To do this, we need to be able to reliably detect and quantitate Pgp expression. Pgp expression is often determined by analysis of mdr1 mRNA [9, 10] or Pgp itself [11]. Blotting methods are inadequate in that they do not permit assessment of the percent of individual cells in a tumor that may express Pgp. By contrast, single-cell detection methods permit identification of the number of cells that express Pgp, but a key question still remains : What is the clinical significance of a low percentage of cells expressing Pgp ?

Others issues relate to the apparent binding sites on Pgp for drugs, such as vinblastine and daunorubicin and modulators of Pgp-MDR, such as verapamil, cyclosporin A, and progesterone. It is well-established that these agents bind to Pgp [12-14], but the actual peptides or amino acids in Pgp that are involved in this binding are unknown. It will be important to determine whether such sites exist or whether these agents — all of which are relatively hydrophobic — fit into a hydrophobic pore or channel produced by the protein. Given that, there appear to be some important structural requirements for the modulators of Pgp-MDR [15], it is likely that specific binding or recognition sites exist. If that premise is correct, then one can ask whether it is possible to design agents that can selectively inhibit tumor cell Pgp with minimal effect on the normal tissue protein.

Department of Biochemical and Clinical Pharmacology, St. Jude Children's Research Hospital, 332 N. Lauderdale, Memphis, Tennessee 38101, USA

At-MDR

The most important question at this point is whether at-MDR has clinical relevance. We know that the mdr1 gene or Pgp are not expressed in all tumors from clinically drug resistant patients [9]. Further, we know that it is relatively easy to select at-MDR cell lines experimentally [16]. We also know that many of the drugs that can select for at-MDR — anthracyclines, epipodophyllotoxins, and aminoacridines — are used widely in the clinic. Accordingly, we suggest that tumor cells expressing the at-MDR phenotype will be found in patients' tumors. We are currently developing functional and molecular biological methods to test this hypothesis. Using Pgp-MDR as a paradigm, we have extensively characterized the biochemical lesions associated with this phenotype [16-20] and these have been summarized elsewhere [6].

Functional assays for MDR

While detection of expression of Pgp and altered topoisomerase II in tumor cells is very important, it is also necessary to determine whether the proteins produced have biological activity and their expression has functional consequences. For example, we know that not all Pgps expressed in tumor cells are functional [21]. Accordingly, we have developed a functional assay that may allow us to determine whether these two forms of MDR are expressed in tumors and whether these phenotypes have relevance to the chemotherapeutic responsiveness of the patient. We have modified an assay that quantitates drug-stimulated topoisomerase II-DNA complexes in intact tumor cells [22, 23]. Since that anti-topoisomerase II drugs will « stimulate » the formation of such complexes [18], and many anti-topo II drugs, especially epipodophyllotoxins and anthracyclines, are substrates for Pgp, it is possible to distinguish between the two phenotypes by measuring the formation of complexes in the absence and presence of verapamil, an inhibitor of the efflux function of Pgp. Thus, as seen in Table 1, VM-26 will stimulate fewer complexes in cells expressing either Pgp-MDR or at-MDR, compared to drug-sensitive cells, but when Pgp-MDR cells are co-treated with VM-26 and verapamil, Pgp will be inhibited, intracellular drug levels will increase, and complex formation will be increased. However, in the at-MDR cells, which express little or no Pgp [6], the effect of verapamil will be either attenuated or non-existent. We have applied this assay to the AML blasts of our patients, and our results will be reported elsewhere. Whether this functional assay will correlate with clinical response remains to be determined.

Conclusion

With the experimental description of several forms of MDR, it is imperative to determine their clinical relevance. To do so, reliable methods are needed

Table 1. Distinguishing between cells that express Pgp-MDR and those that express at-MDR by an intact cell DNA-protein complex formation assay*

Cell Line	Fold-Increase in DNA-Topoisomerase II Complexes	
	30 μM VM-26	30 μM VM-26 + 10 μM verapamil
CEM	7.1	7.7
CEM/VLB$_{5K}$	3.3	8.1
CEM/VM-1	0.9	1.2

*Cells were incubated with ^{3}H-thymidine and ^{14}C-leucine for 18 h to label DNA and protein, respectively. Cells were then washed and incubated with VM-26 $\pm$ verapamil for another 30 min, after which they were washed. DNA-protein complexes were precipitated with K$^+$-SDS and quantitated by liquid scintillation counting, as described [22, 23]

not only to detect these several forms of resistance, but also to determine their functional relevance to the chemotherapeutic responsiveness of the patient. Such efforts will also have importance for the development and clinical utilization of modulators or other agents to overcome these types of MDR.

References

1. Beck WT (1987) The cell biology of multiple drug resistance. Biochem Pharmacol 36 : 2879-2887
2. Moscow JA, Cowan KH (1988) Multidrug resistance. J Natl Cancer Inst 80 : 14-20
3. Endicott JA, Ling V (1989) The biochemistry of P-glycoprotein-mediated multidrug resistance. Ann Rev Biochem 58 : 137-171
4. Van der Bliek AM, Borst P (1989) Multidrug resistance. Adv Cancer Res 52 : 165-203
5. Roninson IB (1991) Molecular and cellular biology of multidrug resistance in tumor cells. Plenum Publishing Corp, New York (in press)
6. Beck WT, Danks MK (1991) Multidrug resistance associated with alterations in topoisomerase II. In : Potmesil M, Kohn K (Eds) DNA topoisomerases in cancer chemotherapy. Oxford University Press, New York (in press)
7. Hindenburg AA, Gervasoni JE Jr, Krishna S, Stewart VJ, Rosado M, Lutzky J, Bhalla K, Baker MA, Taub RN (1989) Intracellular distribution and pharmacokinetics of daunorubicin in anthracycline-sensitive and -resistant HL-60 cells. Cancer Res 49 : 4607-4614
8. McGrath T, Center MS (1988) Mechanisms of multidrug resistance in HL60 cells : evidence that a surface membrane protein distinct from P-glycoprotein contributes to reduced cellular accumulation of drug. Cancer Res 48 : 3959-3963
9. Goldstein LJ, Galski H, Fojo A, Willingham M, Lai SL, Gazdar A, Pirker R, Green A, Crist W, Brodeur GM, Lieker M, Crossman J, Gottesman MM, Pastan I (1989) Expression of a multidrug resistance gene in human cancers. J Natl Cancer Inst 81 : 116-124
10. Noonan KE, Beck C, Holzmayer TA, Chin JE, Wunder JS, Andrulis IL, Gazdar AF, Willman CL, Griffith B, VonHoff DD, Roninson IB (1990) Proc Natl Acad Sci USA 87 : 7160-7164

11. Chan HSL, Thorner PS, Haddad G, Ling V (1990) Immunohistochemical detection of P-glycoprotein : prognostic correlation in soft tissue sarcoma of childhood. J Clin Oncol 8 : 689-704

12. Safa AR, Glover CJ, Meyers MB, Biedler JL, Felsted RL (1986) Vinblastine photoaffinity labeling of a high molecular weight surface membrane glycoprotein specific for multidrug-resistant cells. J Biol Chem 261 : 6137-6140

13. Qian X-d, Beck WT (1990) Binding of an optically pure photoaffinity analogue of verapamil, LU-49888, to P-glycoprotein from multidrug resistant human leukemic cell lines. Cancer Res 50 : 1132-1137

14. Qian X-d, Beck WT (1990) Progesterone photoaffinity labels P-glycoprotein in multidrug-resistant human leukemic lymphoblasts. J Biol Chem 265 : 18753-18756

15. Pearce HL, Safa AR, Bach NJ, Winter MA, Cirtain MC, Beck WT (1989) Essential features of the P-glycoprotein pharmacophore as defined by a series of reserpine analogs that modulate multidrug resistance. Proc Natl Acad Sci USA 86 : 5128-5132

16. Danks MK, Yalowich JC, Beck WT (1987) Atypical multiple drug resistance in a human leukemic cell line selected for resistance to teniposide (VM-26). Cancer Res 47 : 1297-1301

17. Beck WT, Cirtain MC, Danks MK, Felsted RL, Safa AR, Wolverton JS, Suttle DP, Trent JM (1987) Pharmacological, molecular, and cytogenetic analysis of « atypical » multidrug-resistant human leukemia cells. Cancer Res 47 : 5455-5460

18. Danks MK, Schmidt CA, Suttle DP, Beck WT (1988) Altered catalytic activity of and DNA cleavage by DNA topoisomerase II from human leukemic cells selected for resistance to VM-26. Biochemistry 27 : 8861-8869

19. Danks MK, Schmidt CA, Deneka DA, Beck WT (1989) Increased ATP requirement for activity of and complex formation by DNA topoisomerase II from human leukemic CCRF-CEM cells selected for resistance to teniposide. Cancer Commun 1 : 101-109

20. Mickley LA, Bates SE, Richert ND, Currier S, Tanaka S, Foss F, Rosen N, Fojo AT (1989) Modulation of the expression of a multidrug resistance gene (mdr-1/P-glycoprotein) by differentiating agents. J Biol Chem 264 : 18031-18040

21. Fernandes DJ, Danks MK, Beck WT (1990) Decreased nuclear matrix DNA topoisomerase II in human leukemia cells resistant to VM-26 and m-AMSA. Biochemistry 29 : 4235-4241

22. Trask DK, DiDonato JA, Muller MT (1984) Rapid detection and isolation of covalent DNA/protein complexes : application to topoisomerase I and II. EMBO J 3 : 671-676

23. Zwelling LA, Hinds M, Chan D, Mayes J, Sie KL, Parker E, Silberman L, Radcliffe A, Beran M, Blick M (1989) Characterization of an amsacrine-resistant line of human leukemia cells. J Biol Chem 264 : 16411-16420

Acknowledgements. This work is supported in part by research grants CA-30103, CA-40570 and CA-47941, Cancer Center Support (CORE) grant CA-21765, all from the National Cancer Institute, Bethesda, MD, and in part by American Lebanese Syrian Associated Charities.

Pharmacokinetic study of Neo-Adjuvant chemotherapy combining Carboplatin, Cisplatin and 5-Fluorouracil in head and neck squamous cell carcinoma

R Fety, J Vignoud, P Cappelaere, A Pineau, P Viau

Neo-adjuvant chemotherapy combining 5-Fluorouracile (5-FU) and platinum compounds, Cisplatine (CP) and Carboplatine (CB), offers a high response rate in squamous cell carcinoma of head and neck [1, 2]. However, pathologic complete remission rate rarely exceed 30 %. So, new treatment strategy are needed to improve the overall long term survival in patients with this disease. Of interest is the fact that the toxicity pattern of CP is very different from that of CB : nephrotoxicity, ototoxicity and peripheral neurotoxicity are the toxic effects of CP, while myelosuppression effect is rare compared to CB. Considering that the antitumor activity is dose-dependant and that the toxicities do not overlap, it appears possible that the use of a combination of CP + CB associated with 5-FU may improve the antitumor activity by increasing the platinum dose while reducing the toxicity. According to these data, in vitro [3] and clinical [4-6] studies have been performed. However, there is no information about pharmacokinetic (PK) of platinum and 5-FU during these combinations. In this report, we compared PK of total (TT), ultrafilterable (UF) platinum and 5-FU in plasma of patients treated with CP + 5-FU or CB + CP + 5-FU combination in order to correlate treatment, related response and toxicity.

Materials and methods

Patients

One hundred and fourteen patients with histologically proved epidermoid cancer of head and neck were entered into this study.

Chemotherapy

Ninety-two patients received CP + 5-FU : CP (100 mg/m²) was given first as a 2 h infusion and 5-FU (4 g/m²) was given over 96 h immediately after CP administration. This regimen was repeated every 2 weeks for 3 courses.

Twenty-two patients received CB + CP + 5-FU : CB (200 mg/m²) was given first as a 30 min infusion. High volume fluid hydratation with 0.9 % NaCl followed. CP (100 mg/m²) was given over 2 h infusion 5 h after CP administration. 5-FU (4 g/m²) was given over 96 h immediately after CP. This regimen was repeated every 3 weeks for 2 courses.

Centre René Gauducheau, Nantes, France

Pharmacokinetic study

Blood was drawn at differents times over the perfusion and 24 h (CP and/or CB) or 96 h (5-FU) post infusion.

Analysis of platinum compounds

Plasma samples were immediately centrifuged on Amicon Centrifree for 20 min at +40 °C. Each fraction was stored at −20 °C until analysis. Platinum (TT and UF) was analysed by atomic absorption spectrophotometry.

Analysis of 5-FU

Blood samples were centrifuged for 10 min. The plasma was removed and frozen at −20 °C until analysis. 5-FU concentration was determined by HPLC [7]. AUC values were determined using trapezoidal method.

Results

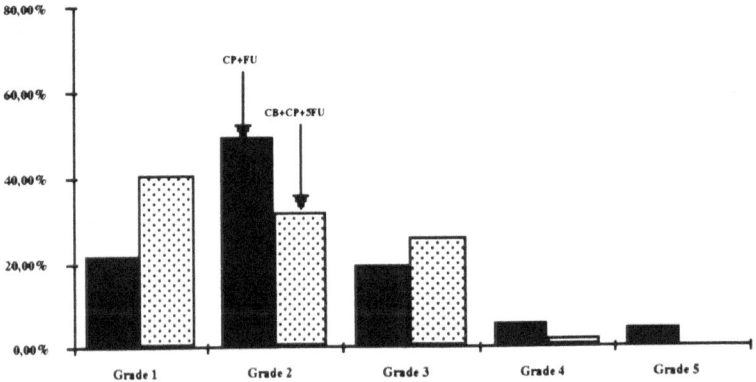

Fig. 1. Hematological toxicity

Conclusion

The present study provided evidence that the combination therapy with CB + CP + 5FU : *1)* induce no change in 5-FU pharmacokinetic ; *2)* induce increase of platinum exposition (AUC) which could be correlated with increase of clinical response ; *3)* induce increase in residual platinum concentrations probably related with greater than expected myelosuppression. In the further development of chemotherapy using CB + CP + 5-FU combination, new modalities of administration have to be studied in order to decrease hematological toxicity.

Table 1. PK parameters

	CP + 5FU	CB + CP + 5FU
AUC TT (μg/ml*h)	73 + 15	132 + 28
AUC UF (μg/ml*h)	4.0 + 0.2	39 + 9
Residual platinum (μg/ml)	2.2 + 0.5	3.5 + 0.8
AUC 5FU (ng/ml*h)	40 827 + 16 100	42 235 + 18 590

Table 2. Tumoral response

	CP + 5FU	CB + CP + 5FU
Global response	70,0%	76,9%
Complete response	20,1%	26,9%

References

1. Amrein P, Weitzman S (1985) Treatment of squamous-cell carcinoma of the head and neck with cisplatin and 5-Fluorouracil. J Clin Oncol 12 : 1632-1639
2. Cappelaere P, Vignoud J, Fargeot P, Metz R, Chauvergne J, Meeus L, Schneider M, Chazard M (1990) Palliative chemotherapy with a combination of carboplatin and fluorouracil of epidermoid carcinoma of the upper aerodigestive tract. Bull Cancer 77 : 1099-1105
3. Hida S, Okada K, Yoshida O (1990) Advantages in combination chemotherapy using cisplatin and its analogues for human testicular tumor xenografts. Jp J Cancer Res 81 : 425-430
4. Klastersky J, Sculier J, Dabouis G, Bureau G, Libert P, Ravez P, Vandermoten G, Thiriaux J, Lecomte J, Cordier R et al (1990) A randomized trial of twoplatinum combinations in patients with advanced non-small cell lung cancer : a preliminary report. Seminars in Oncol 17 : 20-24
5. Piccart M, Nogaret J, Marcelis L, Longrie H, Ries F, Kains J, Gobert P, Domange A, Sculier J, Gompel C (1990) Cisplatin combined with carboplatin : a new way of intensification of platinum dose in the treatment of advanced ovarian cancer. J Nat Cancer Inst 82 : 703-707
6. Trump D, Grem J, Tutsch K, Willson J, Simon K, Alberti D, Storer B, Tormey C (1987) Platinum analogue combination chemotherapy : cisplatin and carboplatin — a phase I trial with pharmacokinetic assessment of the effect of cisplatin administration on carboplatin excretion. J Clin Oncol 5 : 1281-1289
7. Christophidis N, Mahaly G, Vajda F, Louis W (1979) Comparison of liquid and gas-liquid chromatography assays of 5-fluorouracil in plasma. Clin Chem 25 : 83-87

The influence of tumour stage on in vitro sensitivity of renal carcinoma cells to Mitozantrone

MO Symes, CMP Collins, T Lai, PJB Smith

Of patients presenting with renal cell carcinoma, some 25 % have metastatic disease and 74 % of these will die of the disease within one year. Mitozantrone has been used to treat patients with metastatic renal carcinoma [1, 2] but with minimal success. It is questionable, however, whether useful plasma levels of mitozantrone were achieved in one of these studies.

In this study carcinoma cells were separated from the nephrectomy specimens in 20 patients with renal cell carcinoma (RCC) and were cultured with various concentrations of mitozantrone. The resulting inhibition of (^{75}Se) selenomethionine uptake by the tumour cells was used to assess anti-tumour activity.

Materials and methods

Cell culture

Following enzymatic disaggregation of the solid tumour, the mixed cell suspension was centrifuged on a continuous density gradient, Nycodenz^R (Nycomed UK) column to obtain a discrete band of neoplastic cells. Characteristically this band was composed of 95 % carcinoma cells [3]. The carcinoma cells were cultured for 24 h in RPMI 1640 with 10 % v/v newborn calf serum, 1 % glutamine and antibiotics. Separate aliquots of cells from each RCC were cultured in medium alone or in the presence of 0.1, 1.0, 5.0 or 10 μg/ml Mitozantrone (Lederle). Thereafter, the RCC were washed and maintained for a further 48 h in methionine free Eagles MEM with with 0.5 μCi/ml (^{75}Se) selenomethionine. Incorporation of isotope, as a measure of protein synthesis, was then determined using a gamma counter.

Tumour classification

Tumours were classified according to their clinical stage and also by histological grade. Stage I tumours were confined to the renal parenchyma, Stage II showed extension to but not across the renal capsule, Stage III showed penetration of the renal capsule and Stage IV had distant metastases.

Histological Grade I tumours had nuclei indistinguishable from normal tubular cells, Grade II showed pyknotic and irregular nuclei without conspicuous

University Depts of Surgery and Pathology Bristol Royal Infirmary, Bristol BS2 8HW, UK nucleoli, Grade III showed enlarged, irregular nuclei often with large nucleoli but without bizarre forms and Grade IV had numerous bizarre giant nuclei [4]. 8/20 (40 %) of the tumours were Stage IV and of these 7/8 (87.5 %) were histological Grade IV.

Results

The effect of Mitozantrone on the percent inhibition of ^{75}SeM uptake was assessed with respect to tumour stage (Fig. 1). These results are summarised in Table 1. This details the proportion of drug exposed RCC cultures which showed a > 50 % reduction in isotope uptake, by comparison with the corresponding renal carcinoma cells maintained in medium alone.

Table 1.

STAGE	I	II	III	IV
Concentration of Mitozantrone ng/ml				
0.1	—	0/3	1/3	1/4
1.0	0/2	0/4	1/5	8/8
5.0	0/2	0/4	0/4	8/8
10.0	0/2	1/1	1/3	7/8

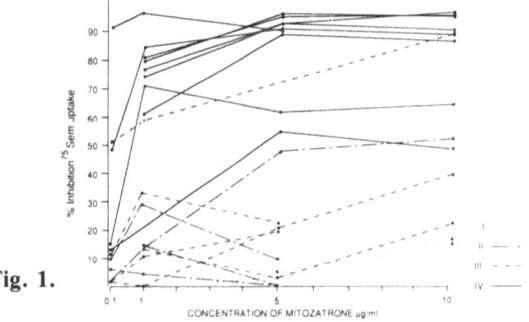

Fig. 1.

Of Stage IV tumours, with distant metastases, 7/8 (87.5 %) were histological Grade IV while the remaining tumour was Grade III.

Discussion

Stage IV tumours of histological Grade IV showed the greatest drug sensitivity. This may be due to their higher proliferation index or to the relatively reduced expression of the MDR gene product p 170. This determines multi-drug resistance in RCC and is least expressed in undifferentiated tumours [5]. Studies to assess the proliferation index and the expression of p 170 are currently in progress.

The present findings suggest that Mitozantrone may be of value in selected patients — those with metastases whose tumours are of histological Grade IV.

References

1. Van Oostrom AT, Fossa SD, Pizzocaro G, Bergerat JP, Bono AV, De Pauw M and Sylvester R (1984) Mitozantrone in advanced renal cancer : a phase II study in previously untreated patients from the EORTC genito-urinary cancer cooperative group. Eur J Cancer 20 : 1239-1241
2. Gams RA, Nelson O and Birch R (1986) Phase II evaluation of mitozantrone in advanced renal cell cancer. A South Western cancer study group trial. Cancer Treatment Reports 70 : 921-922
3. Ford TC, Lai T and Symes MO (1987) Morphological and functional characteristics of mouse mammary carcinoma cells separated on Nycodenz columns. Br J Exp Path 68 : 453-460
4. Skinner DG, Colvin RB, Vermillion CD, Pfister RC and Leadbetter WF (1971) Diagnosis and management of renal cell carcinoma. Cancer 28 : 1165-1177
5. Kanamaru H, Kakeni Y, Yoshida O Nakanishi S, Pastor I and Gottesman MM (1989) MDRI levels in human renal carcinomas : correlation with grade and prediction of reversal of doxorubicin resistance by quinidine in tumor explants. JNCI 81 : 844-849

Circadian chemotherapy against stage IIIB-IV non-small-cell lung cancer (NSCLC) with 5-Fluorouracil (5-FU), folinic acid (FOL) and cisplatin (CDDP) via a multichannel programmable pump. Preliminary results

M Vincent*, F Levi**, B Girodet*, E Laennec*, P Poirie*, B Guibert*, JM Ardiet***, A Boisson*, L Van-Straaten*

Non-small-cell lung cancer (NSCLC) is the most common malignancy diagnosed both in the European Community and the United States. It is also the leading cause of cancer-related deaths in men. According to the new system UICC, stages IIIB and IV are generally considered as incurable. Five year survival rate is 5-10 %.

The CDDP-5-FU combination has been frequently used and has achieved results similar as other protocols. It has also allowed concurrent radiation therapy for stage IIIB disease [1, 2].

FOL increases the therapeutic index of 5-FU against colorectal cancer by increasing the intracellular concentration of reduced folates [3]. But folates adjunction has often resulted in an increased gastrointestinal toxicity (mucositis and diarrhea). Circadian chemotherapy can reduce toxicity : least dosing time for CDDP bolus injection is between 16-20 h [4, 5], 24 h modulation of continuous of FUDR with peak between 15-21 h is less toxic than flat delivery [6], continuous 5-FU with peak delivery at 4 h allows too largely increase dose intensity as compared to flat infusion [7].

Computerized automated portable infusion reduce nursing workload for inpatient care, allow high quality outpatient care and reduce toxicity through circadian modulation of infusion rate.

We hereby report the preliminary results of circadian chemotherapy against stage IIIB and IV NSCLC with 5-FU, FOL, CDDP via a multichannel programmahle pump (Aguettant laboratory Lyon).

Patients and methods

The objectives of the study are to estimate toxicity (daily for 5d, on d10 and on d21 ; WHO criteria), response rate (standard criteria) and duration, resectability after 3 courses (stage IIIB only), survival, possibility of carrying this protocol in outpatient (with oral hydratation).

Eligibility criteria were : histologically proven stage IIIB or IV NSCLC according UICC classification, Karnofsky Index > 60, age under 71 years, infor-

Department pneumology and oncology, St Joseph Hospital, Lyon. ** Chronobiologie laboratory cancer (cnrs i-6212), Paul Brousse Hospital, Villejuif. ***Leon Berard Center, Lyon

med consent, at least 1 mesurable lesion, implanted venous access port, no prior treatment. Ineligibility criteria were : coronaropathy, renal or hepatic failure, cerebral metastasis with intracranial hypertension, psychological, geographic circumstances that do not warrant proper staging treatment of follow-up conditions.

All patients had an initial staging with history and physical examination, chest x-ray, thoracoabdominal and cerebral CT-scan, bronchial endoscopy, bone scan, routine chemistries, pulmonary spirometry. First evaluation during fourth course included CT-scan and repeat of all initial pathologic test. Patients with stable disease (SD) or progression (PROG) subsequently underwent palliative treatment, stage IV with minor response (MR), partial response (PR) or complete response (CR) received 4 more courses, stage IIIB after MR, PR or CR had surgery if resectable. Non resectable and operated patients received combination of circadian chemotherapy CDDP-5-FU-FOL (2 courses) and radiotherapy. A second evaluation was performed after 6-8 courses (stage IV). MR or PR patients had 4 more courses and CR patients stopped treatment.

Treatments were automatically administered via a programmable pump (Aguettant*) (Table 1).

Table 1.

Drug given	Dose : mg/m²/day × 5 days	Times of infusion (hr)	Peak delivery (hr)
FOL	300	22.00 - 10.00	4.00
5 FU	600	22.00 - 10.00	4.00
CDDP	12,5	10.00 - 22.00	16.00

Table 2. Preliminary results for 10 patients after 4 fours courses : response rate : 5/10

Nom	Age	Sex	Histology	Stage	Response	Surgery	Radiotherapy
JOU	55	M	SCC	IIIB	SD	no	yes
MOR	54	M	ULC	IIIB	PR	no	yes + ch.*
ALL	66	M	SCC	IV (lung)	PR	no	no
BEA	54	M	ULC	IIIB	PR	no	yes + ch.*
LAR	56	M	ULC	IIIB	SD	no	yes + ch.*
DUF	62	M	ADK	IIIB	MR	yes	yes + ch.*
SAR	61	M	SCC	IIIB	PR	no	yes + ch.*
ANG	63	M	ADK	IIIB	PROG	no	yes
DAL	46	F	SCC	IIIB	SD	no	yes
ROU	49	M	SCC	IV (bone)	PR	no	no

CH : Chronotherapy, SCC = squamous cell carcinoma, ULC = undifferentiated large cell, ADK = adenocarcinoma

Dose escalation up to 700 mg/m²/d for 5-FU and 16 mg/m²/d for CDDP in the absence of WHO toxicity greater than 2.

Hydration and antiemetic protocol for ambulatory condition after Benhamed [8] ; water : 35 ml/kg/24 h in addition to normal dietary input (1,5 l/24 h)
to obtain urinary output > 3l/24 h. Antiemetics : metoclopromide : 20 mg
supp. twice daily ; Alprazolan : 50 mg capsule at 22 h. If creatininemia > 130
micromole/l : parenteral hydratation.

Results

From March 1990 until January 1991, 19 patients have been included. Ten
patients are evaluable to date since they have received four courses. (Figs. 2,
3, 4, 5, 6).

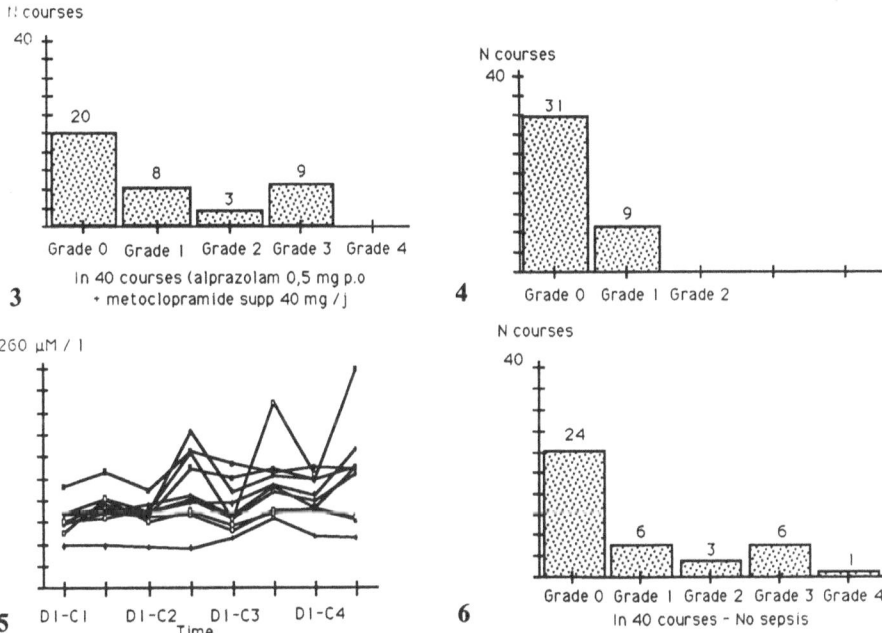

Fig. 3. Toxicity : nausea and vomiting

Fig. 4. Toxicity : creatinine

Fig. 5. Serum creatinine evolution

Fig. 6. Toxicity : granulocytes

Discussion

The response rate in these 10 evaluable patients was good (5/10 PR). Both
patients with metastatic disease achieved PR. One patient with MR changed

from stage IIIB to IIIA and became resectable. We continue this trial to include thirty patients.

CDDP chronotherapy-induced emesis and renal toxicity could not be properly handled with oral hydration and minimal antiemetics in these patients. A protocol of continuously infused ambulatory CDDP had been performed by Benhamed [8]. CDDP peak level during chronotherapy may cause nausea and vomiting and alter the efficacy of oral hydration. We have decided to use systematically parenteral hydration for the next patients.

Hematologic and mucosal toxicities were mild despite high doses of 5-FU and FOL which confirms the benefit of chronomodulation as also noticed in colon carcinoma [9].

Conclusion

The response rate to such chronotherapy is encouraging : 5/10 PR, 1 MR (Stage IIIB to IIIA).

Toxicity is acceptable but does not allow outpatient treatment.

This phase II trial will continue until it has included a total of 30 patients.

Supported by Aguettant laboratory and Lederle laboratories.

References

1. Gralla Rj (1990) New directions in non-small cell lung cancer. Semin Oncol 17, 4 : 14-19
2. Riviere A, Abouz D, Ayela P et al (1989) Résultats d'une étude de phase II d'une association de Cis-Platinum et de 5-FU dans les cancers bronchiques epidermoides ou indifferenciés à grandes cellules. Bul Cancer 76 : 1095-1102
3. Machover D, Goldschmidt E, Chollet P et al (1986) Treatment of advanced colorectal and gastric adenocarcinoma with 5-Fluorouracil and high-dose Folinic acid. J Clin Oncol 4 : 685-696
4. Hrushesky WJM (1985) Circadian timing of cancer chemotherapy. Science 228 : 73-75
5. Levi F et al (1990) Chemotherapy of advanced ovarian cancer with 4'-0-tetrahydropyranyl doxorubicin and cisplatin : a randomized phase II trial with an evaluation of circadian timing and dose-intensity. J Clin Oncol Vol 8, N° 4, 705-714
6. Roemeling R et al (1989) Circadian patterning of continuous floxuridine infusion reduces toxicity and allows higher dose intensity in patients with widespread cancer. J Clin Oncol 7 : 1710-1719
7. Levi F et al (1988) Ambulatory 5-day chronotherapy of colorectal cancer with continuous venous infusion of 5-Fluorouracil (cvi-5-FU) at circadian-modulated rate. Proc ASCO 7 : 70
8. Benhamed M, Renaux J, Spielman M, Rouesse J (1986) Cisplatin (CDDP) in continuous intravenous ambulatory infusion : a new method of administration. Cancer Drug Delivery 3 : 183-188
9. Levi F et al (1990) Circadian-rhythm modulated chemotherapy against metastatic colorectal cancer : results of an extended phase II chronotherapy trial with 5-Fluorouracil (5-FU) folinic acid (FOL) and oxalato-platinum (l-ohp) using an ambu-

latory multichannel, programmable in time pump (Intelliject R). Proc. ESMO, Copen-
hagen, Annals of Oncology, supplement to Volume 1, 43 Nov

Abstract. *CDDP-5FU combination is active against NSCLC. FOL increases the therapeutic index of 5-FU against colorectal cancer but often results in an increased toxicity. Computerized automated portable infusion could reduce nursing workload for inpatient care, and allow both high quality outpatient care and reduced toxicity through circadian modulation of infusion rate.*

Ten patients (pts) received 40 courses (c) of chronotherapy (mg/m²/d x 5 days) 5-FU : 600 first c and 700 if no toxicity ; FOL : 300 ; CDDP : 12,5 first c and 16 other c if no toxicity every 3 weeks. Infusion rates were modulated along the 24 h scale (4 a.m for 5-FU and FOL peaks, and 4 p.m for CDDP peak).

Ambulatory conditions were tested with supplementary oral hydration (35 ml/kg/day) to obtain 3l/day diuresis with daily creatininemia. Patients characteristics : 1 f, 9 m median age 58 years (range : 46-66), Karnofsky Index > 60, no prior treatment, 5 squamous cell carcinoma (SCC), 3 undifferentiated large cell RULC), 2 adenocarcinoma (ADK) ; 8 stage IIIB and 2 stage IV inclusion between march 1990 and september 1990. Responses were assessable after 4 c : 5 had partial response (PR > 50 %), (3 SCC, 2 ULC), 1 had minor response (ADK), 3 were stabilised (2 SCC, 1 ULC). 3/5 PR had complete response after chemoradiotherapy realised after 4 c chronochemotherapy.

Further follow-up is required to evaluate survival. Evaluation of toxicity : nausea and vomiting were moderate but increased with mild renal toxicity. According WHO criteria, 9 patients had toxicity grade 1 creatininemia and oral hydratation for ambulatory condition was not sufficient. hematologic toxicity : neutropenia : 6 c grade 3, 1 c grade 4. No septic complication.
Tolerance was good without any septic complication or diarrhea or mucositis, despite the high doses 5-FU and FOL.

CDDP-chronotherapie induced emesis and renal toxicity could not be properly handled with oral hydratation and minimal antiemetics in these patients.

Since such chronotherapie regimen has shown acceptable toxicity and good activity against NSCLC, this phase II trial continues to include thirty patients.

New drugs

Morpholinyl anthracyclines : option for reversal of anthracycline resistance ?

EGE de Vries, JG Zijlstra, NH Mulder

Anthracyclines are potent chemotherapeutic drugs, consisting of a 4-ring aglycon and an aminosugar, which both can be substituted. The most widely used are doxorubicin and daunorubicin, the parent drugs. The efficacy, toxicity and drug resistance may be related to different parts of the anthracycline molecule.

A number of mechanisms are held responsible for the cytotoxicity of the parent compounds. The cytotoxicity can occur at the outer cell membrane. In general however, in order to be cytotoxic, the drug has to enter the cell. Here intercalation of DNA occurs. The anthracycline chromophore fits stereometrically between two base pairs, thus preventing the use of DNA for actions such as replication and transcription. This in turn leads to cell death. A possible other mechanism is the capacity to turn topoisomerases into cellular poisons. This can be one of the ways to induce DNA damage. After exposition of DNA to anthracyclines, DNA breaks can be detected. This can be due, at least in part, to the generation of free radicals by the quinone moiety. None of the above mentioned mechanisms can be pointed to as the principle cause of cytotoxicity. All, probably, participate to a varying extent, depending on the structure of the anthracycline molecule. The effect of the parent compound is limited by myelosuppression, cardiac toxicity and drug resistance.

Intrinsic or acquired resistance in tumors hampers the clinical efficacy of the drug. The cell membrane plays, in contrast to its limited role in cytotoxicity, a very important role as first line of defense in drug resistance. The most extensively studied resistance mechanism is the P-glycoprotein mediated form of multidrug resistance. The P-glycoprotein mediated membrane pump extrudes anthracyclines, which enter the cells by diffusion through the lipid compartment of the membrane. Recently, other membrane pumps have also been described. Some other mechanisms held responsible for anthracycline resistance are a decreased or altered topoisomerase II activity and enhanced detoxifying enzyme activities.

The limitations of the present anthracyclines led to the development of next generation drugs. The morpholinyl substituted anthracyclines have several properties that differ from the parent drug. All are highly lipophylic and therefore diffuse rapidly through the cell membrane. The cyanomorpholinyl substituted anthracyclines can also form DNA-DNA crosslinks. There is topoisomerase I mediated DNA damage and preferential inhibition of ribosomal gene transcription. These mechanisms could contribute to cytotoxicity and are new compared to doxorubicin. There is in-vitro evidence as well as in-vivo in the mouse model that these drugs, although not always, can overcome doxorubi-

Div. Medical Oncology, Dept. Int. Med., University Hospital, Oostersingel 59, 9713 EZ Groningen, Netherlands

cin resistance. Doxorubicin resistant cell lines with resistance due to an alte-red topoisomerase II were also not cross resistant to morpholinyl anthracycli-nes. We found no cross-resistance to cyanomorpholinyl anthracycline in GLC_4-Adr, a doxorubicin resistant P-glycoprotein negative subline from the human small cell lung cancer cell line GLC_4. These drugs are therefore also promising for the treatment of topoisomerase II related resistance. There was, however, cross-resistance in the cisplatin resistant cell line GLC_4-CDDP.

Potential cardiotoxicity due to free radicals, will probably not be of clini-cal importance because morpholinyl anthracyclines are in vitro much more active than the parent drug and will therefore be administered at a much lower dose. The morpholinyl anthracycline structure can possibly be further impro-ved by substitution of other parts of the molecule. Two phase I studies with the 9-alkyl substituted morpholinyl anthracycline MX2 have been reported. The haematological toxicity was dose limiting and no cardiac toxicity occurred [1, 2].

Multidrug resistance associated with P-glycoprotein expression is now the best studied resistance phenomenon. The existence of P-glycoprotein expres-sion in a number of normal tissues as well as in various tumor types has been shown. There are, however, many tumors that show intrinsic or acquired adriamycin resistance without P-glycoprotein expression. The frequency of occurrence of other resistance mechanisms such as topoisomerase II related anthracycline resistance in human tumors is not yet clear. We recently found in e.g. ovarian carcinoma that there is also heterogeneity between tumors in topoisomerase I and II activity ; topoisomerase I was always higher than in benign tumors. Interestingly, topoisomerase I is a newly described target of the morpholinyl anthracyclines.

Until now, clinical trials with anthracyclines and modulators that block the P-glycoprotein pump have had limited success. This is partly due to the fact that full use of some modulators is hampered by side effects of the modula-tors and that it is often not known whether the resistant tumors were actually P-glycoprotein positive. Resistance mechanisms may vary between tumor types as well as within one tumor and various mechanisms may even play a role within one tumor cell. Therefore, next generation anthracyclines with activity against P-glycoprotein multidrug resistant cells as well as against cells with aty-pical (topoisomerase II) mediated multidrug resistance, based on different phar-macokinetics and new mechanisms of action, are interesting for the clinic. Whe-ther the new morpholinyl analogues have a good antitumor activity in the cli-nic next to the promising preclinical data still remains to be proven.

Acknowledgement. Dr EM Acton kindly provided MRA-CN.

References

1. Ogawa M, Tabata M, Horikoshi N, Inoue K, Mukaiyama T, Fukutani H, Hirano A, Muzunuma N, Itami S (1989) Phase I trial of 3'-deamino-3'-morpholino-13-deoxy-10-hydroxycarminomycin hydrochloride (KRN-8602). Proc Am Soc Clin Oncol 8 : A238
2. Majima H (1990) Phase 1 clinical study of MX2 (KRN-8602). Gan-To-Kagaku Ryoho 17 : 359-364

Diarylsulfonylureas : new anticancer agents with novel activities, toxicities and mechanism of action

P Houghton, J Sosinski, J Thakar, J Houghton

The diarylsulfonylureas (DSU's) represent a novel class of antitumor agents that were identified as active against rodent solid tumors, but not against leukemias [1, 2]. We subsequently demonstrated activity against human tumor xenografts [3] and notably against xenografts from colon adenocarcinomas that were refractory to other agents used in clinical therapy. At the same time, preclinical toxicology, undertaken by Eli Lilly and Company, showed that the major toxicities in rodents and primates was limited to hemolytic anemia and methemoglobinemia. Thus, the spectrum of antitumor activity, and pattern of toxicity prompted this laboratory to examine, in detail, the mechanism(s) of action of this class of compound. In this article some of the more interesting preclinical data with DSU's are presented.

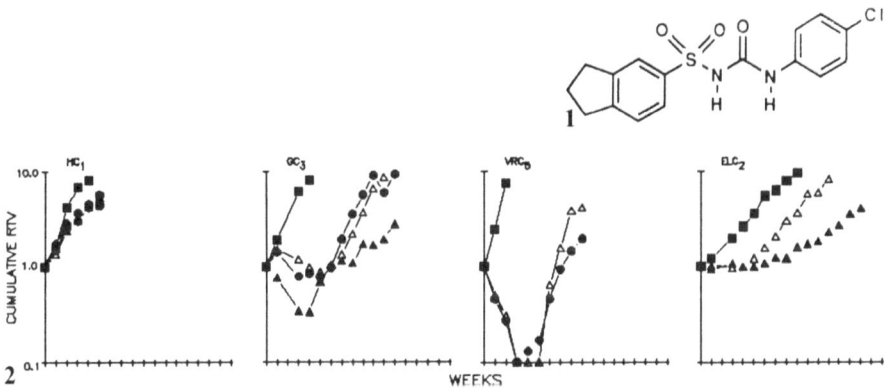

Fig. 1. Chemical structure of N-(5-indanylsulfony)-N'-(4-chlorophenyl) urea (Sulofenur)

Fig. 2. Growth of 4 lines of colon adenocarcinoma xenografts in mice receiving different dosages and schedules (Δ●) sulofenur, or vehicle (■). Each curve represents the mean for 14 tumors

Materials and methods

Human colon tumor xenografts, HCC_1, GC_3, VRC_5 and ELC_2 have been described previously [4]. Tumors were propagated in the subcutaneous space of immuned-deprived CBA/CaJ female mice [4], and treatment was started when

Dept Biochemical and Clinical Pharmacology, St Jude Children's Research Hospital, Memphis, TN 38101, USA

tumors reached and 1cm diameter. Sulofenur was administered by oral gavage twice daily as a suspension in 5 % Emulphor EL-620. For in vitro studies, a cloned cell line derived from the GC_3 tumor (designated GCC_3/cl) was used. Details of clonogenic assays and cellular accumulation studies have been presented previously [5, 6].

Results

Therapeutic activity against xenografts

Responses of four colon adenocarcinoma lines to sulofenur is shown in Figure 2. At the maximal tolerated dose level (200 mg/kg/dose b.i.d x 10 d) sulofenur caused significant regression of GC_3 and VR_5 xenografts, and inhibited growth of ELC_2 xenografts. HC_1 tumors were refractory to this agent. Sulofenur caused complete regressions in each of 9 xenografted lines of childhood rhabdomyosarcoma [8], and also has shown significant activity against osteosarcoma xenografts.

Cellular pharmacology of DSU's

Our initial studies have examined the accumulation and distibution of the analogue N-(4-methylphenylsulfonyl)-N'-(4-chlorophenyl) urea (MPCU). Uptake of [¹]H-MPCU is a temperature dependent, non-saturable process, consistent with passive diffusion [5]. However, drug is concentrated within cells and achieves concentrations 4- to 6-fold greater than the extracellular medium at pH 7.4. Concentration of MPCU is reversibly inhibited by agents that uncouple oxidative phosphorylation [6]. The effect of sodium azide is shown in Figure 3. After removal of azide (arrow), MPCU rapidly accumulated to a higher steady state.

Further experimentation suggested that MPCU (and sulofenur) accumulated in mitochondria, and that sequestration was a consequence of the pH gradient between cytoplasm and the mitochondrial matrix. This was tested directly by examining the effect of ionophores that collapse either the pH gradient or the electonegativity gradient across the matrix membrane. A typical result for nigericin, which collapses the pH gradient, is shown in Figure 4. Further studies with a radiolabeled photoaffinity analogue of MPCU have shown that about 53 % of radiolabel is associated with the mitochondrial fraction subsequent to cell fractionation.

Biological activity of sulofenur

The efficacy against slowly growing xenografts, and the novel pattern of organ toxicity, suggested that sulofenur may be cytotoxic to slowly proliferating, or non-proliferating cells [7]. Conditions were established under which GC_3/cl cells were quiescent ($\leqslant$ 2 % control growth), and these cultures or exponen-

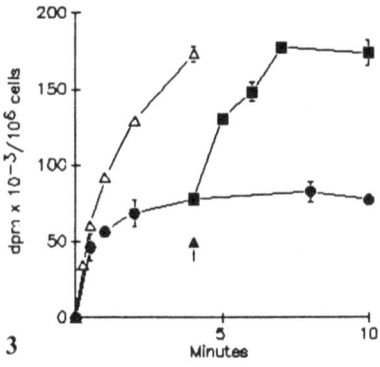

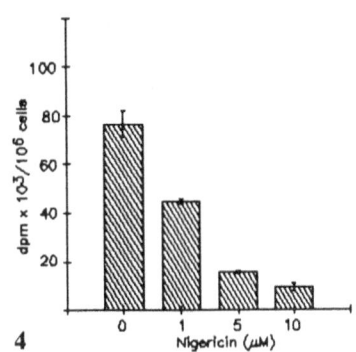

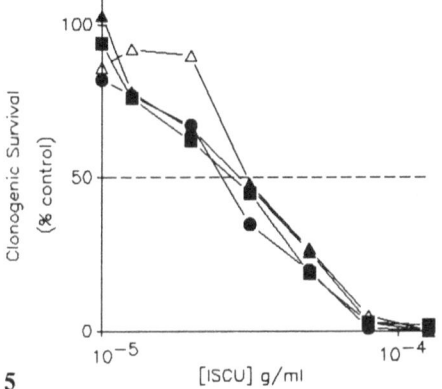

Fig. 3. The effect of azide (10 mM) on the accumulation of [³]H-MPCU. Uptake of MPCU without azide (Δ), in the presence of azide (●), and after removal of azide after 4 min. (■, arrow). From ref [5]

Fig. 4. Accumulation to steady state of [³H]-MPCU in the presence of increasing concentrations of nigericin. From ref [6]

Fig. 5. Colony formation of cells exposed to sulofenur (ISCU) under exponential growth conditions (●), or quiescent conditions and retained in this state for 1 (■), 2 (Δ) or 4 (Δ) days before cloning. From ref [7]

tially growing cultures, were exposed for 24 hours to ISCU. After removing drug, cells were retained in a non proliferating state for up to 4 days, or were refed with growth medium. Colony formation was determined after a further 7 days. As shown in Figure 5 cells were equally sensitive to sulofenur when exposed in proliferative or quiescent phases of growth.

Discussion

ISCU and other DSU's have demonstrated significant therapeutic activity in rodent and human tumor models. The mechanism causing cytotoxicity is unknown, although a secondary target which limits cell growth at high (non-pharmacologic) concentrations is related to uncoupling of oxidative phosphorylation. Of interest is that sulofenur is equally toxic to non-proliferating cells. In man, concentrations of sulofenur that can be achieved are 2- to 4-fold lower than in mice, and are limited by toxicity to red cells [8]. This may be related to more extensive metabolism in man, and the generation of p-chloroaniline, thought to be responsible for the toxicity [9]. Formation of p-chloroaniline is not reponsible for antitumor effects of this class of agent (unpublished data).

Supported by PHS awards CA51949, CA23099, CA21765 (Cancer center Support grant) and by American Lebanese Syrian Associated Charities (ALSAC).

References

1. Grindey GB (1988) Identification of diarylsulfonylureas as novel anticancer agents. 29 : 535
2. Howbert JJ,Grossman CS, Crowell TA, Reider BJ et al (1990) Novel agents effective against solid tumors : the diarylsulfonylureas. Synthesis, activities, and analysis of quantitative structure-activity relationships. J Med Chem 33 : 2394-2407
3. Houghton PJ, Houghton JA, Myers L, Cheshire PJ, Howbert JJ, Grindey GB (1989) Evaluation od N-(5-indanylsulfonyl)-N'-(4-chlorophenyl)-urea against xenografts of pediatric rhabdomyosarcoma. Cancer Chemother Pharmacol 25 : 84-88
4. Houghton JA, Houghton PJ (1980) On the mechanism of cytotoxicity of fluorinated pyrimidines in 4 human colon adenocarcinoma xenografts maintained in immune-deprived mice. Cancer 45 : 1159-1167
5. Houghton PJ, Bailey FC, Germain GS, Grindey GB, Howbert JJ, Houghton JA (1990) Studies on the cellular pharmacology of N-(4-methylphenylsulfonyl)-N'-(4-chlorophenyl)-urea. Biochem pharmacol 39 : 1187-1192
6. Houghton PJ, Bailey FC, Houghton JA, Murti KG, Howbert JJ, Grindey GB. Evidence for mitochondrial localization of N-(4-methylphenylsulfonyl)-N'-(4-chlorophenyl) urea in human colon adenocarcinoma cells. Cancer Res 50 : 664-668
7. Houghton PJ, Bailey FC, Germain GS, Grindey GB, Witt BC, Houghton JA N-(5-indanylsulfonyl)-N'-(4-chlorophenyl)urea, a novel agent equally cytotoxic to non-proliferating human colon adenocarcinoma cells. Cancer Res 50 : 318-322
8. Taylor CW, Alberts DS, Ketcham MA et al (1989) Clinical pharmacology of a novel diarylsulfonylurea anticancer agent. J Clin Oncol 7 : 1733-1740
9. Ehlhardt W (1991) Metabolism and disposition of the anticancer agent sulofenur in mouse, rat, monkey and man. Drug Metab Disp 19 (in press)

Current development of fotemustine : perspectives

D Khayat

Fotemustine is a new 2-chloroethyl-nitrosourea in which 1-amino-ethyl phosphonic acid — a bioisostere of alanine — has been grafted into a nitrosourea radical and whose synthesis was guided by two objectives : to facilitate its cell penetration using active amino acid transport system and to achieve better passage through the blood brain barrier, the octanol-water partition coefficient being within the limits of the maximum antitumor activity as evaluated by structure activity relationship studies [1].

The development of this drug in its various indications, on more than 1,000 treated patients and in studies conducted throughout Europe since 1985 [2], is presented below.

Table 1.

Indication	Study	Evaluable Patients	Response rate (%)	Activity on cerebral metastases (%)
	Fotemustine alone:			
	. Jacquillat	153	24.2	25.0
	. Retsas	24	16.7	8.3
	. Aapro	30	20.0	14.3
	. Schallreuter	19	47.0	35.0
	Combination:			
Melanoma [3,4]	. Avril (+DTIC)	103	27.2	26.3
	. Lopez-Aliaga (+DTIC)	11	36.4	—
	. Aamdal (+DTIC)	42	31.0	20.0
	. Thatcher (+DTIC)	22	41.0	—
	. Israels (+DTIC)	29	24.0	23.0
	. Gore (+DTIC)	14	0	—
	. Avril (DTIC+IFN)	15	20.0	—
	. Khayat (DTIC+VDS)	27	48.0	—
	. Retsas (DTIC+VDS+CDDP)	44	28.0	—

Hôpital Pitié-Salpétrière, Paris, 75013, France

Table 2.

Indication	Study	Evaluable patients	Response rate (%)	Remarks
	Recurrent (Namer)	38	26.3	Median survival 29.8 weeks
	High dose with ABMT (Biron)	17	36.8	—
	Intra-arterial (Poisson)	30	50.0	—
Glioma [5]	Plus radiotherapy (Bourdin) Surgery + Radiotherapy	55	29.0	Median survival 36 weeks
	(Baumgartner)	34	—	1 year survival 52.0%
Non small cell lung cancer [6]	Pre-treated (D1-D8-D15) (Le Chevalier)	17	23.5	
	D1-D8	35	20.0	
	Untreated (Kerbrat)	38	8.0	ST + MR = 40%
Renal	Pre-treated (Kerbrat)	24	4.2	ST + MR = 16%
Carcinoma [7]	After IL2	22	0	
	+ VLB or IFN (Israel)	18	0	
Colon [8]	Rougier-Bleiberg	30	6.8	ST = 43%
	Bleiberg	17	23.5	
	Khayat (liver metastases)			
	. melanoma	13	61.5	
Intra-arterial [9]	. colon	35	20.0	
	. other	18	23.0	
	Banzet (regional perfusion)			
	. melanoma	29	80.0	
	. pelvis	10	—	
Gastric	EORTC	8	—	
Sarcoma	Spielman-EORTC	40	0	
Ovary	EORTC	19	0	
Cerebral metastases	ARTAC	16	18.8	

These data confirm :

• The activity of fotemustine in disseminated malignant melanoma either in monotherapy or in combination with various agents. To be noted the activity on brain metastases observed in all studies.

• The interest of the drug in glioma.

• The benefit in non small cell lung cancer in relapse of conventional first line chemotherapy.

References

1. Hansch C, Smith N, Engle R, Wood H (1972) Quantitative structure-activity relationships of antineoplastic drugs : nitrosoureas and triazene-imidazoles. Cancer Chemother Rep 56 : 443-456
2. Khayat D, Lokiec F, Bizzari JP, Weil M, Meeus L, Sellami M, Rouesse J, Banzet P, Jacquillat C (1987) Phase I clinical study of the new amino acid-linked nitrosourea, S 10036, administered on a weekly schedule. Cancer Research 47 : 6782-6785
3. Jacquillat C, Khayat D, Banzet P, Weil M, Fumoleau P, Avril MF, Namer M, Bonneterre J, Kerbrat P, Bonerandi JJ, Bugat R, Montcuquet P, Cupissol D, Lauvin R, Vilmer C, Prache C, Bizzari JP (1990) Final report of the french multicenter phase II study of the nitrosourea fotemustine in 153 evaluable patients with disseminated malignant melanoma including patients with cerebral metastases. Cancer 66 P (9) : 1873-1878
4. Avril MF, Bonneterre J, Cupissol D, Grob JJ, Kalis B, Fumoleau P, Kerbrat P, Israel L, Fargeot P, Lambert D, Delaunay M, Dreno B, Vilmer C, Bizzari JP, Cour V (1991) Fotemustine and dacarbazine (DTIC) : a combined regimen for malignant melanoma — Final report on 103 evaluable patients. American Society for Clinical Oncology, Houston, 17-21 mai
5. Frenay M, Giroux B, Khoury S, Derlon JM, Namer M (1991) Phase II study of a new nitrosourea, fotemustine, in recurrent supratentorial malignant gliomas. Eur J Cancer (in press)
6. Le Chevalier T, Zabbe C, Gouva S, Cerrina Ml, Quoix E, Riviere A, Berthaud P, Prache C, Berille J (1989) Phase II multicentre study of the nitrosourea fotemustine in inoperable squamous cell lung carcinoma. Eur J Clin Oncol 25 (11) : 1651-1652
7. Chevallier B, Toussaint C, Kerbrat P, Bonneterre J, Mousseau M, Audhuy B, Droz JP, Vignoud J, Coste M, Benoliel C, Berille J (1991) Final report : phase II study of fotemustine in advanced renal cell carcinoma (RCC) ; an assessment of Elson prognostic factors American Society for Clinical Oncology, Houston, 17-21 mai
8. Bleiberg H, Becquart D, Michel J, Cavalli F, Gerard B (1990) Phase II trial of fotemustine in advanced colorectal cancer. Eur J Cancer 26 (11/12) : 1260-1261
9. Khayat D, Cour V, Aigner C, Vignoud J, Audhuy B, Monnier A, Lerol A, Bouillet T, Brion G, Dumesnil Y, Cohen-Aloro G, Bizzari JP, Weil M, Jacquillat C (1990) Final report of a phase II study of hepatic intra-arterial fotemustine : 66 evaluable patients (pts). American Association for Cancer Research, Washington, 23-27 mai

CPT-11 : an analog of Camptothecin in early clinical development

A Mathieu-Boué*, G Chabot**, I Barilero**, S Culine***, M de Forni****, D Gandia**, M Clavel*****, JP Armand**, M Marty**, R Bugat****

CPT-11 is a water-soluble analog of camptothecin synthesized by Yakult Honsha Co. Ltd (Japan). CPT-11 and its main metabolite SN-38 are active against a variety of human cancer cell lines, even in resistant cell lines [1], as well as in murine tumor models [2]. Their mechanism of action is presumed to be through inhibition of TopoIsomerase I. A previous Japanese Phase I study of CPT-11 established the MDT at 250 mg/m² as a single dose. The dose limiting toxicity was leukopenia with mild anemia and thrombocytopenia [3]. The recommended dose for Phase II trials was 200 mg/m² every 3 weeks. Phase II trials started in Japan with different therapeutic schedules, and showed interesting response rates in lung cancers and others tumors including colorectal, gastric, cervical, ovarian [4,5] and hematological malignancies [6].

The on going French Phase I studies (started in July 1990), are exploring 3 different schedules of 30 min infusions :

— 1 single dose weekly, (minimum 3) ; 1 single dose every 3 weeks (minimum 3) ; and 1 dose every day for 3 days, every 3 weeks (minimum 3).

We report here the toxicities, responses, and pharmacokinetics available to date.

Patients and methods

The criteria of eligibility were as follows : histologically confirmed malignancy refractory to standard therapy ; no chemotherapy or radiotherapy in the previous month ; no evidence of serious cardiovascular, hepatic, or renal dysfunction ; a life expectancy of more than 3 months ; a performance status of 0-2 (ECOG) ; age 18-75 ; and, hematological and biochemical parameters had to be within normal range. A written informed consent was obtained from all patients included in this study.

CPT-11 was dissolved in normal saline (250 ml) and administered intravenously over 30 min.

CPT-11 and SN-38 plasma concentrations were determined by HPLC. Briefly, after a solid-phase extraction using C18 columns, the methanolic extract was evaporated and reconstituted in the mobile phase (acetonitrile : phosphate buffer-heptane sulfonic acid ; 34 : 66).

* Laboratoire Roger Bellon, Neuilly sur Seine ** Institut Gustave-Roussy, Villejuif *** Hôpital Saint-Louis, Paris **** Centre Claudius-Régaud, Toulouse ***** Centre Léon-Bérard, Lyon France

Separation was accomplished with a C18 column, and fluorescence detection was set at 380 nm (excitation) and 500 nm (emission).

Results and discussion

To date 37 patients were entered with the following characteristics : 17 females, 20 males, the median age was 53.5. One patient was found not eligible soon after inclusion because of abnormal hepatic test. All patients, except 2 were pretreated.

The main side effects were nausea, vomiting, diarrhea, myelosuppression, alopecia, and fatigue. Myelosuppression was mainly leukopenia and granulocytopenia, and seemed dose — related, so far.

Other toxic effects were : stomatitis, allergy (with negative rechallenge), erythema, vertigo, local irritation, pain, tachycardia, hypotension, abnormal hepatic tests, and myalgia with transient elevation of CPK, but negative rechallenge.

Among evaluable patients for efficacy we observed several stable diseases including 1 case each of renal carcinoma, melanoma, sarcoma, cholangio carcinoma, and breast cancer. These patients happened to be among those who received the highest doses (400-705 mg/m², total dose).

To study pharmacokinetics of CPT-11, a sensitive HPLC assay with fluorescence detection was developed allowing simultaneous quantification of both CPT-11 and its main metabolite SN-38.

Plasma elimination of CPT-11 was triphasic with an alpha half-life of 6 min, a beta half-life of 2.3 h and a terminal gamma half-life of 17 h (Table 1). This prolonged terminal half-life could be of therapeutic advantage for this S-phase specific agent. Unlike camptothecin, CPT-11 pharmacokinetics (AUC) was correlated with toxicity in 2 patients to date. Cytotoxic concentrations of the active metabolite SN-38 were also reached (10-40 ng/ml).

Table 1. CPT-11 Pharmacokinetics in patients

Dose mg/M²	N	Cmax ng/ml	Half-lives (h) Alpha	Beta	Gamma	AUC ng.h/ml	Vdss L/M²	Clearance L/M²/h
50	2	664	0.31	3.6	16.4	2684	140	18.9
66	6	1552	0.10	1.5	11.7	4279	115	18.6
75	6	1733	0.03	2.8	22.5	8064	103	10.2
85	1	1225	0.30	3.3	7.7	8190	71	10.4
100	7	2566	0.07	2.2	18.2	8190	153	18.8
MEAN			0.09	2.3	17.0		124	16.1
(SE)			(.02)	(.2)	(2.9)		(15)	(2.0)

Conclusion

The French Phase I trials of CPT-11 are still going on and the MDT is not reached yet. The main toxic effects are digestive and myelosuppression. Interesting responses observed to date have be confirmed in Phase II trials.

References

1. Tsuruo T, Matsuzali T, Matsushita M et al (1988) Antitumor effect of CPT-II, a new derivative of camptothecin, against pleiotropic drug-resistant tumors in vitro and in vivo. Cancer Chemother Pharmacol 21 : 71-74
2. Kunimoto T, Nitta K, Tanaka T et al (1987) Antitumor activity of 7-ethyl-10-[4-(1-piperidino)-1-piperidino] carbonyloxy-camptothecin, a novel water-soluble derivative of camptothecin, against murine tumors. Cancer Res 47 : 5944-5947
3. Suminaga M, Furue H, Taguchi T et al (1989) Phase I study of CPT-11, a derivative of camptothecin. 16th International Congress of Chemotherapy, Jerusalem, Israel, p 51
4. Futuoka M, Negoro S, Niitani H et al (1990) A phase II study of a new camptothecin derivative, CPT-II in previously untreated non-small cell lung cancer (NSCLC) (meeting abstract). Proc Am Soc Clin Oncol n° 873 9 : p 226
5. Taguchi T (1990) Phase I and II Clinical Studies of CPT-11 Program and Abstracts of the Third Conference on DNA Topoisomerases in Therapy, New York, n° 48, p 33
6. Ohno R, Okada K, Masaoka T et al (1990) An early Phase II study of CPT-11 : a new derivative of Camptothecin, for the treatment of leukemia and lymphoma. J Clin Oncol 8 : 1907-1912

Abstract. CPT-11 is a water-soluble analog of camptothecin synthesized by Yakult Honsha Co. Ltd (Japan). CPT-11 and its main metabolite SN-38 are active against a variety of human cancer cell lines as well as in murine tumor models. Their mechanism of action is presumed to be through inhibition of TopoIsomerase I. A previous Phase I study of CPT-II established the Maximum Tolerated Dose (MTD) at 250 mg/m², with leukopenia as the limiting toxicity. Japanese Phases II trials showed interesting response rates in lung cancers and other tumors including colorectal, gastric, cervical, ovarian and hematological malignancies. The ongoing French Phase I studies are exploring 3 different schedules of 30 min infusions. The main side effects observed so far included nausea, vomiting, diarrhea, myelosuppression, alopecia and fatigue. The MDT has not been reached yet. Although stable diseases have been observed, no objective response has been achieved yet. To study pharmacokinetics of CPT-11, a sensitive HPLC assay with fluorescence detection was developed allowing simultaneous quantification of both CPT-II and its main metabolite SN-38. Plasma elimination was triphasic with a relatively long mean terminal half-life of 17 hours that could be of therapeutic advantage for this S-phase specific agent.

Modulation of glutathione and associated enzymes as a therapeutic strategy

K Tew, P Ciaccio, M Clapper, R Krigel, S Kuzmich, F LaCreta, R Ozols, P O'Dwyer, J Schisselbauer

Since tumor cell resistance to anticancer drugs is one of the primary factors limiting disease response, recent protocols attempt to modulate existing drugs with relatively non-toxic agents as a means of increasing therapeutic effect. The involvement of GSH and GST in resistance to alkylating agents is now well established. Preclinical data is supportive of the concept that interference with GSH and associated pathways is a viable approach to enhancement of alkylating drug efficacy.

Materials and methods

HT29 human colon carcinoma cell lines were grown as monolayers. The EA resistant HT/M line was established by mutagenization and maintained in drug except during experiments to measure colony forming ability. Quantification and identification of GST isozymes was achieved by GSH-affinity purification, followed by SDS-PAGE and Western blot using a battery of polyclonal antibodies against GST isozymes. Estimates of transcriptional activity were based upon Northern and slot blots of mRNA transcripts using cDNA clones coding for a human anionic GST.

Pharmacokinetic analyses either in cultured cells or in human plasma were measured using sensitive HPLC procedures. BSO was derivatized with phenylisothiocyanate prior to separation of the S and R isomers on reverse phase HPLC with nor-leucine as the internal standard ; EA is extracted in acidified ethyl-acetate and evaporated under a stream of nitrogen. Using 4-(2,4-dichlorophenoxy) butyric acid as an internal standard, EA was determined using UV absorption of eluant following reverse phase chromatography.

Results

Non-toxic levels of EA were previously found to increase the antitumor effects of chlorambucil and melphalan against cells in culture [1] or SCID mice bearing human colon tumors [2]. In vitro incubations of chlorambucil with GSH lead to the formation of both the mono- and di-glutathionyl conjugate of the drug. The rate and extent of formation of these metabolites is enhanced 2 to 5-fold by the presence of GST isozymes ($\alpha > p > \mu$).In order to gain insight

Department of Pharmacology, Fox Chase Cancer Center, 7701 Burholme Avenue, Philadelphia, PA 19111, USA into the mechanism of EA, HT29 cells (HT/M) were selected for resistance to the drug. Characterization of GST showed microheterogeneous forms of the π isozyme detected in both WT and HT/M. In the continuous presence of EA, GST activity and GSH levels were increased approx. 3-fold in HT/M. The presence of the drug was a requirement for the elevated GST/GSH. In vitro metabolism of EA with purified GST from each cell line was characterized by a biphasic disappearance of the parent drug.

Cross-resistance to various agents is shown in Table 1. The data are consistent with the enhanced thiol detoxification of certain electrophilic drug species.

Table 1. Cross-Resistance patterns of WT and EA-resistant cells

Cell Line	EA	Melphalan	BCNU	5 FU	Adriamycin (nM)
WT	26	3	90	0.48	11
HT/M	48 (1.8)	11 (3.7)	140 (1.4)	0.64 (1.4)	14 (1.3)

Values are IC_{50} in μM except where stated. Parentheses show fold resistance at IC_{50}'s.

Resistance to melphalan could be partially reversed by depletion of GSH by BSO, suggesting that spontaneous conjugation accounted for a proportion of conjugate formation.

Induction of GST by EA occurred at the transcriptional level. Northern and slot blot analyses revealed approx. Three-fold increase in the 1.2 kb transcript for GST π in HT/M compared to the WT. No gene amplification was apparent. The Phase I trial data showed a MTD of 75 mg/m² q 6 h x 3. Inhibition of GST was found in peripheral mononuclear cells and the major dose limiting toxicity was metabolic and electrolyte disturbance. Preliminary pharmacokinetics in a patient receiving 100 mg EA p.o. indicated first order elimination of the drug. Rapid absorption and high protein binding were apparent, with a concentration maximum of 0.25 μg/ml at 48 min. Based on our earlier data in CLL patients resistant to chlorambucil [3], a Phase II trial has been designed (Table 2).

Table 2. GST Activity in Lymphocytes from CLL Patients

Lymphocyte sample	Specific Activity (nmol/min/mg)
CLL, nontreated	51.3 ± 8.5
CLL, treated, nonresistant	67.4 ± 6.9
CLL, treated, resistant	103 ± 13.6
Normal B + T cells	47.5 ± 8.7

Phase II Protocol for Chlorambucil and
Ethacrynic Acid in Refractory CLL

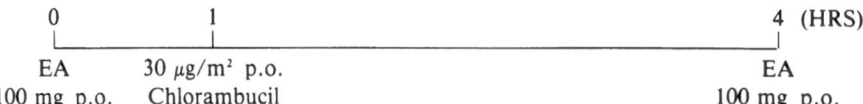

In a Phase I trial of melphalan and BSO [4] 10 patients have received 2 cycles of treatment ; cycle 1 BSO iv q 12 h x 6, 1.5 g/m² ; cycle 2 one week later BSO as cycle 1 with iv melphalan 15 μg/m², 1 hr after the fifth dose. Toxicities associated with the combination were : nausea/vomiting, grade III-IV neutropenia (6/10) and grade IV thrombocytopenia (2/10). Plasma disappearance of BSO isomers was biphasic, S-BSO αt1/2 = 17.9 min, βt1/2 = 3.4 hr ; R-BSO αt1/2 = 19.4 mins, βt1/2 = 3.5 hr. An 80 % decrease in PMN GSH levels occurred in 5/8 patients and in tumor ascites of 2 patients.

Modulation of GSH and associated GST enzymes can reverse resistance in preclinical models and can be used with manageable side-effects in Phase I trials. Further clinical development of these modalities is warranted.

References

1. Tew K, Bomber A, Hoffman S (1988) Ethacrynic acid and piriprost as enhancers of cytotoxicity in drug resistant and sensitive cell lines. Cancer Res 48 : 3622-3625
2. Clapper M, Hoffman S, Tew K (1990) Sensitization of human colon xenografts to melphalan using an inhibitor of glutathione S-transferase. J Cell Pharmacol 1 : 71-78
3. Schisselbauer J, Silber R, Papadopoulous E, LaCreta F, Tew K (1990) Characterization of lymphocyte glutathione S-transferase isozymes in chronic lymphocytic leukemia (CLL). Cancer Research 50 : 3569-3573
4. LaCreta F, Brennan J, Padavic K, Hamilton T, Tew K, Young R, Comis R, Ozols R, O'Dwyer P (1991) Phase I clinical, biochemical and pharmacokinetic study of buthionine sulfoximine (BSO) in combination with melphalan (L-PAM). ASCO abstract, in press

Abstract. The use of relatively non-toxic modulators of cancer drugs is becoming an accepted technique for reversing acquired resistance expressed by many tumor cells. Resistance to alkylating agents, especially nitrogen mustards may be mediated by increased intracellular glutathione (GSH) and/or glutathione S-transferase (GST) isozymes, resulting in increased detoxification potential. Buthionine sulfoximine (BSO) depletes GSH through competitive inhibition with -glutamyl cysteine synthetase, a key enzyme in the synthesis of the tripeptide. Ethacrynic acid (EA) depletes GSH and inhibits GST isozymes. In preclinical and more recently clinical situations, these drugs are effective modulators of resistance.

Lung

Neo-Adjuvant chemotherapy (N-CT) followed by concomitant chemotherapy and radiotherapy (CC-CT) for locally advanced non-small cell lung cancer (NSCLC)

JJ Illarramendi, JJ Valerdi, FJ Dominguez, E Martinez, MA Dominguez

N-CT principles may display different roles in the management of NSCLC. The value of N-CT before radiotherapy (RT) means an important point of clinical research, since many patients could benefit from even small improvements in survival or tumor control.

RT alone has a doubtful value in locally advanced NSCLC, and no survival benefit has been shown for this treatment in a recently performed randomized trial [1]. Since CC-CT sems to improve tumor control in various epithelial neoplasms [2], the contribution of N-CT for NSCLC could be enhanced by choosing CC-CT as a potentially more active treatment than RT alone.

We have undertaken this study to ascertain the feasibility and preliminary results of a program that combines N-CT and CC-CT in order to attempt a better local and systemic control of neoplasms.

Material and methods

Forty-one patients (33 epidermoid, 5 adenocarcinoma, 3 large cell). Median age : 66 years (37-77). Performance status ECOG 0-1 : 41/41. Clinical stage (UICC) IIIb 37/41 and II or IIIa in 4/41 (these patients were unfit for surgery). Most patients (31/31) had a bronchoscopic diagnosis, and a routine staging study that included thoraco-upper abdominal CT scan and bone scintigraphy in all the patients. Entry criteria also required patient consent as well as absence of renal, heart or bone marrow failure.

Therapy included Cisplatin (120 mg/m^2), Mitomycin (10 mg/m^2) and Vindesine (3 mg/m^2) administered at day 1. Vindesine (3 mg/m^2) was also weekly injected for the next three weeks (days 8, 15, 22). From 28th to 32th day Cisplatin (20 mg/m^2/day) was given as continous infusion for 5 days, concomitant with the first days of RT. Radiation was used with standard megavoltage techniques, to a total dose of 60 Gy/6 weeks.

Results

Sixteen out of 37 (43 %) were regarded as radiologic responders to N-CT, with 40.5 % partial (PR) and 2.7 % complete (CR) responses. The rate of responses in higher after completion of CC-CT, with 92 % responses (50 % CR, 42 %

Serv. of Hematology and Oncology, Hospital Virgen del Camino. Servs. of Radiation Oncology and Pneumology, Hospital de Navarra, Navarre Health Service-Osasunbidea, Pamplona, Spain

PR). We must point out that radiologic assessment of response was very difficult after CC-CT, because fibrotic masses around the hilar region were visible in many CT scans, and it proved difficult to ascertain the true nature of these masses in many patients. Radiologic response could be only evaluated in 12 patients.

Bronchoscopic response was also evaluated in a large number of patients with a previous positive bronchoscopy. After CC-CT, 61 % of the patients were regarded as CRs (no endoscopic and pathologic data related to the previous neoplasm) and there were 30.7 % PRs (clear image improvement, but endoscopic or pathologic signs of active tumor).

The overall toxicity displayed by this therapeutic schedule was not very severe, although 2 patients died of neutropenic sepsis, and more than 2 grade (WHO scale) leukopenia was present in 70 % patients. Moderate to severe esophagitis, emesis and alopecia were also present in more than half of the patients.

With 36 months median follow up, median survival was 19 months. 60 % and 22 % survived for 12 and 24 months, respectively.

Discussion

The therapy schedule developed in this report was well tolerated. Toxicity was not severe, and neutropenia represents the most dangerous adverse effect. We have not found Mitomycin-associated pneumonitis in this series, although several cases of this complication have been seen by us in other patients. However, the therapeutic index of Mitomycin is far from clear and the potential appearance of severe pneumonitis must be recognized.

A higt rate of bronchoscopic responses was achieved with this program, although our data on radiologic responses must be taken with care because many patients were found not to be candidates for response evaluation. This increased antineoplastic effect has been also found in other reports of concomitant chemoradiotherapy [3]. There is some consensus of the potential role, in survival, of the rate of CRs achieved by different therapeutic programs.

This treatment schedule is short, with no long-term toxicity. The role of maintenance CT after N-CT has been questioned is a recently performed randomized trial [4].

Cisplatin seems to be a useful drug for this approach, combining antineoplastic potential and radiosensibilizing properties [5]. Trials employing other concomitant drugs have often failed to obtain positive results [6].

Survival results in this study compare well with other series not using N-CT or CC-CT. A recent trial has demonstrated the potential survival benefit of the use of N-CT before RT. Our program does not seem to have a major impact on survival, and only larger and controlled studies will ascertain if there is a survival benefit from N-CT plus C-CT in NSCLC.

References

1. Johnson DH, Einhorn LH, Bartolucci A et al (1990) Thoracic radiotherapy does not prolong survival in patients with locally advanced, unresectable non-small cell lung cancer. Ann Intern Med 113 : 33-38
2. Vokes EE, Weichselbaum RR (1990) Concomitant chemotherapy : rationale and experience in patients with solid tumors. J Clin Oncol 8 : 911-934
3. Schaake-Kooning C, Maat B, Van Houtte P et al (1990) Radiotherapy combined with low dose cisplatin in non operable, non metastatic, non-small cell lung cancer : a randomized three arms study of the EORTC Lunc Cancer and Radiation Therapy Cooperative groups. Int J Radiat Oncol Biol Phys 19 : 967-972
4. Tourani JM, Timsit JF, Delaisement C et al (1990) Two cycles of cisplatin-vindesine and radiotherapy for localized non-small cell carcinoma of the lung (stage III). Cancer 65 : 1472-1477
5. Douple EB (1988) Keynote address : platinum-radiation interactions. NCI Monograph 6 : 315-319
6. Vokes EE, Vijayakumar S, Hoffman P et al (1990) 5-Fluorouracil with oral leucovorin and hydroxyurea an concomitant radiotherapy for stage II non-small cell lung cancer Cancer 66 : 437-442

Multimodality therapy of non-small cell lung cancer (NSCLC)

KS Sridhar and RJ Thurer

Conventional treatment with external RT is suboptimal in unresectable NSCL [1]. The survival may be improved by aggressive intraoperative and perioperative interstitial brachy RT [2]. We developed a chemotherapy (CT) program incorporating 5-FU and Cisplatin as radiation sensitizers in combination with Etoposide [3, 4]. Our objective of multimodality was to eradicate the tumor in the chest and micrometastases by a combination of pre and postoperative CT, radical surgical excision and perioperative RT [4]. We report the safety, tolerance, and efficacy of this intensive multimodality treatment administered with a curative intent for patients with stage III.

Patients and methods

The selection criteria were : pathologically proved NSCLC, stage III B or marginally resectable stage IIIA, performance status 0-2, normal, renal, hepatic, and hematopoietic functions, no myocardial infarction in the preceding 6 months, and an informed consent. Preoperative CT consisted of Cisplatin 100 mg/m^2 given I.V over 4 h on day 1. This was preceded and followed by intensive antiemesis and hydratation. This was followed by the administration of Etoposide 80 mg/m^2 I.V over 1 h on days 2,3 and 4. 5-FU was administered on days 2 through 5 as a continuous infusion 960 mg/m^2/day x 3. The 5-FU infusion was interrupted to administer Etoposide. From days 2 through 5, patients were given prophylactic antiemetics consisting of prochlorperazine, lorazepam and diphenhydramine [5]. Recent data suggest that phenothiazines such as Prochlorperazine may increase CT drug retention [6].

In absence of tumor progression, the patients were retreated with CT on or about the 22nd day.

Patients with tumors showing reduction on the serial chest x-rays after the first and second cycle of CT received a third cycle of CT.

In absence of systemic metastasis and adequate lung function tests, the patients were surgically explored. In general, an effort was made to excise all tumors with negative margins and to sample all the appropriate lymph nodes.

^{125}I and/or ^{192}Ir were used to treat positive or close surgical margins [2, 4]. External RT was used in patients with positive or close margins, those treated with brachy RT and patients with histologically documented Nl or rN2 disease. External RT fields consisted of AP-PA portals to cover the primary tumor volume and regional lymph nodes (mediastinum, bilateral supraclavicular areas

University Of Miami School Of Medicine, and Veterans Administration Medical Center, (D 8-4)
P.O. Box 016960, Miami, Florida 33136, USA

and ipsilateral hilum). If only external RT was delivered, a secondary coned-down field was by rotation to avoid excessive spinal cord dose. Patients received a total of 9-10 Gy per week (180-200 cGy fractions 4 to 5 days per week), bringing the RT dose to the primary tumor to 60 Gy or higher. The total dose delivered to the spinal cord did not exceed 50 Gy. The total dose in patients treated with brachy RT consisted of a minimum additional 45 Gy to the mid plane using an AP - PA portal. Post-operative adjuvant CT was advised to the patients who had an objective response to pre-operative CT. We administered a total of 6 cycles of CT pre and post-surgery. Patients who received 2 cycles of CT pre-surgery were advised 4 cycles post-surgery and those patients who received 3 cycles pre-surgery received 3 cycles post-surgery.

Results

We report data on 25 patients who have either died or have a minimum follow-up of one year. There were 17 partial responders to preoperative CT. On surgical exploration, 16 patients were found to have residual tumor compatible with a partial response and one patient was tumor free. Radiologic assessment of lack of response is inaccurate in patients who gained weight, had symptomatic relief and improvement in performance status despite stable disease. Less tumor was found on surgical pathologic evaluation than that assessed by the radiologic studies. Of the 25 patients evaluable, 23 were explored, and 19 were rendered disease free. After the use of preoperative CT, the number of patients who required brachy RT was lower than what we had expected. Patients who had a good response to CT generally did not need brachy RT. Post-operative RT was used in 14 patients. Fifteen patients accepted post-operative adjuvant CT. Eleven patients are alive and tumor free and this includes 5 patients with a minimal follow-up of 4 years. The projected 5 year survival is about 35 %. These include patients with left vocal cord paralysis, tumor extending into the spine, and lymph node proven mediastinal disease pre-CT. There have been 10 deaths due to tumor and in 5 of these patients, brain metastases was the first site of failure. However, in none of these patients was the brain metastasis the sole cause of death. Patients relapsed with other sites of systemic metastases within a couple of months of brain metastasis. Four patients died tumor free, 1 due to pulmonary embolism, within 30 days post-surgery.

References

1. Johnson DH, Einhorn LH, Bartolucci A et al (1990) Thoracic radiotherapy does not prolong survival in patients with locally advanced, unresectable non-small cell lung cancer. Ann Intern Med 113 : 33-38
2. Hilaris BS, Gomez J, Nori D et al (1985) Combined surgery, intraoperative brachytherapy, and post-operative external RT in stage III non-small cell lung cancer. Cancer 55 : 1226-1231
3. Sridhar KS, Varki J, Donnelly E et al (1987) Toxicity of FED CT in non-small cell lung cancer. Amer J Clin Oncol 10 : 499-506

4. Sridhar KS, Thurer R, Kim Y et al (1988) Multimodality treatment of non-small cell lung cancer : response to cisplatin, VP-16, and 5-FU CT ; and to surgery and RT. J Surg Oncol 38 : 193-215
5. Sridhar KS, Donnelly E (1988) Combination antiemetics for cisplatin CT. Cancer 61 : 1508-1517
6. Krishan A, Sridhar KS, Sternheim W et al (1987) Patterns of anthracycline modulation in human tumor cells. Cytometry 8 : 306-314
7. Gralla RJ (1990) New directions in non-small cell lung cancer. Seminars in Oncol 17 : 14-19

Abstract. Stage III NSCLC is a chemosensitive tumor. Pre-operative CT appears to increase the resectability and reduce the need for pneumonectomy. Local tumor progression during pre-operative CT is rare. Patient acceptance and tolerance of pre-operative CT is excellent. Relief of subjective symptoms and weight gain are good indicators that the radiologic studies may be underestimating the tumor regression. Nearly 70 % of patients with marginally resectable NSCLC, can undergo potentially curative resection after pre-operative CT. Nearly 75 % of responders to pre-operative CT undergo resection [7]. In a few of these patients, no residual tumor can be identified by histopathologic examination. Adjuvant CT subsequent to post-operative RT is less well tolerated and accepted. In patients with non-squamous NSCLC, brain metastases is often the first site of recurrence. Brain metastases are indicators of future systemic metastases in other sites and death. The median survival of about 17 months and the projected 5 year survival of 35 % are remarkable and suggest that patients with stage III NSCLC should be managed by neo-adjuvant CT. Patients not amenable to a total resection should receive RT subsequent to CT.

Combined modality therapy for stage III non-small cell lung cancer : the University of Chicago experience

JD Bitran, EE Vokes, PC Hoffman, E Ellis, W Gradishar, C English, HM Golomb

The prognosis of patients with advanced locoregional stage (IIIA and IIIB) non small cell lung cancer (NSCLC) is quite poor. Over the past two decades, there is little evidence to suggest that the median survival or the 3 or 5 year survival rates for such patients have significantly improved. Despite the use of radical pneumonectomies with mediastinal dissection or radical radiotherapy, the majority of patients with Stage III NSCLC will succumb to metastatic disease. The five year survival rate for patients with stage IIIB NSCLC is less than 10 % [1]. More recently, efforts to improve this grim outlook for patients with stage III NSCLC have focused on bimodality and multimodality therapies including radiotherapy followed by chemotherapy, neo-adjuvant chemotherapy followed by surgery or radiotherapy or concurrent chemotherapy and radiotherapy. The rationale for such approaches in that chemotherapy might reduce the relatively lower tumor burden in patients with stage III NSCLC (as compared to patients with stage IV NSCLC) and that this decrease in the tumor burden would allow the local therapy (i.e. radiotherapy, surgery) to be more effective. Additionally, the use of chemotherapy concurrently with radiotherapy would permit synergistic effects between radiotherapy and chemotherapeutic agents that are radiosensitizers and possibly increase tumor cell kill. (It is recognized that the toxic effects of radiotherapy will be enhanced on normal tissues).

Since 1975, we have performed a series of phase II studies employing radiotherapy and chemotherapy or more recently, multimodality therapy in patients with stage III non small cell lung cancer in an attempt to identify promising new treatment approaches that could then be tested in randomized phase III trials. The sequential nature of these studies has been radiotherapy followed by chemotherapy (RT → CT). neo-adjuvant chemotherapy followed by surgery and/or radiotherapy (CT → S → RT, CT → RT) and conconcurrent chemotherapy and radiotherapy (CCTRT) [2-6]. In this report, we summarize our studies conducted over a 15 year period.

Patients and methods

From January 1, 1975 to December 31, 1990, 174 patients with stage IIIA and B NSCLC have been entered into 4 consecutive phase II studies employing che-

Department of Medicine, Section of Hematology/Oncology, University of Chicago Medical Center, Chicago, IL, USA

motherapy and radiotherapy with or without surgery. Of the 174 patients, there were 129 men and 45 women with a median age of 58 years (range 34-80 years) and a median PS of 1 (0-3). Many of these trials have been previously reported [4-6]. In brief, the first two trials employed initial radiotherapy 3,000 cGy/10 fraction and 4,200 cGy/14 fractions via anterior and posterior portals encompassing the pulmonary lesion and mediastinum followed by chemotherapy consisting of Cyclophosphamide, Adriamycin, Methotrexate, and Procarbazine (CAMP) or employing the CAMP regimen with high doses of Methotrexate with Leucovorin rescue (CAMP-L). The third generation study explored neo-adjuvant chemotherapy with Vindesine, Etoposide, and Platinol for 6 weeks (2 cycles) followed by surgery (4 patients) and/or radiotherapy, 5,400 cGy/27 fractions via a 4 mV or 6-mV linear accelerator with a portal that included the primary tumor, ipsilateral helium, mediastinum, and supraclavicular fossae [5]. The fourth generation trial employed concurrent chemotherapy and radiotherapy with continuous infusion 5-FU with high dose Leucovorin (L), and Hydroxyurea (H), and concomitant radiotherapy, 6,000 cGy/30 fraction by a 4 mV or 6-mV linear accelerator on alternate week basis (week on, week off). The portal included the primary tumor, the ipsilateral hilum, mediastinum, and supraclavicular fossae via oblique fields [6].

Our recent study commencing in October 1988 entered 23 patients, stage IIIA (11 patients), stage IIIB (12 patients) on a trial consisting of neo-adjuvant chemotherapy consisting of Mitomycin, Vinblastine, and Platinol, [7] followed by 5-FU, L, H with concomitant radiotherapy 6,000 cGy/30 fractions via a 4 mV or 6-mV linear accelerator as described above.

All patients have been followed for a minimum of a year and a median follow-up of 5 years (range 1-11 years). All events, toxicity, death from other causes, death from lung cancer, have been included in event-free survival and overall survival.

Results

Of the 174 patients entered in these 5 consecutive trials, the median survival regardless of the treatment employed was 9.0 months, the 1 year survival rate is 40 %, and the 5 year survival rate ranges from 4 to 10 % (Table 1). Of the 174 patients, 24 patients (14 %) are currently alive beyond 1 year, range 1-10 years). Of the remaining 150, 61 patients (24 %) failed to achieve any type of objective response. Relapse occurred in 89 patients ; 27 patients (33 %) relapsed locally within the radiotherapy portal, 21 patients (23 %) relapsed solely in distant sites, and 41 patients (46 %) relapsed in both local and distant sites. Toxicities and complications of therapy have been previously reported [4-6].

The characteristics of the 24 patients who are alive longer than 1 year are as follows : 14 patients with stage IIIA NSCLC, 10 patients with stage IIIB disease, 16 patients had adenocarcinoma, 7 had large cell carcinoma and 1 patient had squamous cell carcinoma, PS-0, 18 patients, PS-1, 6 patients. No patient had a performance status greater than 1.

Table 1. University of Chicago phase II Trials in Stage IIIA and B Small Cell Lung Cancer

Protocol*	No. of Pts	Event Free Survival	Median Survival	5 yr Survival	Reference
RT →CAMP	101	7.7	8.8	10%	[4]
RT →CAMP VEP →S ① →RT	27	8.0	8.0	4%	[5]
VEP → RT CCTRT (5FU/L/HU)	23	6.0	12.0	12% at 2 yrs	[6]
MVP →CCTRT MVP →S →CCTRT	23	NYR+	NYR+	projected 30 % at 1 yr	

*For details of the protocols, see references 4-6, and text ; CCTRT = Concurrent chemotherapy and radiotherapy ; RT Radiotherapy ; S = Surgery ; + Not yet reached

Discussion

We undertook the current analysis to determine the long term survival rate in patients with stage IIIA and B NSCLC who were treated in a series of phase II studies conducted over a 15 year period. Of the 174 patients entered on these sequential phase II trials there are 24 patients who are alive, disease-free at 1 year or greater with a projected 5 year and 7 year survival rate of 14 %. While it is difficult to compare these phase II trials with one another because of slightly different eligibility criteria, all of these patients were uniformly staged in an identical manner at a single institution. As shown in Table 1, the median survival was remarkably uniform at 9-12 months. Yet, the long term survival rate varied by trial.

While these trials are sequential and cannot be compared with one another, one might ask whether we have accomplished any progress in the treatment or outcome of patients with stage III NSCLC over a fifteen year period of sequential clinical trials. The obvious answer to this question is apparently not. Additionally, if one reviews the published phase II to other neo-adjuvant published trials in stage III NSCLC (Table 2), it is apparent [7-14] that differences in results or outcome are based on differing eligibility criteria, differing proportions of stage IIIA and IIIB patients entered on study as opposed to real difficulties based on treatment employed. The exception to this generalization is the report by Dillman et al [15]. This is the first to compare initial chemotherapy followed by radiation therapy to radiation therapy alone (Table 2). While the increase in median survival is modest, the differences observed in the median survivals (14 months for chemotherapy and radiation, 10 months for radiation alone) are statistically significant (p = 0.0066). These

Table 2. Phase II and Phase III Neo-Adjuvant and chemotherapy trials in NSCLC

Neo-adjuvant - Phase III

Regimen	No. of Pts	Objective Response	Median Survival		Reference
CAP→S→RT	41	25%	32		8
CAP×2→RT	30	43%	9		9
CAP×3→RT	39	51%	11		10
EP→RT	30	20%	<12		11
BEP×2→RT	30	36%	19		13
V+P,Velban- +P, MVP×2→S →RT	41	73%	20		12
MVP×3–4 →S→RT	22	73%	19		14

. . . .

Neo-adjuvant - Phase III

Velban+P× 2 → RT	155	36%	14 } p = 0.066		15
v s					
RT alone			10		

CAP = Cyclophosphamide, adriamycin, and platinol ; S = Surgery ; RT = Radiotherapy ; EP = Etoposide + Platinol ; BEP = Bleomycin, Etoposide + Platinol ; V+P = Vindesine, Platinol ; P = Platinol ; MVP = Mitomycin-C, Velban, Platinol

results require obvious confirmation, however, they do represent a starting point for additional studies in patients with unresectable stage IIIA and stage IIIB non small cell lung cancer.

References

1. Perez CA, Pajak TF, Rubin P, Simpson JR, Mohiuddin M, Brady LW et al (1987) Long-term observation of the pattern of failure in patients with unresectable non-oat cell carcinoma of the lung treated with definitive radiotherapy. Cancer 59 : 1874-1881
2. Spain RC, Jost J, Kircher T, Spen JF, Anderson PN, Zinn CJ et al (1987) neo-adjuvant mitomycin, cisplatin, and infusion vinblastine with reduced pulmonary toxicity in stage III non-small cell lung cancer. In : Salmon SE (ed) Adjuvant Therapy of Cancer V., Grune and Stratton, Inc. 165-177
3. Taylor SGW, Trybula M, Bonomi PD, Faber LP, Lee MS, Reddy S et al (1987) Simultaneous cisplatin fluorouracil infusion and radiation followed by surgical reaction in regionally localized stage III, non-small cell lung cancer. Am Thorac Surg 43 : 87-91
4. Madej PJ, Bitran JD, Golomb HM et al (1984) Combined modality therapy for stage IIIMO non small cell lung cancer : a 5 year experience. Cancer 54 : 50-58

5. Vokes EE, Bitran JD, Hoffman PC et al (1989) neo-adjuvant vindesine, etoposide, and cisplatin for locally advanced non-small cell lung cancer. A final report of phase II study. Chest 96 : 110-113

6. Vokes EE, Vijayakumar S, Hoffman PC, Ferguson MK, Bitran JD, Krishnasamy S, Jacobs R, Golomb HM (1990) Five-Fluorouracil with oral leucovorin and hydroxyurea and concomitant radiotherapy for stage III non-small cell lung cancer. Cancer 66 : 437-442

7. Kris MG, Gralla RJ, Wertherm MS et al (1986) Trial of combination mitomycin, vindesine, and cisplatin in patients with advanced non-small cell lung cancer. Cancer Treat Rep 70 : 1091-1096

8. Skarin A, Jachelson M, Sheton T et al (1989) neo-adjuvant chemotherapy in marginally resectable stage IIIMO non-small cell lung cancer : long-term follow-up in 41 patients. J Surg Oncol 40 : 266-274

9. Fram R, Skarin A, Balikian J et al (1985) Combination hemotherapy followed by radiotherapy for inpatients with regional stage III unresected no small cell lung cancer. Cancer Treat Rep 69 : 587-590

10. Eagan RT, Rund C, Lee RE et al (1987) Pilot study of induction therapy with cyclophosphamide, doxorubicin, and cisplatin and chest irradiation prior to thoracotomy in initially operable Stage IIIMO non-small cell lung cancer. Cancer Treat Rep 71 : 895-900

11. Cox JD, Samson MK, Herskovic AM et al (1986) Cisplatin and etoposide before definitive induction therapy for inoperable squamous carcinoma, adenocarcinoma, and large cell carcinoma of the lung : a phase I-II study of the Radiation Therapy Oncology Group. Cancer Treat Rep 70 : 1219-1220

12. Martini N, Kris MG, Gralla RJ et al (1988) The effects of pre-operative chemotherapy in the resectability of non-small cell lung carcinoma with mediastinal lymph node metastases (N_2M_0). Ann Thoracic Surgery 45 : 370-379

13. Osoba O, Rusthaven JJ, Evans WK et al (1986) Combined chemotherapy and radiation therapy for non-small cell lung cancer. Semin Oncol, 13 (Supp 3) : 121-124

14. Spain RC (1988) neo-adjuvant mitomycin C, cisplatin, and infusion vinblastine in locally and regionally advanced non-small cell lung cancer : problem and progress from the perspective of long-term follow up. Semin Oncol 15 : 6-15

15. Dillman RO, Seagren SL, Propert K et al (199) A randomized trial of induction chemotherapy plus high dose radiation versus radiation alone in stage III non-small cell lung cancer. N Engl J Med 323 : 940-945

High incidence of CNS metastases in long-term survivors (LTS) stage III (T4/N2) non-small cell lung cancer (NSCLC). Patients treated with Neo-Adjuvant chemotherapy

J Fleck, D Godoy, J Camargo

It has been already shown that neo-adjuvant chemotherapy, for non-small cell lung cancer, is very effective in reducing intrathoracic tumor bulk [1-6], trying, simultaneously, a better control of distant micrometastases. Surgical resection and irradiation can than be used as subsequent local consolidation therapy.

In 1988 we began a prospective study in stage III NSCLC patients, using MVP (Mitomycin C, Vinblastine, Cisplatin) neo-adjuvant chemotherapy, followed by consolidation therapy. Effective local and systemic control were achieved with this aggressive combined treatment. Unfortunately, a high incidence of CNS metastases was observed in our LTS.

Thirty-five stage III (T4-N2) non-small cell lung cancer patients were treated with MVP neo-adjuvant chemotherapy. Objective response was observed in 17 patients (48 %). However, only 7 patients (20 %) were eligible for surgery. One of these patients was in histological complete remission and was followed. The other 6 patients with histological residual disease and those 10 patients in clinical partial remission who were not eligible for surgery were additionally treated with 3 courses of PE (Cisplatin, Etoposide) every 3 weeks alternated with 3 courses of radiotherapy (1,500 cGy) administered in 5 twice-daily fractions of 150 cGy. Ten of those 17 patients who achieved objective response with MVP chemotherapy were in a maintained complete remission after a minimum follow-up of 18 months (LTS). Five of these 10 LTS patients developed CNS metastases and in 4 patients CNS was the only site of relapse. They were treated with CNS irradiation and dexamethasone and had a medium survival of 3 months.

The high incidence of CNS metastases (50 %) in our stage III (T4/N2) NSCLC LTS patients could be a consequence of better systemic and local control. We believe that prophylactic cranial irradiation (PCI) should be considered in a prospective randomized trial for stage III (T4/N2) NSCLC patients who were maintained in complete clinical remission after aggressive combined treatment.

Patients and methods

Eligibility criteria for study entry required patients with histopathologically confirmed non-small cell lung carcinoma. The histologic sub-types should be adenocarcinoma or squamous cell carcinoma. Patients with large cell carcinoma

Universidade Federal do Rio Grande do Sul, Pavilhao Pereira Filho, Hospital de Clinicas de Porto Alegre, Porto Alegre, RS Brazil Avenida Mostardeiro 333, Sala 403 Porto Alegre, RS, Brazil CEP 90410

were not included. Patients were staged according to the new International Staging System (ISS) [7]. The stages should be IIIa (N2), as a consequence of metastases to subcarinal or ipsilateral mediastinal lymph nodes or IIIb (T4) defined as mediastinal organ invasion. No patients with pleural effusion was included. Patients had to be ambulatory (Karnofsky performance scale above 60 %). They should not have been previously treated and should not present more than 5 % weight loss. Adequate bone marrow, renal, respiratory and cardiac function were also required. Leukocyte count should be over 3,000/mcl, platelet count over 100,000/mcl and serum creatinine below 1,5 mg/dl. A signed informed consent should be obtained.

Thirty-five stage III NSCLC patients entered the study. Stage IIIa (N2) represented 40 % of the accrual (14/35) and stage IIIb (T4) included 60 % of the patients (21/35). According to the histologic classification they were almost equally divided in adenocarcinoma (18/35) and squamous cell carcinoma (17/35).

The patients were sequentially treated with MVP neo-adjuvant chemotherapy and later on with consolidation combined modality treatment including surgery, radiation therapy and chemotherapy (Fig. 1). After MVP, patients in clinical complete remission (CR) and partial remission (PR) were subjected to mediastinal lymph node evaluation. Those with negative lymph nodes were subjected to surgery. Patients with no post-operative histological residual disease were just followed. Patients who were not eligible for surgery and those with post-operative histological residual disease were subjected to combined modality treatment with 3 courses of chemotherapy (Cisplatin + Etoposide) alternated with 3 split courses of multi-fraction radiation therapy. Each course of radiation therapy included 150 cGy twice-daily fraction for 5 days.

The MVP neo-adjuvant chemotherapy used consisted of Mitomycin C 8 mg/m^2, Cisplatin 120 mg/m^2 and Vinblastine 4.5 mg/m^2. Mitomycin C and Cisplatin were administered IV days 1,29 and 71. Vinblastine was given IV day 1 and each 2 weeks for a total of 6 doses. PE was used as a consolidation program alternated with split courses of radiation therapy. Cisplatin 30 mg/m^2 and Etoposide 100 mg/m^2 were administered IV days 1-3, each 3 weeks for a total of 3 courses.

As previously described [8] lung toxicity was avoided using dexamethasone 20 mg IV previously to each course of Mitomycin. C avoiding more than 3 courses of Mitomycin C or simultaneous use of irradiation and chemotherapy.

Results

Objective response to MVP which means CR and PR were obtained in 17/35 patients (49 %). There was a trend for a higher response rate in stage IIIa than stage IIIb NSCLC patients. However, the numbers were still too small to obtain significance (Table 1).

Only seven patients were eligible for surgery (20 %). They were, predominantly, stage IIIa (N2) (6/7 patients). The resection rate was significant higher for stage IIIa (N2) than stage IIIb (T4) NSCLC patients (Table 2). We observed one histologic complete remission after only three courses of MVP chemotherapy and this patient was just followed.

Fig. 1 : Treatment schema for stage III NSCLC patients

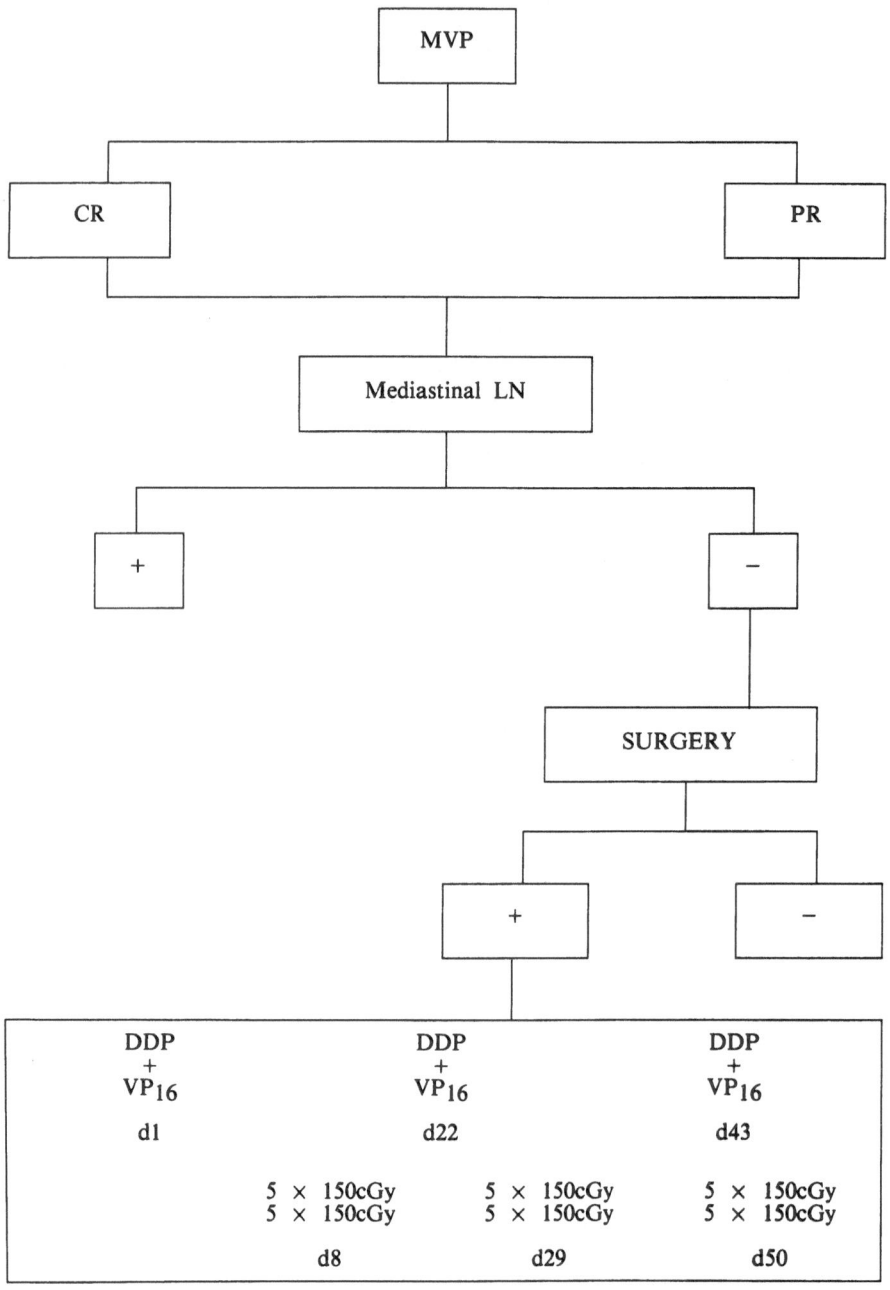

Table 1. Response to MVP Neo-Adjuvant chemotherapy

Objective Response	17/35 (49%)
IIIa (N2)	9/14 (64%)
IIIb (T4)	8/21 (38%)

Table 2. Surgery of stage III NSCLC patients

Resection	7/35 (20%)
IIIa (N2)	6/14 (43%)*
IIIb (T4)	1/21 (5%)

*p = 0.009

Sixteen of 17 NSCLC patients who responded to MVP chemotherapy were eligible for consolidation with PE chemotherapy and irradiation, which included 10 patients in PR after MVP chemotherapy and not subjected to surgery (these patients had measurable disease) and 6 patients in complete clinical response after MVP plus surgery, but with histological residual disease (these patients had non-measurable disease). In the 10 patients with measurable disease we observed a trend for a better response in stage IIIa (N2) than stage IIIb (T4) with consolidation combined treatment (Table 3). However, the number of patients was too small to show any significant difference.

Table 3. Response to consolidation therapy (PE + RT) stage III NSCLC patients with measurable disease

Objective response	7/10 (70%)
IIIa (N2)	3/3 (100%)
IIIb (T4)	4/7 (57%)

Ten out of the 17 NSCLC patients who responded to MVP chemotherapy were maintained in freedom from progression (FFP) after a minimum follow-up of 18 months (LTS). Five of these ten patients (50 %) developed CNS metastases, and in 4 patients CNS was the first and only site of relapse. These 4 patients were treated with CNS irradiation and Dexamethasone and had a medium survival of 3 months. All the 4 patients died as a consequence of CNS metastases. Despite an exhaustive search, including chest and abdominal CT and bone scan, no metastases were clinically detected outside the CNS. Unfortunatly, no autopsy study were performed.

Discussion

The biological behaviour of NSCLC is still under investigation, specially after the increasing use of neo-adjuvant chemotherapy. Our preliminary results indicated that CNS metastases could be a major prognostic limitation in stage III NSCLC patients successfully treated with agressive combined treatment. Forty percent of our LTS patients relapsed exclusively in the CNS after a minimum follow-up of 18 months. All these patients died as a consequence of CNS relapse.

Several randomized studies using PCI in small cell lung cancer (SCLC) patients have shown a significant reduction in CNS relapse rate [8-12]. These studies included a heterogeneous patient population that was comprised of patients who dit not achieved CR and of patients with extensive disease. This heterogeneity in SCLC patients could explain the absence of significant improvement in survival observed in all these studies. The only group of patients who theoretically could enjoy improved survival with PCI would be that group of patients achieving a CR. A proposed Eastern Cooperative Oncology Group protocol is presently randomizing, SCLC patients achieving CR to receive or not receive PCI. Similary, we believe that stage III NSCLC patients who achieve a CR after aggressive combined treatment should be considered for a prospective randomized trial to evaluate the usefullness of PCI.

As previously described [13], PCI could be associated with a high incidence of neurological complications, specially when the patients were treated simultaneously with chemotherapy and PCI doses higher than 3,000 cGy. In an attempt to avoid a dangerous liaison [14] PCI should be administered to stage III NSCLC patients only after the completion of all systemic and local treatment and only to patients in complete remission.

References

1. Gralla R, Kris M, Martini N, Stampleman L, Burke T (1987) Adjuvant chemotherapy approaches in non-small cell lung cancer. In : Salmon SE (ed) Adjuvant therapy of cancer V. Grune and Stratton, New York, p 147
2. Spain R (1988) neo-adjuvant mitomycin C, Cisplatin, infusion vimblastine in locally and regionaly advanced non-small cell lung cancer : problems and progress from the perspective of long term follow-up. Sem Oncol 15 : 6-15
3. Pincus M, Reddy S, Lee M, Bonomi P, Taylor S IV, Rowland K, Faber L, Warren W, Kittle C, Hendrickson F (1988) Pre-operative combined modality therapy for stage III Mo non-small cell lung carcinoma. Int J Rad Oncol Biol Phys 15 : 189-195
4. Umsawasdi T, Valdivieso M, Barkley T, Chen T, Booser D, Chiuten D, Dhingra H, Murphy W, Carr D (1988) Combined chemoradiotherapy in limited-disease, inoperable non-small cell lung cancer. Int J Rad Oncol Biol Phys 14 : 43-48
5. Osoba D, Rusthoven J, Evans W, Turnbull K (1986) Combined chemotherapy and radiation therapy for non-small cell lung cancer. Sem Oncol 13 : 121-124
6. Livingston R, Griffin B, Higano C, Laramore G, Rivkin S, Goldberg R, Schulman S (1987) Combined treatment with chemotherapy and neutron irradiation for limited non-small cell lung cancer : a southwest oncology group study. J Clin Oncol 5 : 1716-1724
7. Mountain C (1986) A new international staging system for lung cancer. Chest 89 : 225-232

8. Aisner J, Whitacre M, Van Echo D (1982) Combination chemotherapy for small cell carcinoma of the lung. Continuous versus alternating non-cross resistant combination. Cancer Treat Rep 66 : 221-230

9. Beiler D, Kane R, Bernath A (1979) Low dose elective brain irradiation in small cell carcinoma of the lung. Int J Rad Oncol Biol Phys 5 : 944-945

10. Jackson D, Richards F, Cooper M (1977) Prophylactic cranial irradiation in small cell carcinoma of the lung. A randomized study. JAMA 237 : 2730-2733

11. Maurer L, Tulloh M, Weiss R (1980) A randomized combined modality trial in small cell carcinoma of the lung. Comparison of combination chemotherapy-radiation therapy versus cyclosphosphamide-radiation therapy, effects of maintenance chemotherapy and prophylactic whole brain irradiation. Cancer 45 : 30-39

12. Syedel H, Creech R, Paganon M (1981) Combined modality treatment of small cell undifferentiated carcinoma of the lung. A cooperative study of the RTOG and the ECOG. Int J Rad Oncol Biol Phys 7 : 41

13. Fleck J, Einhorn L, Lauer R (1990) Is prophylactic cranial irradiation indicated in small-cell lung cancer ? J Clin Oncol 8 : 209-214

14. Turrisi A (1990) Brain irradiation and systemic chemotherapy for small-cell lung cancer. Dangerous liaisons ? J Clin Oncol 8 : 196-199

Combined modality therapy for stage IIIA (clinical N2) non-small cell carcinoma of the lung (NSCLC)

S Darwish, V Minotti, R Rossetti, M Lupattelli, L Crinò,
E Maranzano, F Checcaglini, P Fiaschini, E Bucciarelli, O Pensa,
U Mercati, M Tonato

Prognosis for locoregionally advanced NSCLC patients is poor. Five year survival rates of less than 10 % are reported for patients with mediastinal lymph-node involvement [1]. Efforts to improve this poor prognosis have recently focused on multiple therapeutic modalities including neo-adjuvant chemotherapy [2-6] and give the best reproducible response rates. Since 1988 a phase II trial of this neo-adjuvant chemotherapy combination has been used in patients with clinically apparent N2 to assess response rate, complete resection by surgery and the feasibility of combined treatment.

Material and methods

From August 1988 to December 1990, 42 patients with histologically confirmed NSCLC and stage IIIA disease entered this study : 37 males, 5 females, median age 58 yrs (range 45-70), median PS = 90 % ; 34 squamous cell carcinomas, 7 adenocarcinomas and 1 large cell carcinoma. All patients had clinical N2 stage defined by the presence of bulky ipsilateral lymphoadenopathy evident on chest-x-ray, nodes > 2 cm at CT scan, or evidence of tracheal, carinal or main bronchus compression by nodes at bronchoscopy. Inclusion criteria were : age below 70, performances status 80-100 (KPS), respiratory function compatible with surgical resection, normal baseline renal and cardiac functions.

Treatment

Treatment was Cisplatin 120 mg/m² on day 1, Etoposide 100 mg/m² on days 1-3 for 2 or 3 cycles every 21 days. In 8 patients chemotherapy was combined with radiotherapy on a split course schedule (1,500 cGY in 5 fractions over 5 days concomitantly with 1st and 2nd cycle). Responses were graded according to standard response criteria. Patients achieving major response (CR or PR) or with technically resectable stable disease were surgically explored in an attempt to resect all primary disease and perform mediastinal lymph-node dissection.

Divisions of Medical Oncology, Radiotherapy, Surgery, Pathology, Perugia Hospital, 06100 Perugia, Italy

Results

Response to initial chemotherapy was determined by restaging CT scan prior to surgery. Forty-one patients were evaluable for 2 cycles. The overall response rate to neo-adjuvant chemotheray was 81 % (34/42) (Table 1). Four patients (10 %) had complete response and 30 (71 %) partial response. All 8 patients who received chemotherapy plus radiotherapy had partial response. Thirty-one patients (2 CR, 27 PR, 2 SD) underwent surgical resection and 26 patients (62 %) had complete resection. No tumour was in the resected specimen of 5 patients. Mild myelosuppression was the main toxicity. There was 1 sepsis and 3 episodes of febrile neutropenia. Ten patients died : 4 from progressive disease, 3 from surgical complications (1 gastro-intestinal bleeding 2 wks after surgery ; 1 bronchus-pleural fistula 4 months after pneumonectomy as a consequence of infective complication ; 1 ventricular fibrillation the day after surgery), 1 after start of chemotherapy for an undetermined cause, 1 for second tumour, and 1 for myocardial infarction. Five patients relapsed ; 1 distant relapse (brain) and 4 local relapse. Median follow-up was 8 months (range 1-24). The 1.5 yr survival probability of operated and non-operated patients was 83 % and 55 %, respectively.

Table 1. Resection rate by chemotherapy

| | Chemotherapy response | | | | |
	Complete	Partial	SD	Progr.	Tot.
Completed therapy	4	30	5	2	41
Surgically explored	2	27	2	0	31
Complete resection	2	23	1	0	26
No tumour in resected specimen	1	4	0	0	5

Discussion

This pilot trial with neo-adjuvant chemotherapy in a selected and homogenous group of patients with regionally advanced NSCLC shows that the PE regimen was very active with an 81 % objective response rate and 10 % CR rate. This high activity may be tumour burden with respect to patients with metastatic NSCLC. No technical difficulties during surgery were encountered in this study, even in patients who had received chemotherapy plus radiotherapy. Toxicity was primarily moderate myelosuppression and did not result in severe morbidity. Though 3 patients died from surgical complications, we consider surgery-related mortality acceptable. Our preliminary results support data of other authors that high complete resection (62 % in our study) is obtained after a major response to pre-operative chemotherapy. A similar study with MVP chemotherapy [2] (Mitomycin, Vinca alkaloid and high-dose Cisplatin) gave a high response rate in stage IIIA, clinical N2 NSCLC patients. Our follow-up was not long enough to estimate survival (median follow-up was 8 months, range 1-24). However, preliminary survival analysis shows some difference between the 31 operated and 11 non-operated patients, with a 1.5 yr actuarial survival of 83 % and 55 %, respectively.

References

1. Martini N, Flehinger BJ (1987) The role of surgery in N2 lung cancer. Surg Clin NA 67 (5) : 1037-1049
2. Pisters KMW, Kris MG, Grallat RJ, Martini N (1990) Pre-operative chemotherapy in stage IIIA non-small cell lung : an analysis of a trial in patients with clinically apparent mediastinal node involvement. In : Sidney and Salmon (ed) Adjuvant therapy of cancer. Sanders, Philadelphia, p 132
3. Skarin A, Jochelson M, Sheldon T et al (1989) neo-adjuvant chemotherapy in marginally resectable stage III Mo non-small cell lung cancer. Long-term follow-up in 41 patients. J Surg Oncol 40 : 266-274
4. Vokes EE, Bitran JD, Hoffman PC et al (1989) neo-adjuvant vindesine etoposide and cisplatin for locally advanced non-small cell lung cancer. Final report of a phase 2 study. Chest 96 : 110-113
5. Cisplatin and etoposide in bronchogenic squamous cell carcinoma and adenocarcinoma. A study by the EORTC lung cancer working party (Belgium). Cancer 50 : 2751-2756
6. Crinò L, Darwish S, Corgna F et al (1988) Treatment of advanced non-small cell lung cancer (NSCLC) : the « Umbria » cooperative study. Seminars in Oncology 15 (supp 7) : 52-55

Abstract. Forty-two patients (pts) with marginally resectable, regionally advanced NSCLC (stage IIIA, clinically apparent N2 extent) received neo-adjuvant chemotherapy with higt-dose Cisplatin and Etoposide (PE). Eight pts received chemotherapy plus radiotherapy. Total response rate to primary PE was 81 % (34/42) : 4 complete response (CR), 30 partial response (PR). Thirty-one pts underwent surgery and 26 were completely resected (62 % of all patients). Five pts had no tumour in resected specimen. The combined treatment was well tolerated : mild myelosuppression was the main toxicity and 3 pts died from surgical complications. With a median follow-up of 8 months, the 1.5 yr actuarial survival of operated and non-operated pts was 83 % and 55 % respectively. Although further follow-up is required, these data show that high complete resection rates can ben obtained following PE neo-adjuvant chemotherapy and that surgery is feasible with low morbidity and mortality.

Phase II pilot study of Ifosfamide-Cisplatine-Etoposide association as Neo-Adjuvant chemotherapy in locally advanced non-small cell lung cancers

JL Pujol*, JF Rossi**, T Le Chevalier***, JP Daurès*,
JY Douillard****, P Rouanet**, JB Dubois**, H Mary*,
R Arriagada***, P Godard*, FB Michel*

Locally advanced non-small cell lung cancers (NSCLC) have a poor prognosis following surgery alone when this has been possible, because of a high rate of local and metastatic relapses [1-3]. Probability of 5 years survival for these patients ranges between 5 and 15 % [4-6]. Thus, locally advanced NSCLC for which resection is potentially possible but poorly curative are usually designated as marginally resectable [7]. Adjuvant post-operative chemotherapy or radiation therapy hardly seem to improve survival [8]. Therefore, other modality treatments might be proposed to improve survival.

A multicentric phase II pilot study of neo-adjuvant Ifosfamide, Cisplatin, and Etoposide in locally advanced non small cell lung cancer was performed in 4 institutions. This study was carried out in order : 1) to determine the complete and partial response rate following Ifosfamide, Cisplatin and Etoposide (IPE) combination, 2) evaluate the pathological complete resection rate obtained by surgery for responder patients, and 3) evaluate surgical morbidity after neo-adjuvant chemotherapy.

Patients and methods

Patients of both sexes with locally advanced and histologically proven NSCLC were entered into the study. Prerequesites for inclusion were : age < 75 years, WHO performance status (PS) ≤ 2, weight loss ≤ 10 %, respiratory function compatible with surgical resection, normal baseline renal and cardiac functions, baseline neutrophil count ≥ 2,000/ μL and platelet count ≥ 100,000/ μL.

None of them had received prior therapy. Patients with gross mediastinal involvement, i.e. more than 2 ipsilateral nodal stations with mediastinal lymph nodes greater than 20 mm on computed tomographic scan, and widened carina or main bronchus distorsion suggestive of subcarenal lymph nodes, were considered as locally advanced NSCLC and were included directly into the study ; patients for whom this staging procedure failed to demonstrate mediastinal involvement had cervical mediastinoscopy.

Chemotherapy consisted of daily administration of the following treatment : Etoposide 100 mg/m², Cisplatin 25 mg/m², Ifosfamide 1.5 g/m², and Mesna 1.8 g/m² for 4 days. A cycle started every 21 days. Patients were evaluated for

* Centre Hospitalier Universitaire, Montpellier, ** Centre Régional de Lutte contre le Cancer, Montpellier, *** Institut Gustave Roussy, Villejuif, **** Centre René-Gauducheau Nantes, France

response at the start of each cycle of chemotherapy by clinical examination and chest x-ray. Based on the response after the second cycle of chemotherapy, patients with evidence of major response underwent a new complete staging procedure to evaluate response precisely and a resection was planned at that time, whereas other patients underwent a third cycle before complete staging procedure.

For patients who achieved CR or PR a thoracotomy was scheduled two weeks after hematologic recovery with an attempt at curative resection and mediastinal lymph node dissection. A complete resection was defined as resection of all macroscopic disease and normal histology of the margin. Surgery was completed by radiation therapy for all patients and by two additional cycles for pathologically proven N2 patients. Patients with stable or progressive disease were not planned for surgery.

Results and discussion

Between September 1987 and September 1989, 33 patients took part into the study. Patient characteristics are shown in (Table 1).

Table 1. Patients characteristics

No. of treated patients	33
Sex Male/female	31/2
Mean age ± SD (range)	56 ± 10 (42 – 74)
Histology	
Squamous cell carcinomas	22
Adenocarcinomas	5
Large cell carcinoma	6
Mediastinal extent	
by computed tomographic scan	23
by biopsy results	9
by pulmonary angiography	1
Prestudy stage grouping	
T3N2M0	30
T2N3M0	2
T4N2M0	1

Objective responses to IPE chemotherapy were obtained in 23/33 patients. Among them a complete response (CR) was achieved in 5 patients (15 %) and a partial response (PR) in 18 patients (55 %). Stable disease (SD) was observed in 3 patients and progressive disease (PD) occurred in 7 patients. Progression during the chemotherapy program consisted of metastases in 5 patients and local progression in the two others.

IPE chemotherapy hematologic toxicity was moderate to severe but manageable. Mean nadir neutrophil counts were 0.91 x 103/ μL for the first cycle, 1.21 x 103/ μL for the second cycle and 0.46 x 103/ μL for the third cycle.

Frequency of grade 3-4 hematologic toxicity increased from cycle 1 to cycle 3 and led to a chemotherapy dose reduction in 4 patients. Among the patients with neutropenia, 10 developed a grade 2-3 infection requiring antibiotics. Blood tranfusions were given to 6 patients owing to grade 3-4 anemia. The death-related toxicity was due to a grade 4 thrombopenia-induced central nervous system hemorrhage. Other notable toxicities were nausea and vomiting in 93 % of the patients requiring rehydration in 3 patients.

Thoracotomy was performed in 21 patients. No surgery was planned for 2 PR patients for whom gross mediastinal involvement remained in spite of primary tumor objective response. Of the 21 patients who underwent thoracotomy a resection was possible in 20 patients. A complete resection was achieved in 18 patients without technical difficulties. Only incomplete resections were possible in 2 patients because of upper mediastinum tumor involvement in one and microscopic left atrium margin involvement in the other. No macroscopic lung or lymph nodes were observed in the 5 patients with CR. For these patients, histological analyses of lung and lymph node surgical samples were negative. A complete resection was achieved after chemotherapy in the 2 patients who underwent a prestudy investigative thoracotomy. Surgery induced no morbidity. Mean follow-up was 1 year. Probability of survival from day 1 of treatment were 37 and 30 % at 12 and 18 months respectively.

Conclusion

We conclude that IPE chemotherapy is an active treatment of locally advanced NSCLC with a 70 % objective response rate and 15 % CR rate ; in responder patients surgery is feasible allowing a 55 % complete resection rate and negative histology in all clinical CR patients, and no surgery-related morbidity and mortality were observed after neo-adjuvant chemotherapy. However, it is not possible to conclude whether or not neo-adjuvant chemotherapy can reverse unresectable NSCLC in resectable ones. This study allowed us to start in March 1990 a phase III randomized study to compare neo-adjuvant chemotherapy followed by surgery with surgery alone, in an attempt to determine whether enhenced response and resection rates could increase survival of NSCLC patients treated by IPE neo-adjuvant chemotherapy.

References

1. Mulshine JL, Glatstein E, Ruckdeschel JC (1986) treatment of non-small cell lung cancer. J Clin Oncol 4 : 1704-1715
2. Cox JD, Yesner RA (1981) Causes of treatment failure and death in carcinoma of the lung. Yale J Biol Med 54 : 201-207
3. Aisner J, Forastiere A, Aroney R (1983) Patterns of recurrence for cancer of the lung and esophagus. Cancer Tret Symp 2 : 87-105
4. Naruke T, Suemasu K, Ishikawa S (1978) Lymph node mapping and curability at various levels of metastasis in resected lung cancer. J Thorac Cardiovasc Surg 76 : 832-839

5. Pearson FG, DeLarue NC, Ilves R, Todd TRJ, Cooper JD (1982) Significance of positive superior mediastinal nodes identified at mediastinoscopy in patients with resectable cancer of the lung. J Thorac Cardiovasc Surg 83 : 1-11

6. Martini N, Flehinger BJ, Zaman MB, Beattie EJ (1983) Results of resection in non-oat cell carcinoma of the lung with mediastinal lymph node metastases. Ann Surg 198 : 386-397

7. Sherman DM, Neptune W, Weichselbaum R et al (1978) An aggressive approach to marginally resectable lung cancer. Cancer 41 : 2040-2045

8. The Lung Cancer Study Group, prepared by Lad T, Rubenstein L, Sadeghi A (1988) The benefit of adjuvant treatment for resected local advanced non-small cell lung cancer. J Clin Oncol 6 : 9-17

Initial intensive drug chemotherapy (CT) followed by extensive irradiation for limited small cell lung cancer (LSCLC). Improved response rate and survival. A pilot study

R Levy, JM Tourani, C Le Maignan, P Even, JM Andrieu

Best therapeutic results in limited small cell lung cancer (LSLSC) are usually achieved by a combination of standard doses of CT and RT. The complete response rate and the three-year survival, however, rarely exceed 80 % and 20 % respectively. Failure can be attributed to the occurrence of micrometastases and to the emergence of chemoresistant clones causing visceral and local relapses. Considering 1) the Goldie and Coldman's hypothesis that implies the early and simultaneous use of all active agents at optimal dosage in order to limit the occurrence of chemoresistance. 2) the prognostic value of initial response to CT and 3) the dose response effect we have thus set up a pilot study consisting of an initial short intensive five drug CT followed by an extensive RT.

Patients

Sixteen patients with LSCLC (homo and controlateral hilar nodes, homolateral pleural effusion, ipsilateral supraclavicular nodes) were included in this study. Median age was 53 years and median Karnofsky index was 80 %. Fourteen patients had mediastinal involvement, 2 had pleural effusion, 2 had ipsilateral supraclavicular involvement. The initial investigation included : chest x-ray, fiberoptic examination with biopsies, thoracic, abdominal and brain computed tomographic scans, bone scintigraphy, bone marrow biopsy.

Treatment

After being hooked up to a central line patients received 3 cycles of CT given at 30 day interval. Each cycle combined : Cisplatin 40 mg/m²/day (d) d1, d2, d3 ; Cyclophosphamide 750 mg/m²/d, d4, d5 ; Adriamycin 50 mg/m²/d, d5 ; Vindesine 2 mg/m²/d, d1 and d5 ; Etoposide 100 mg/m²/d, d1, d2, d3. No modification in the doses of CT according to hematological toxicity was foreseen. One month after the 3rd cycle of CT, RT was delivered (1.8 Gy/d five time each week : 55 Gy to the mediastinum, the primary tumor, 45 Gy to the ipsi and controlateral supraclavicular area, 22 Gy to the whole homolateral lung and 34 Gy (prophylaxis) to the brain and the entire spinal axe (L5-S1).

Laennec Hospital, 42, rue de Sèvres, 75340 Paris Cedex 07, France

Results

The complete response rate judged by the same exams as in the initial investigation (including histology) was 100 % after the 3 cycles of CT. All patients were still in complete response after RT. The median survival was not reached at 32 months and the two-year actuarial survival was 78 % with a median follow-up of 24 months. Two patients died of local relapse and 2 of extrathoracic relapse. The median time to relapse was 9 months (range 4-17). The 12 remaining patients are still disease free. Main toxicities were hematologic (median duration of aplasia : 9 days) and gastro intestinal (8 grade II, 3 grade III). No treatment-related death occurred. To our knowledge, no other CT schedule (conventional or alternate non cross resistant) with or without RT has given these results. Of note is that the so called high dose CT protocols usually exploit the dose effect for one agent only or are limited to one cycle. Based upon these promising data, initial high dose CT in LSCLC deserves a further multicentric evaluation with dose intensification.

Cisplatin, 5-Fluorouracil + Leucovorin and Vindesine, in non-small cell lung cancer : a phase II study

H de Cremoux*, N Azli**, S Voisin***, I Monnet*, P Ruffié**, M Riggi**, L Vergnes**, J Huet***, JC Saltiel***, E. Cvitkovic**

Vindesine (VDS) and 5-Fluorouracil (5-FU) administered by continuous infusion have shown an increased therapeutic index in many solid malignancies. On the basis of our encouraging results obtained by the association of Cisplatin (CDDP, bolus) and VDS with 5-FU by continuous infusion, in unresectable non small cell lung cancer (NSCLC) [1], we tested VDS and 5-FU by continuous infusion in combination with CDDP and high doses of leucovorinin in order to enhance the anti tumoral effect of 5-FU [2].

Patients and methods

From 11/89 to 11/90, 56 previously untreated patients with histologically proved NSCLC were entered in this study. In all cases the carcinoma was thought unresectable or marginally resectable. Measurable target(s) (CT scan) and performance status ≥ 70 % were mandatory for inclusion in this study. Staging was performed according to the TNM system of the American joint committee on cancer [3].

Patients characteristics were as follows : median age 57 (range : 34-71) ; 49 patients were males (87 %) ; performance status = 70 % : 8 patients, > 70 % : 48 patients. Histology : squamous cell carcinoma 33 patients (59 %), adenocarcinoma 12 patients (21 %), large cell carcinoma 11 patients (20 %). TNM classifications : stage IIIa : 16 patients (28 %), stage IIIb : 12 patients (21 %), and stage IV : 28 patients (50 %).

Patients received every 3 weeks : VDS (0.8 mg/m²/day by 24 h continuous infusion, day 1-4), 5-FU (600 mg/m²/day by 24 h continuous infusion day 1-4), leucovorin (150 mg/m² by 20 min infusion every 6 h day 1-4 starting 12 h before 5-FU) and CDDP (100 mg/m² over 30 min on day 1).

Results

Evaluation was done after 3 cycles according to the WHO criteria.

Response rate

Forty-six patients are evaluable for response (7 too early, 1 toxic death). Median

---

* CHI Créteil, 40 av de Verdun, 94000, Créteil. ** IGR (La Grange), 77176 Savigny le Temple. *** CH Corbeil, 91100 Corbeil Essonne. France

follow-up is 7 months (range 1-12). 17/46 patients achieved PR (37 %) (95 % CI 25 %-57 %) (CR 1, PR 16), 11/26 patients with limited disease (40 %) and 6/23 patients with extensive disease (26 %), without difference according to histology.

Surgical resection

Six patients (1 patient stage IV, 5 patients stage IIIa) could had surgical resection (1 lobectomy with no residual tumor, 1 lobectomy + parietectomy, 4 pneumonectomy with 2 bronchopleural fistula lethal in 1 patient). With one exception (1 patient in stage IV, 5 patients stage IIIa), all patients had a Stage IIIa lung carcinoma. Eighteen patients had radiotherapy.

Toxicity

Forty-seven patients are evaluable for toxicity according to the WHO criteria (147 evaluable cycles). Neutropenia grade 3 : 23 cycles (17 patients), grade 4 : 36 cycles (28 patients) ; thrombopenia grade 4 : 1 cycle ; mucositis grade 3 : 20 cycles (15 patients), grade 4 : 5 cycles (6 patients) ; peripheral neuropathy grade 1 : 6 cycles ; hypoaccousia : 5 patients. A catheter-induced venous thrombosis was clinically observable in 5 patients. Treatment was stopped in 2 patients (poor performance status), and there was 1 toxic death (sepsis). Sixteen cycles were delayed because of neutropenia, with no dose reduction.

Conclusion

These results confirm that FA/5-FU and VDS given by continuous infusion with CDDP may offer equivalent activity as other active regimen.

In the absence of simultaneous and comparative study the actual effect of Leucovorin in this schedule remains unknown. However, this effect may be low : indeed in a previous similar study (without Leucovorin, 5-FU : 800 mg/day) we observed a similar response rate [2].

That only patients in stage IIIa could have surgical resection enlightens the surgical relevance of the AJCC TNM and questions about the feasibility of resection after PR induced by chemotherapy in locally more advanced cancer (stage IIIb).

References

1. Riggi M, Cvitkovic E, Voisin S et al (1990) Phase II trial of CDDP bolus and continuous infusion (CI) of vindesine (VDS) and 5-Fluorouracil (5-FU) in non small cell lung cancer (NSCLC). Proc ASCO 9 : 915 (Abstr)
2. Bleyer WA (1989) New vista for leucovorin in cancer chemotherapy. Cancer (suppl) 63 : 995-1007
3. AJCC (1988) Manual for staging of cancer. Third Ed, Lippincot Ed

Faster response and survival advantage with Neo-Adjuvant Cisplatin and 5-Fluorouracil infusion versus Cisplatin and Bleomycin in advanced non-small cell lung cancer

L Thiberville, C Faure, J Bouillard, J Clavier, Ph David,
JP Duhamel, J Heintz, Ph Hubscher, JF Muir, G Ozenne,
P Quillec, G Nouvet

Recent studies have shown that,

1) platinum-based chemotherapy combinations are able to prolonge survival of patients with metastatic non small cell lung cancer [5] ;

2) induction chemotherapy before radiation improves survival of non resectable, locally advanced non small cell lung cancer [1].

However, since only half of the non small cell lung tumors are sensitive to chemotherapy, and because most patients will ultimately receive thoracic radiotherapy, we must choose a chemotherapy regimen with a tolerable toxicity, that is able to provide a high response rate, a rapid tumor response and a synergism with radiotherapy. For these reasons we undertook in october 1987 a prospective randomised trial to compare two induction platinum-based chemotherapy regimens followed by thoracic radiotherapy or surgery if possible, in initially non resectable, advanced non small cell lung cancer. This study was stopped in november 1989, after the first interim analysis, because of a surprising response rate difference between the two arms.

Eligibility

To enter the study patients had to have an histologically proved non small cell lung cancer, initially non resectable, because of a poor pulmonary function, or because of the locoregional or metastatic extent. They had to be younger than 75, had to have at least one evaluable or measurable lesion, an ECOG performance status of 0 to 2, and no previous treatment to the primary tumor. Patients with brain metastasis, previous cardiac ischemia history, hepatic or renal failure, interstitial pneumonitis and concurrent neoplasm could not be included.

Treatment schedules

In each center, patients were randomised in two arms, using a random permuted block method. Arms differed only in the initial chemotherapy regimen. In both arms, patients received 2 cycles of induction chemotherapy with a 3 weeks intercourse.

Chemotherapy regimens were :

— in group A : *Cisplatin* 100 mg/m² per cycle in a continuous infusion

Commission de cancérologie de la société de pneumologie de l'Ouest de la France over 5 days and *5-Fluorouracil* 4 g/m² per cycle in a continuous infusion over 4 days (d. 2 to d. 5) ;

— in group B : *Bleomycin*, 25 mg/m² per cycle in a continuous infusion, took the place of 5-FU.

The response to the chemotherapy was assessed early in the third week after the second course. Due to the precocity of this response assessment, a « minor response » criteria was added to the WHO criteria [4]. Minor response was defined as less than 50 % and more than 25 % reduction of the tumor mass or a re-expansion of a previously collapsed lobe without appearance of a new lesion.

Patients achieving an objective response or a minor response received two other courses of the same treatment, whereas chemotherapy was stopped for the non responders. After the completion of chemotherapy, localised tumors were treated by surgery if possible or by thoracic radiotherapy (55 to 60 Gys, 200 cGys daily 5 days per week for 6 weeks).

Study design, statistics

In the initial design of the study, a sample size of 240 patients was required on the basis of a 80 % power for detecting a 20 % difference in the response rate after two courses of chemotherapy and a 50 % change in the two years survival rate (α risk = 5 %). This study was closed in november 1989 after the first interim analysis of the data because of an impressive difference in the response rate at 2 courses between the 2 arms. At the end of this study 112 patients had been included and 110 were eligible following the inclusion criteria. To date, we have more than one year of follow-up for the last patient included, and half of the data were reviewed by two independant observers.

Patient characteristics

The characteristics of the 110 eligible patients are shown in Table 1. One patient in each arm was dropped out of the study because of a small cell histology in one case and a concurrent carcinoma of the œsophagus in one case. Thirteen patients had a metastatic disease, 9 in the 5-FU group, 4 in the Bleomycin group. Almost all patients had a squamous cell lung carcinoma. There were no significant differences between the two treatment groups in any of the characteristics listed.

Chemotherapy and radiotherapy related toxicities

Severe treatment related toxicities (WHO grades > 3) were :

— *in the 5-FU arm :* 7 hematologic toxicities (neutropenia, thrombopenia) with 3 toxic deaths after the first cycle, one reversible acute cardiac failure (no sequeale) ;

Table 1. Characteristics of the patients

	CDDP/5FU	CDDP/bleomycin
pts included	57	55
eligible	56	54
median age (years)	60,6	59,2
(range)	(41-78)	(38-74)
sex: M/F	53/3	54
disease extent		
st I/II	4	10
st III	43	39
st IV	9	4
ECOG PS		
0,1	38	46
2	18	7
sq. cell histology	54	52
weight loss (kg)	3,6	5,1

— in the bleomycin arm : 2 hematologic toxicities, 2 bleomycin related pneumonitis before radiotherapy (one death).

Response to chemotherapy

Thirteen patients, 7 in the 5-FU group and 6 in the Bleomycin group were not evaluable for response because of early death or because they received only one course of chemotherapy. The rates of response after the second course of chemotherapy in each treatment group are shown in Table 2. There was no complete response. Response rate to CDDP-5-FU is much higher than to CDDP-bleomycin. This difference in objective response rate between the two arms is highly significant ($p < 0,01$).

Table 2. Tumor response to chemotherapy (2 courses)

	CDDP/5FU	CDDP/bleomycin
No of evaluable pts	48	49
complete response	0	0
partial response	22	5
(confidence limits)	(27-52%)	(2-17%)
minor response	15	14
no change	9	20
progression	2	10
early deaths	3	1

Adjuvant treatment, survival

After the completion of chemotherapy, 40 patients with localised tumor in the 5-FU arm, and 36 patients in the bleomycin arm received radiotherapy. However, only 24 patients in the 5-FU arm and 19 patients in the bleomycin arm received a total dose of more than 55 Gys. Surgery was possible in 10 cases in the 5-FU arm (9 complete resection) and in 6 cases in the bleomycin arm (2 complete resection). Post operative death occured in 3 cases. No significant difference exists between the two arms in terms of doses of radiotherapy effectively received or in the resectability rate.

Overall median survival is 35.5 weeks with a longer survival for the responders patients, as in most study. As shown in Figure 1, median survival and two years survival rate are significantly higher in the 5-FU group (38.7 w) than in the Bleomycin group (33.5 w) (p < 0,03). However, median survival difference is only 5 weeks and it is possible that the two years survival rate difference observed may be due to more chemotherapy or a higher rate of resectability in the 5-FU arm, whereas this point did not reach statistical significance. Along this line, an univariate prognostic factor analysis shows that beside N and M status and chemotherapy regimen, complete resectability of the tumor is effectively a prognostic factor of longer survival in this study.

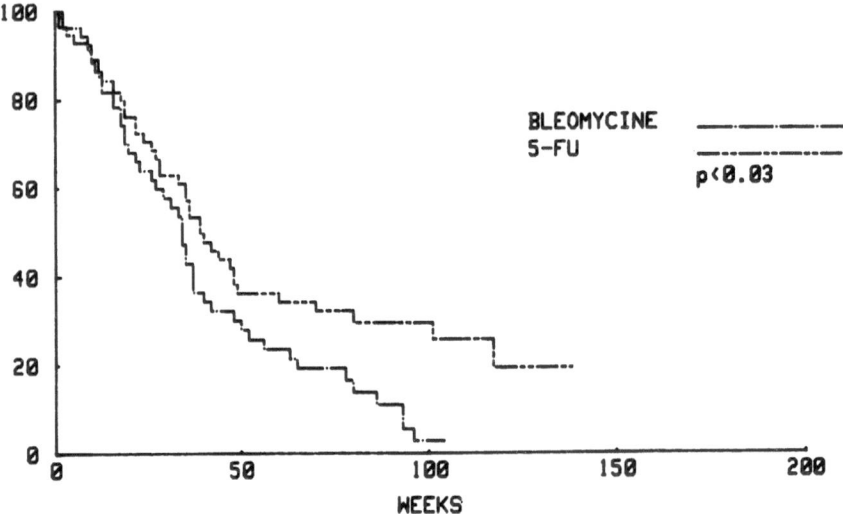

Fig. 1. Probability of survival (%)

Conclusions

This study shows that advanced squamous cell lung cancers achieve earlier response to Cisplatin and 5-FU than to Cisplatin and Bleomycin. The response rate observed with 2 courses of Cisplatin and Bleomycin in this study is surprisingly low [2, 3] and may be related to the cytotoxic effect of CDDP alone. It is possible that the cytotoxic effect of Bleomycin requires more than two cycles of chemotherapy to occur. However, in a « neo-adjuvant point of view », late response to the primary treatment is questionable and may not be of clinical value. Although no complete response occured in this study, the rapid response rate and the survival advantage obtained with the CDDP-5-FU arm suggest that this schedule may be a useful neo-adjuvant approach of advanced non small cell lung cancer.

References

1. Dillman RO, Seagren SL, Propert KJ, Guerra J, Eaton W, Perry MC, Carey RW, Frei III EF, and Green MR (1990) A randomized trial of induction chemotherapy plus high-dose radiation versus radiation alone in stage III non-small-cell lung cancer. N Engl J Med 323 : 940-945
2. Israel L, Aguilera J, Breau JL (1981) Traitement des cancers epidermoides par bleomycine et platine en administration prolongée. Serie préliminaire de 80 cas avec 75 % de reponse objectives. Nouv Presse Med 10 : 1817-1824
3. Karp SJ, Young TE, Bakowski MT, Spittle MF (1986) Combination chemotherapy of squamous cell carcinoma of the bronchus with cisplatinum and bleomycin followed by radiotherapy : results of a pilot study. Journal of the royal society of medicine 79 : 588-592
4. Miller AB, Hoogstraten B, Staquet M, Winkler A (1981) Reporting results of cancer treatment. Cancer 47 : 207-214
5. Rapp E, Pater JL, Willan A, Cormier Y, Murray N, Evans WK, Hodson DI, Clark DA, Feld R, Arnold AM, Ayoub JI, Wilson KS, Latreille J, Wierzbicki RF, Hill DP (1988) Chemotherapy can prolonge survival in patients with advanced non small cell lung cancer. Report of a canadian multicenter randomized trial. J Clin Oncol 6 : 633-641

Abstract. We present the preliminary results of a randomized, multicentric phase III trial, comparing 2 cisplatinum-based induction chemotherapy regimens (CDDP-5-FU versus CDDP-Bleomycin) followed by high dose thoracic radiotherapy or surgery in advanced, initially inoperable non small cell lung cancer. Response was assessed 15 days after the second course of chemotherapy and determined the subsequent treatment : radiotherapy for the non responders or two other courses of chemotherapy followed by radiotherapy for the responders. Overall median survival is 35,5 weeks. After the second course of chemotherapy, 22/56 eligible patients in the CDDP-5-FU arm achieved a partial response versus only 5 /54 in the CDDP-Bleomycin arm (p < 0.01). Whereas thoracic radiotherapy doses did not differ in both arms, survival was shorter in the Bleomycin group (median 33.5 w.) than in the 5-FU group (median 38.7 w.) (p < 0.03). We conclude that non small cell lung cancer respond earlier to CDDP-5FU than to CDDP-Bleomycin. This rapid response and the survival advantage observed with the CDDP-5-FU regimen suggest that this schedule may be a useful neo-adjuvant approach of advanced non small cell lung cancer.

Multimodality treatment for small cell bronchial carcinomas (SCLC)

E Ulsperger and K Karrer

Following discussions of our previous results of postoperative adjuvant chemotherapy for SCLC at the 13th Int. Congress of Chemotherapy in Vienna
1983 the ISC (Int.Soc.of Chemotherapy) — Lung Cancer Study Group was
formed and the ISC-protocols for small cell lung cancer were formulated for
prospective randomized ISC-studies I-IV [1]. Our preliminary evaluation presented for discussions concentrated on results of our neo-adjuvant protocol
(ISC-Studies III) compared to some results of our adjuvant ISC-study I, II [2].

Methods

Patients, clinically staged as T1-3N + M0 are included. They become randomized for two different chemotherapy-regimens (CT1 or CT2). After application of 2-3 courses of these chemotherapies, surgical removal of the primary
tumor (T) and resection of the mediastinal lymph nodes are performed, if response to chemotherapy became evident. After surgery for cure the cytostatic
treatment continues up to a half year after randomization. CT1 consists of :
Cytoxan 1,000 mg/m^2, Adriamycin 50 mg/m^2, Vincristine 1.4 mg/m^2, administered i.v. on day 1 of onset of treatment, administered at 3 - week intervals.
CT2 consists of : combination A : Cytoxan 1,500 mg/m^2, CCNU 100 mg/m^2
and MTX 15 mg/m^2 is given on day 1 of onset of treatment, followed after
an interval of 4 weeks by combination B : Cytoxan 1,000 mg/m^2, Adriamycin
40 mg/m^2 and Vincristine 1 mg/m^2, followed after 4 weeks by combination C :
Ifosfamide 1.6 g/m^2, VP-16 120 mg/m^2 both given for five days. This is repeated a second time. The first preliminary evaluation per January 1991 after study
closure by the end of December 1990 is based on 147 randomized patients from
15 centers (Table 1).

Patients characteristics

From 147 randomized patients 8 were not evaluable because they had no SCLC
or received no initial chemotherapy. From 139 eligible patients 123 were men
with a median survival time (MSVT) of 12,0 months and 16 women with 15.2
MSVT ; 99 patients already died after a MSVT of 11.9 months, 18 living
patients had 19.7 months median observation time (MOST). Twenty-two

The ISC Lung Cancer Study Group Institute for Epidemiology of Neoplasms of the Univ, Vienna
and 5th Med. Dept. and Oncology, KH Lainz, Vienna, Austria

Table 1.

Participants of the cooperative isc-study III

Country/City	Surgery	Medical Oncology	Radiology	Pathology
A Vienna	H. Denck, N. Pridun	M. Neumann, N. Vetter	G. Alth	E. Lintner
RC Shanghai	O. Wang, Y. Chow	M. Liao, J. Chao	M. Lin	Z. Lin
I Forli	Lattuneddu, Dell'Amore	Galassi, Campanini	Fiorentini	Padovani
A Vienna	Wolner, Eckersberger	W. Schlick	K. Kärcher	H. Holzner
USSR Moskau	Pirogov, Davydov, Al-Ansari	Perevodchikova, Garin Smirnova, Gorbunova	Z. Mikhina	Y. Solovyev
RA B. Aires	A. Imposti	M. Bruno, N. Brocato	N. Ruggeri	G. Galippi
I Cosenza		V. Zottola, S. Barbera		N. Takayanagi
Jp Toyama	Y. Kusajima	Y. Mizukami	M. Sugihara	
RC Shenyang	H. Li, D. Chen, L. Han			
A Gaisbühel	G. Zimmermann	J. Rothmund, M. Amann	Oser	G. Breitfellner
Jp Kawasaki	H. Osada	M. Koike	M. Endoh	Sodemoto, Kakimoto
I Firenze	C. Crisci	N. Nozzoli, S. Nutini		Dini, Santucci
RA B. Aires	Della Torre, Campana	H. Pepe, L. Tabares	M. Filomia	Kaufer de Chiocca
I Bologna	P. Sette		L. Cacciari	
BRD Donaustauf		F.von Bültzingslöwen		

ISC-Study Center : K.Karrer, H.Hansluwka, E.Ulsperger, T. Waldhör, W.Theuer, Inst.f.Epidemiol. of Neoplasms of the Univ. Vienna/A ; T.Shields, Northw. Univ. Chicago/USA

Reference-Pathologists : H.J. Holzner, Inst. for Pathology of the University of Vienna/A
K.-M. Müller, Inst. for Pathology of the Univ. of Bochum/Germany

patients were lost to follow up. Thirty-six patients received surgery for cure, 25 died (MSVT 16.1 months), while 9 patients are still alive (19.1 MOST). Comparing the cT stages according to the TNM classification at the onset of treatment with the pT stages, defined after preoperative chemotherapy and surgery, there were identical stages in 14 patients, enlarged stages in 11 and decreased stages in 11 patients, while in 4 of these patients the primary tumor was histological no more evident. The comparison regarding the lymphnode involvement of those patients showed identical cN and pN stages in 14 patients, enlarged stages in only 7 and a lower stage in 15 patients, in 8 of these patients no more lymph node metastases were histologically evident.

Results

From 139 patients randomized after chemotherapy 4 showed complete (CR) and 72 partial remissions (PR), 50 patients had stable (SD) and 13 progressive diseases (PD) and were estimated at the judgement for surgery. The 36 resected patients consitst of 3 CR, 26 PR, 6 SD and 1 PD.

The life table survival rates (SVR) of the entire study population of 139 patients are 50 % at 12, 16 % at 24 and 8 % at 36 months. The survival rates of 76 responders (CR and PR) to chemotherapy — 29 of these received also surgery-, (61 % at 12, 22 % at 24 and 14 % at 36 months) showed a significant better survival ($p > 0.01$) compared to the 63 nonreponders (SD and PD)(32 % at 12, 8 % at 24 and 0 % at 36 months).

Comparing the survival rates of 29 responders to chemotherapy who were resected (showing a SVR of 73 % at 12, 42 % at 24 and 18 % at 36 months), with those 47 responders, who received for unforseen circumstances no surgical resection but continuation of cytostatic treatment (53 % at 12, 16 % at 24 and 8 % at 36 months), we found a significant survival improvement in the Breslow test ($p = 0.02$). Thirty-four patients of the adjuvant study protocol with pTN2 stages, who received surgery first followed by adjuvant chemotherapy, which is in summary comparable to 15 pTN2 patients treated by the neo-adjuvant modality, show a SVR of 45 % at 12, 29 % at 24 and 19 % at 36 months, while the neo-adjuvant treated patients had a SVR of 54 % at 12, 23 % at 24 and 7 % at 36 months.

Discussion and conclusion

The observed SVR seem to be definitely above those of patients treated by chemotherapy and radiotherapy without surgery, as known from the literature and from our studies as well [3, 4]. This seems to be particularly important for patients with definitely histologically proved pTN2 stages. The rationale of the studies was primarily to prove the advantage of surgery but not to estimate if pre- or postoperative chemotherapy is preferable. The continuitation of these investigations is not only justified but emphatically indicated. Therefore, we feel obliged to invite more colleagues to join our cooperative group.

References

1. Karrer K (1990) The importance of surgery as the first step in multimodality treatment of small cell bronchial carcinoma. Int J Clin cell lung cancer. Lung Cancer 6 : 73-83
2. Karrer K, Denck H, Karnicka H, Orel J, Drings P (1990) Surgery for cure followed by multimodality treatment for small cell bronchial carcinoma. Suppl J Cancer Res Clin Oncol 116 : 110
3. Ulsperger E, Shields T, Karrer K (1990) The role of surgery in small cell lung cancer. Lung Cancer 6 : 73-83
4. Karrer K (1990) Is the progress in cancer treatment results adequate or are we confronted with a more or less worldwide stagnation ? J Cancer Res Clin Oncol 116 : 425-430

Special lectures

Neo-Adjuvant chemotherapy : new approaches involving alkylating agent modulation

E Frei III

The modulation of chemotherapeutic agents has a long history. A modulator is best defined as an agent that modifies the biochemical pharmacology of the modulee in the direction of the improved therapeutic index. Modulation has been perhaps most intensively studied with Fluorouracil wherein a variety of potential modulators have been evaluated. Within the past several years it has been found that leucovorin has a profound effect on the biochemistry and cytotoxicity of Fluorouracil. This effect has been realized in the clinic in metastatic colorectal cancer, in head and neck cancer (PFL program), and perhaps in breast cancer.

We have found in the PFL program that the use of high dose Leucovorin along with Fluorouracil and Cisplatin, all given by continuous infusion, produces a complete response rate of 65 % in patients with advanced stages III and IV head and neck cancer. Since Cisplatin and the alkylating agents are probably the most commonly employed and effective in the treatment of solid tumors (including head and neck cancer and lung cancer) we embarked on a program four years ago of alkylating agent modulation.

Discussion

Much is known about the cellular pharmacology of the alkylating agents, including Cisplatin, that is subject to the potential for modulation.

Nitrogen mustard and phenylalanine mustard are actively transported into cells by a choline and amino acid transporter system respectively. Resistant cells may lose this transport capacity. One can compete out these alkylating agents with the normal substrates. However, improvement in therapeutic index with this approach has not yet been possible.

Once the alkylating agents enter the cytoplasm they are exposed to millimolar concentrations of glutathione, a tripeptide sulfhydryl containing compound, which is capable of combining with and inactivating free radicals including some of the alkylating agents. It has been found that some alkylating agent resistant lines have increased levels of glutathione. Glutathione biosynthesis can be inhibited by buthoxamine sulfoxamide (BSO). BSO *in vitro* and experimentally *in vivo* will decrease GSH levels some 90 %, thus converting GSH elevated resistant cell lines and indeed sensitive cell lines to increase in sensitivity to alkylating agents. Clinical studies of BSO have been initiated by Dr. Ozols and others.

Dana Farber Cancer Institute, 44 Binney Street Boston, MA 02115, USA

462 E Frei III

The conjugation of GSH with the alkylating agents is expedited by the enzyme system, glutathione transferases in accordance with the general formula. There are three major isozymes of glutathione which have varying, though somewhat overlapping, substrate patterns and substrate affinities. These affinities include some of the alkylating agents. Inhibition of glutathione transferase by piriprost, or by ethacrynic acid has been shown *in vitro* and *in vivo* to increase the sensitivity of the tumor cell to the alkylating agent. It is of interest that reduction in GSH and/or GST by modulation produces the aforementioned biochemical effect not only in tumor cells but also in normal cells.

Nevertheless, there is imparted greater cytotoxicity to tumor cells and improvement in the therapeutic index in a number of preclinical systems. Ethacrynic acid has been introduced in the clinic in phase I studies as a modulator of GST and therefore of alkylating agent activity. Conversely one can increase GSH levels in normal cells and protect the animal against alkylating agent cytotoxicity. Thus Teicher has demonstrated with Glutathione Ethylester a marked protection of several inbred strains of mice to cytotoxicity with, for example, BCNU. Of interest is the fact that now in two solid tumors the tumor itself is not protected from the alkylating agent.

As the alkylating agents enter the nucleus they approach and finally ligand to the target molecule DNA. It has long been known that radiotherapy requires oxygen for its cytotoxic effect. This also has been known for Adriamycin, for Bleomycin, and for thioTEPA. Teicher has found that the red blood cell substitute for Fluorocarbon (Fluosol DA) plus oxygen breathing will improve radiotherapy of experimental solid tumors presumably by controlling the hypoxia. Song has demonstrated directly that hypoxia is corrected. Of interest is the fact that the 2-5 fold improvement in therapeutic index occurs with essentially all of the alkylating agents including Cisplatin with Fluosol using this technique. The Fluosol particles are less than 1 % the size of red blood cells and therefore have access to hypovascular solid tumors. Clinical studies of Fluosol and X-ray are underway and clinical studies of Fluosol and chemotherapeutic agents have been initiated.

The oxygen mimic group of compounds, the nitroimidazoles, have long been of interest to radiotherapists as radiosensitizers. The nitroimidazoles result in a series of metabolic products including at least one that is cytotoxic and one that produces an oxygen-like effect when tagged by X-ray. Of interest is the observation that the nitroimidazole similarly improved the therapeutic index of alkylating agents. The new nitroimidazole is Etanidazole which achieves modulating concentrations at acceptable dose limiting neurotoxicity.

Of very substantial interest was the observation that Etanidazole plus Fluosol were synergistic in-vivo in terms of anti-tumor effect.

So much for DNA damage. Now about DNA repair :

A major determinant of alkylating agent sensitivity and of some alkylating agent resistant lines relates to inhibition of DNA repair. Such inhibition, other things being equal, will increase the cytotoxicity of a given compound. One specific repair mechanism for BCNU is removal of the monoligand by the cysteine containing methyl transferase. It has been shown in several systems that administration of Methylguanine, which competes for this enzyme, will inhibit the repair process and produce an experimental anti-tumor effect.

Topoisomerase II plays an important role in DNA confirmation. The inhibition of topoisomerase II by novobiocin and by etoposide will increase cytotoxicity from alkylating agents. It is postulated that topoisomerase II untangles DNA in a way that increases accessibility of repair enzymes. Thus inhibition of topoisomerase II would indirectly inhibit DNA repair and thus modulate alkylating agents.

It has been found that resistance to chemotherapeutic agents generally is not monofunctional but rather multifunctional. For example, cell line resistance to alkylating agents will often express low level resistance to 2 or 3 of the mechanisms which I have described. Thus, one modulator may partially increase the sensitivity to alkylating agents, but a combination of modulators may be required to optimize this effect.

The neo-adjuvant chemotherapy for head and neck cancer is primarily directed at improving local control. This can be accomplished by modulation strategies as described above and as exemplified in the PFL program.

In patients with stage III A and B lung cancer, neo-adjuvant chemotherapy with Cisplatin plus Vinblastine followed by radiotherapy improves survival over radiotherapy alone. In this case the big problem is hematological micrometastatic disease. The interpretation of the survival curve suggests that chemotherapy control over micrometastatic disease in this protocol was responsible for the improved survival. Since control of systemic disease is the major problem in lung cancer, improvement in systemic disease has to be a prime target of our research. Experimentally, this can be achieved with the modification of aklylating agents. This applies in varying degrees to other tumors as well.

Conclusion

At the Dana-Farber we have mounted a multifaceted laboratory and clinical program directed at the modulation of alkylating agents and it is our hope that such modulation and perhaps combined modulation will improve the effect of chemotherapeutic agents and, hopefully, eventually the curative effect of the neo-adjuvant approach.

The impact of molecular genetics on the detection of residual malignant disease

EJ Freireich

We have a broad spectrum of treatment techniques which can render patients with diagnosable malignancy free of disease (N.E.D. or C.R). Such patients depending on the characteristics of the original tumor are at variable risks of recurrence of disease. It is clear that patients in complete remission can benefit from adjuvant treatment given during the disease free period. The basis for such adjuvant therapy depends on the probability that the patient will develop recurrent disease. The prescription of adjuvant treatment results in offering treatment to some patients who are already cured of their disease in an effort to prolong the disease free period for patients who have residual disease. Thus, a pressing problem in the field of adjuvant therapy is the development of techniques for the objective detection of residual disease which would serve as a guide to the treating physician and would maximize the benefit/risk ratios for each individual patient.

The rapidly developing fields of cytogenetics and molecular genetics have already demonstrated the potential for greatly improving our ability to detect residual malignancy. Virtually all malignancies have chromosome abnormalities which can be detected by cytogenetic, flow microspectrophotometric, and molecular genetic techniques [1]. Even more important is the fact that there are specific genetic lesions associated with specific diagnoses. The long sought after unique characteristic of the cancer cell when contrasted to host's normal somatic cells has been identified at least for a significant fraction of systemic tumors.

Chronic granulocytic leukemia (CML) as a model of developing objective criteria for therapy intervention. CML was the first malignancy found to be associated with a specific cytogenetic change, a reciprocal translocation of genetic material between chromosomes 9 and 22, the Philadelphia chromosome (Ph^1). The translocation results in a new and unique hybrid gene, the BCR/abl gene. This hybrid gene is transcribed and the hybrid message has been identified. This message is translated into a unique protein which has unique tyrosine kinase activity [2]. While the specific function of this protein has not yet been fully elucidated, it has been demonstrated in the rodent that transfection of the human BCR/abl gene into rodent myeloid stem cells can result in a myeloproliferative disease which has all of the hallmarks of CML in man [3]. These results indicate that this genetic event is fundamental to the biology and natural history of this disease.

These findings have proved to be of crucial importance to the treatment of CML. Although it is possible to treat such patients into a status of complete hematological remission so that no hematological or cytological criteria

The University of Texas M.D. Anderson Cancer Center Houston, 77030 Texas, USA

allow identification of the disease, cytogenetic study of the metaphases of the bone marrow reveals that the metaphases still contain the Ph^1 chromosome which predicts that these patients have residual disease, which is confirmed by the fact that the patients have recurrence and progression to a more malignant form of blastic transformation. Innovative therapeutic strategies such as intensive combination chemotherapy, interferon therapy, and allogeneic bone marrow transplant have been developed which results not only in complete hematological and cytological remissions, but also in cytogenetic complete remissions where all of the metaphases in the patient's bone marrow lack the Ph^1 chromosome. The discovery of the technique of the polymerase chain reaction (PCR) for amplifying minimal residual transcripts of the BCR/abl gene has greatly extended the ability to detect residual disease [4]. Although the final data are not in, many of the patients who are in cytogenetic complete remission have persistent BCR/abl transcripts in their peripheral blood measured by the PCR. By making probes which hybridize to the BCR/abl gene, it is possible to visualize this chromosomal aneuploidy by immunofluorescent techniques, so-called chromosome painting or fluorescence in-situ hybridization (FISH). Recent studies have shown that using FISH, it is possible to identify the hybrid gene in interphase cells as well as cells in metaphase. For CML, the objective of therapy has become to render patients disease free by the criteria of the absence of the Ph^1 chromosome by cytogenetics. The biological implications of residual disease detected by the PCR or by the FISH studies remain to be worked out. However, these techniques offer enormous potential for identifying patients who are in need of additional treatment.

Studies in acute leukemia

A high percentage of patients with acute myeloblastic leukemia (AML) have cytogenetic aneuploidy. But unlike the situation in CML, there is enormous heterogeneity. The heterogeneity is so extensive that it was believed to be random damage to the chromosomes. We now recognize that there are non-random chromosome aneuploidies which identify unique biological subsets of AML. At least one-third of AML patients fit into six diagnostic categories which are specifically associated with unique disease outcome [5]. We have recently found that patients who achieve complete hematological and cytological remission also achieve complete cytogenetic remission. However careful study of metaphase plates of patients in remission have revealed a fraction of patients who have residual metaphases and these patients have developed recurrence of their AML. Again, as with CML, the objective of treatment is the development of complete cytogenetic remission.

For one subset of AML, the disease call acute promyelocytic leukemia which is characterized by a reciprocal translocation between chromosomes 15 and 17, there is with currently available chemotherapy a cured fraction of between 30-50 %. Therefore, the problem of detecting residual disease is extremely important. It has recently been observed that such patients, which constitute approximately 6 % of AML patients, show dramatic biological changes when they are treated with all-trans retinoic acid. This has led a number of workers to discover that, the gene for the alpha receptor of retinoic acid (RAR) is located at the breakpoint on chromosome 17. This has led to the discovery of another unique hybrid gene in patients with this disease [6]. The breakpoints are localized in the second intron of the alpha RAR gene and the appropriate probes have demonstrated that virtually all patients with the 15, 17 translocation have a rearrangement of this gene. The transcript of this gene has also been identified and is currently being actively studied. The importance of this observation is that a normal biological can induce differentiation in tumor cells which have this unique hybrid gene. Not only will this gene be useful for detection of residual disease, but it forms a potential basis for therapeutic intervention and for the development of therapeutic agents [7, 8].

Solid tumors

Do the findings in lymphoma and leukemia have application to the management of the more frequently diagnosed solid tumors, those of breast, lung or colon ? A striking recent development is the observation of the frequency of the mutations in the p53 gene in these common malignancies. Many authors have suggested that this is a final common pathway for tumorigenesis to occur in these solid tumors. The p53 gene functions as a suppressor of replication and in these tumors, the occurence of tumor formation is associated with either deletion of one allele with mutation in the other allele, or mutation in both alleles of this gene in many of the common malignancies [9]. The p53 gene, like the other important suppressor gene for retinoblastoma, has been cloned and sequenced and therefore the transcription and translation products can be identified. By applying the technique of FISH for both cells in metaphase and for interphase cells, it should be possible to apply the observations made on the leukemic disorders to the problem of detection of residual disease for the solid tumors [10]. Moreover, once the protein products of these unique or deleted genes are identified, the possibility that these products of the unique genes can be detected in body fluids or in serum or plasma, offers a rich area for clinical research [11].

References

1. Mitelman F (1991) Catalog of chromosome aberrations in cancer. Alan R Liss Inc, New York
2. Daley G, Van Etten R, and Baltimore D (1990) Induction of AML in mice by the P210 BCR/abl gene of the Philadelphia chromosome. Science 247 : 824
3. Lugo T, Pendergast A-M, Müller A, and Witte O (1990) Tyrosine kinase activity and transformation potency of ABCR-abl oncogene products. Science 247 : 1079
4. Lee M-S, Chang K-S, Freireich E, Kantarjian H, Talpaz M, Trujillo J, and Stass S (1988) Detection of minimal residual bcr/abl transcripts by a modified polymerase chain reaction. Blood 42 : 893
5. Freireich EJ (1990) The impact of cytogenetics and molecular genetics on diagnosis and treatment. In : Freireich EJ (ed) New approaches to the treatment of leukemia. Springer Verlag, Berlin, Heidelberg, p 173

6. Chang K-S, Trujillo J, Ogura T, Castiglione C, Kidd K, Zhao S, Freireich E, and Stass S (1991) Rearrangement of the retinoic acid receptor gene in acute promyelocytic leukemia. Leukemia (in press)

7. Dauwerse J, Kievits T, Beverstock G, van der Keur D, Smit E, Wessels H, Hagemeijer A, Pearson P, van Ommen, G-J, and Breuning M (1990) Rapid detection of chromosome 16 inversion in acute nonlymphocytic leukemia, subtype M4 : regional localization of the breakpoint in 16p. Cytogenet Cell Genet 53 : 126

8. Tkachuk D, Westbrook C, Andreef M, Donlon T, Cleary M, Suryanarayan K (1990) Detection of bcr-abl fusion in chronic myelogenous leukemia by two-color fluorescence hybridization. Science 250 : 559

9. Nigro J, Baker S, Preisinger A, Jessup J, Hostetter R, Cleary K, Bigner S, Davidson N, Baylin S, Devilee P, Glover T, Collins F, Weston A, Modali R, Harris C, and Vogelstein B (1989) Mutations in the p53 gene occur in diverse human tumour types. Nature 342 : 705

10. Liu P, Siciliano J, and Siciliano M (1991) Efficient method for the production of in-situ hybridization probes that simultaneously paint and band human chromosomes. Submitted

11. Rowley J (1990) Molecular cytogenetics : rosetta stone for understanding cancer-twenty-ninth GHA Clowes memorial award lecture. Cancer Research 50 : 3816

Hairy cell leukemia : current treatment strategies

HM Colomb

Hairy cell leukemia is a chronic lymphoproliferative malignancy first described by Bouroncle et al over 30 years ago [1]. The typical patient is a middle-aged man with complaints of fatigue or weakness ; symptoms of splenic pain, bleeding or bruising, or recurrent infections are less common at presentation [2]. Splenomegaly without peripheral adenopathy occurs in 70-80 % of newly diagnosed patients [2]. Pancytopenia is present in approximately two-thirds of patients, although 10 % of patients present with a leukocytosis resulting from a high circulating hairy cell count. Representing less than 2 % of adult leukemias, hairy cell leukemia has become the focus of intense interest over the past few years as a result of therapeutic advances.

At this point in time, curative treatment for hairy cell leukemia has not been documented, although complete responses to treatment have been obtained. The intent of therapy has been to relieve symptoms and to prevent the frequent complications of progressive disease. Treatment indications for hairy cell leukemia include severe anemia (HCT < 25 %), thrombocytopenia ($< 50,000/$ μl), marked granulocytopenia (< 500 neutrophils/ μl), splenic pain or rupture, recurrent infections, bone involvement, vasculitis and bulky retroperitoneal disease. Up to 15 % of newly diagnosed patients will never require therapy [3]. These patients are typically 10 years older than the median age of 52, and have less splenomegaly, fewer circulating hairy cells and more granulocytes at the time of presentation.

The large majority of patients will require some form of treatment for their disease, either at the time of diagnosis or within several years of presentation. The options for treatment have expanded greatly in the past five years, allowing the clinician to tailor therapy to each individual situation. Splenectomy may still be a therapeutic modality offered to some patients, with good results in the vast majority of cases. Alpha-interferon has been used extensively in the treatment of hairy cell leukemia with excellent control of the cytopenias but is rarely, if ever, curative. Deoxycoformycin appears to have greater curative potential. Treatment of short duration with 2-Chlorodeoxyodenosine results in a high percentage of complete remissions. Hematopoietic growth factors may ameliorate the leukopenia associated with hairy cell leukemia and its treatment. The integration of these treatment modalities is the focus of this paper.

Department of Medicine, Section of Hematology/Oncology, University of Chicago Medical Center, Chicago, USA

Treatment Choices

Splenectomy

The pattern of hematologic response to splenectomy has been well characterized. The platelet count is the most likely to respond, often rising within days after surgery. The anemia and granulocytopenia may improve gradually over the course of weeks to months after the splenectomy [2, 4]. In a group of 170 patients who underwent splenectomy, the median platelet count doubled, the median granulocyte count tripled and the median hemoglobin rose by 1 mg/dl [2].

Interferon

The use of alpha-Interferon in the treatment of hairy cell leukemia was first recommended by Quesada et al in 1984 [5]. Partially purified alpha-Interferon at 3×10^4 units SC was given daily to 7 patients. Normalization of the peripheral blood counts occurred in all patients. Three complete remissions were reported and 4 patients entered a partial remission.

The ability to eradicate hairy cells from the bone marrow led to the use of new definitions of response. A complete remission was reported only if hairy cells were absent from the marrow, organomegaly resolved, and the peripheral blood counts were restored to the following values : a hemoglobin > 12 g/dl, an absolute neutrophil count > 1.500 cells/μl, and a platelet count > 100,000/μl. A partial remission was defined as a decrease in the hairy cell infiltration of the marrow by 50 % with restoration of peripheral blood counts as defined for a complete remission. Some authors have also included a minor response category, which requires the normalization of at least one blood count without deterioration in any other cell line.

Examples of the responses seen with interferon alfa-2b is shown by the following recently updated study [6]. One hundred ninety-five patients were entered onto a multi-institutional study of interferon alfa 2b from 1983-1986 ; follow-up was completed through June 1989. A complete remission was documented in 7 patients, a partial remission in 152 patients, a minor response in 10 patients, and no response in 26 patients. One-hundred fifty-nine of the 195 patients treated (81 %) had a normalization of their peripheral blood counts by the criteria used. To date, 17 patients have died. Only 3 of the 159 patients (2 %) with a PR or CR have expired. Three of 10 MR patients have expired and 11 of 26 NR patients have expired. Of the 11 who expired, 7 did so before receiving an adequate duration of treatment. Three of the NR patients died within 1 week of starting interferon from intracranial hemorrhages secondary to severe thrombocytopenia (present prior to initiation of interferon) and 4 NR patients died of infectious deaths within 2 months of initiating interferon therapy secondary to severe neutropenia (present prior to initiation of interferon). Of the 17 NR's who remained alive and on-study for at least 6 months, only 2 eventually died, both after failing subsequent pentostatin therapy.

Deoxycoformycin

Kraut et al [7] recently updated their experience at Ohio State with a report of 23 patients with hairy cell leukemia treated with 4 mg/m^2 every two weeks (two patients received lower doses due to renal insufficiency). Twenty of these 23 patients went into a complete remission after a median of eight doses of dCF. One partial remission and one minor response were seen, with only one patient failing to respond. Five relapses have occurred at a median of 13.5 months ; only one of these patients has required retreatment with dCF, which resulted in re-induction of a complete remission. The National Cancer Institute has recently published the outcome of 66 patients with hairy cell leukemia treated with dCF by the Special Exception mechanism [8]. Through this mechanism, clinicians may obtain dCF through application to the Division of Cancer Treatment of the NCI. Three different dosing schedules were used, although most patients were treated with 4mg/m^2 of dCF every week or every other week, with a 56 % complete remission rate and a 23 % partial remission rate. A median of 8.5 doses was given before a complete remission occurred. Prior treatment with interferon or a splenectomy did not appear to influence the overall response rate ; a tendency towards a slightly higher complete remission rate was noted in non-splenectomized patients. No relapses have yet been noted at a median follow-up of seven months.

2-Chlorodeoxyadenosine

A new inhibitor of adenosine deaminase, 2-chlorodeoxyadenosine, has been reported to have activity in hairy cell leukemia [9]. A single course of 2-chlorodeoxyadenosine at 0.1 mg/kg/day for seven days by continuous infusion was given to six patients. Three patients had complete responses to therapy ; it was still to early to evaluate the other three patients. The complete remissions were durable, lasting 2 years, 1.5 years and one month. More recently, the authors have updated their results and reported on 12 patients [10]. All the patients responded to treatment ; 11 had complete remissions. None of the patients have relapsed and the median duration of remission was 15.5 months. There were no serous toxic reactions. This may become the most effective and least toxic therapy for HCL.

Conclusion

It is quite likely that future HCL patients severely affected with thrombocytopenia and/or neutropenia will be candidates for initial treatment with 2-Chlorodeoxyadenosine, Pentostatin, or a combination of Interferon plus growth factor rather than with Interferon alone which takes a median of 6-8 weeks to induce a hematologic response.

References

1. Bouroncle BA, Wiseman BK, Doan LA (1958) Leukemic reticulœndotheliosis. Blood 13 : 609-630
2. Golomb HM, Ratain MJ, Vardiman JW (1986) Sequential treatment of hairy cell leukemia : a new role for interferon. In : DeVita VT Jr (ed) Important Advances in Oncology. Lippincott, Philadelphia p 311-321
3. Golomb HM (1987) The treatment of hairy cell leukemia. Blood 69 : 979-983
4. Flandrin G, Sigaux F, Sebahoun G, Bouffette P (1984) Hairy cell leukemia : clinical presentation and follow-up of 211 patients. Seminars in Oncology 11 (Suppl. 2) 458-471
5. Quesada JR, Reuben J, Manning JT, Hersh E, Gutterman JU (1984) Alpha interferon for induction of remission of hairy cell leukemia. N Engl J Med 310 : 15-18
6. Golomb HM, Fefer A, Golde DW, Ozer H, Portlock C, Silber R, Rappeport J, Ratain MJ, Thompson J, Bonnem E, Spiegel R, Tensen L, Burke JS, Vardiman JW Survival experience of 195 patients with hairy cell leukemia treated in a multi-institutional study with interferon alfa-2b. Leukemia and Lymphoma (in press)
7. Kraut EH, Bouroncle BA, Grever MR (1989) Pentostatin in the treatment of advanced hairy cell leukemia. J Clin Onc 7 : 168-172
8. Grem JL, King SA, Cheson BD, Leyland-Jones B, Wittes RE (1989) Pentostatin in hairy cell leukemia : treatment by the special exception mechanism. J Natl Cancer Inst 81 : 448-453
9. Piro LD, Carrera CJ, Carson DA, Beutler E (1988) Complete remissions in hairy cell leukemia after treatment with 2'-chlorodeoxyadenosine (Abstract). Blood 72 (Suppl 1), 220 a
10. Piro LD, Carrera CJ, Carson DA, Beutler E (1990) Lasting remissions in hairy cell leukemia induced by a single infusion of 2-chlorodeoxyadenosine. N Eng J Med 322 : 1117-1121

Dose intensification and autologous stem cell support in breast cancer

GN Hortobagyi

Experimental studies demonstrate the existence of a close correlation between the dose of a cytotoxic agent and the response of cancer cells to therapy [1]. This correlation has been confirmed for mammary cancer in the nude mouse model, with transplanted human xenografts [2]. The slope of this dose response curve varies from to agent, and is also dependent to a large extent on the drug sentivity of the tumor model utilized. In preclinical tumors models, relatively modest differences in dose-intensity correlate with substantial differences in response rate and survival, and in many of the models, may represent the difference between cure, or the appearance of overt metastatic disease and death. In *in vitro* systems the possible range of drug concentrations is very large, limited only by the solubility of the agent, or the cytotoxicity of the diluent utilized. On the other hand, in *in vivo* systems dose intensification can be limited by the development of drug related toxicity. In clinical practice the maximally tolerated dose, or dose-intensity is employed based on these principles developed in preclinical models.

Several retrospective analysis have addressed the dose-response correlation of chemotherapy for metastatic breast cancer. Some of these analyses have shown a direct correlation with higher response rate and survival, while others have not [3]. Similar retrospective analysis have also been performed for adjuvant chemotherapy trials. Again the results have been conflicting. One of the most systematic approaches to the evaluation of dose-intensity was developed by Hill Hryniuk [4]. His system takes into consideration the dose, and the frequency of administration of the individual agents used in the combination. Thus, dose-intensity is expressed in terms of the quantity of each drug delivered per unit of time (mg/m^2/week). This method standardizes dose-intensity and allows inter-trials comparisons, as well as comparisons across different regimens. Dr Hryniuk's evaluation of multiple clinical trials where the CMF or the CAF combinations were used for the treatment of metastatic breast cancer demonstrated a clearcut, and steep, dose-response correlation. This correlation was shown for response rate, and survival. His analyses demonstrated something similar for adjuvant chemotherapy trials.

The retrospective evaluation of dose-intensity has been criticized on account of limitations, and statistical pitfalls. Nevertheless, the results of these analyses were interesting enough to suggest that the concept of a dose-response curve should be tested prospectively.

There are at least 9 prospective, randomized trials with chemotherapy for metastatic breast cancer where either a single-agent, or a combination of cyto-

The University of Texas MD Anderson Cancer Center, Department of Medical Oncology, Breast Medical Oncology Service, 1515 Holcombe Boulevard, Houston, 77030 Texas, USA

toxic agents was used and where a difference in dose-intensity was correlated with response rate and survival [3]. The single-agent trials demonstrated a steep dose response for doxorubicin, while the combination regimens also showed a correlation between higher dose-intensity and higher response rate in most, but not all trials. The correlation of dose-intensity with survival was less convincing, although it reached statistical significance in some of the trials. Prospective trials to test the dose response correlation are ongoing in adjuvant therapy, but the results of these trials are not available as yet.

Increases in dose-intensity for most cytotoxic agents used for the treatment of breast carcinoma are limited by the appearance of drug-related toxicity. The most common dose-limiting toxicity is myelosuppression. The first approach to prevent myelosuppression, or accelerate hematologic recovery targeted the harvesting and reinfusion of autologous bone marrow. This technique has been demonstrated to be effective and safe. More recently, peripheral stem cell harvest and reinfusion was added to autologous bone marrow grafting ; the development of hematopoietic growth factors (rhG-CSF, rhGM-CSF) has been the latest addition to this field. Higt-dose regimens supported by autologous stem cells were first tested in patients with advanced, refractory, metastatic breast cancer [5]. Although high overall response rate were observed, complete remission rates were low, and response durations in the order of 3 months. No long term survivors were identified. The same high-dose regimens, when administered to patients with minimal, or no prior chemotherapy produced markedly superior results. The overall responses rates approached (Table 1). In addition, almost 20 % of patients treated with high-dose chemotherapy and autologous marrow support survived without recurrence beyond 2 years. The next step included the use of high-dose chemotherapy with autologous stem cell support as consolidation of objective responses obtained with standard-dose chemotherapy. While this strategy is still being evaluated, preliminary results suggest that complete remission rates between 50 and 70 % are regularly observed, and that 20-30 % of patients survive without progression beyond two years [6, 7]. As a corollary to the progression and the development of this field towards more favorable subgroups, high-dose chemotherapy with autologous stem cell support is being evaluated in high-risk breast cancer, including patients with more than 10 positive axillary nodes of those with inflammatory, or locally advanced breast cancer.

It is clear that there is a strong correlation between dose-intensity and response to therapy. It is also clear that the first step towards curative treatment of most metastatic cancers has been the achievement of a high complete remission rate. To continue developing this field, better preparatory regimens, and remission maintenance strategies need to be developed. At this time, definitive therapies to assess the benefit of high-dose chemotherapy consolidation with autologous stem cell support must be completed.

Table 1. HDCT + ABMT for Metastatic Breast Cancer

Chemotherapy	No. of Pts.	% CR	% CR + PR
Refractory Breast Cancer			
Single agent	49	12	51
Combination alkylators	111	16	70
Combination others	77	22	67
Untreated Breast Cancer			
Induction	55	47	75
Consolidation	193	54	90

References

1. Schabel FM (1975) Animal models as predictive systems. In : Cancer chemotherapy-fundamental concepts and recent advances. Year Book Medical Publishers, Inc, Chicago, p 323
2. Giovanella BC, Stehlin JS (1978) Heterotransplantation of human cancers into nude mice. Cancer 42 : 2269
3. Henderson IC, Hayes DF (1988) Dose-response in the treatment of breast cancer : a critical review. J Clin Oncol 6 : 1501
4. Hryniuk W, Bush H (1984) The importance of dose intensity in chemotherapy of metastatic breast cancer. J Clin Oncol 2 : 1281
5. Antman K, Gale RP (1988) Advanced breast cancer : high-dose chemotherapy and bone marrow autotransplants. Ann Interm Med 108 : 570
6. Peters WP, Jones RB (1989) Dose intensification using high-dose combination alkylating agents and autologous bone marrow support for the treatment of breast cancer. In : Dicke KA, Spitzer G (eds) Autologous bone marrow transplantation, Proceedings of the fourth international symposium. The University of Texas MD Anderson Cancer, Houston, p 389
7. Spitzer G, Dunphy F (1989) High-dose intensification for stage IV hormonally-refractory breast cancer. In : Dicke KA, Spitzer G (eds) Autologous bone marrow transplantation, Proceedings of the fourth international symposium. The University of Texas MD Anderson Cancer, Houston, p 399

The current status of therapy for aggressive non-Hodgkin lymphoma

J Armitage

An important advance in the management of patients with aggressive non-Hodgkin lymphoma is the recognition that there are discernable subgroups of patients that share clinical characteristics and for whom certain principles of therapy should be applied their management. The remainder of this manuscript will be devoted to briefly reviewing several of these important subgroups of patients with aggressive non-Hodgkin lymphoma.

Minimal, localized lymphoma

Patients with minimal, localized lymphoma (i.e. nonbulky stage I or nonbulky stage II with adjacent sites of involvement) have an extremely good outlook when managed appropriately. When stage I diffuse large cell lymphoma is proven by laparotomy 80 %-90 % of patients can be cured with radiotherapy. However, staging laparotomies will not be appropriate in the older adults who represent most of the patients with this subtype of lymphoma. Several randomized clinical trials documented the fact that clinically staged patients with localized lymphoma had a lower relapse rate when given « adjuvant » chemotherapy following local radiotherapy. More recently, it has been shown that primary, or « neo-adjuvant », chemotherapy given for only 3 cycles followed by local radiotherapy has a very high (i.e. approximately 90 %) cure rate clinically staged patients [1]. It appears that similar outcomes can be achieved with a full course of chemotherapy alone.

Disseminated aggressive non-Hodgkin lymphoma

It is not clear that one chemotherapy regimen is superior for patients with disseminated aggressive non-Hodgkin lymphoma. A number of chemotherapy regimens have been proven to be efficacious, but all have potentially serious side effects. It is my opinion that, in the absence of participation in a study asking an important question, each oncologist should choose a regimen in which he or her has the most confidence and become expert in its use. Doing this should reduce unnecessary treatment related toxicity and optimize the cure rate [2]. At the present time complete remissions can be achieved in the majority of patients with aggressive non-Hodgkin lymphoma utilizing effective chemotherapy regimens and the majority of patients who achieve a complete remis-

University of Nebraska Medical Center, 600 South 42 Street, Omaha, NE 68198-3332, USA

sion appear to be cured. Certain subgroups of patients should have prophy-lactic therapy to the central nervous system, usually with intrathecal chemo-therapy, added to their treatment. Although there might be some debate over exactly which patients should be so treated, the data is probably best establis-hed for those with epidural involvement and sinus involvement by lymphoma.

True high grade lymphomas

These tumors, with an unusually aggressive clinical course and rapid progres-sion, occur proportionally more frequently in children than in adults. Chil-dren seem to have a better outlook than in adults. Lymphomas that fit in this category include lymphoblastic lymphoma and small noncleaved cell lymphoma. Previous reports suggest that adults with lymphoblastic lymphoma and small noncleaved cell lymphoma can be divided into two categories. Patients with nonbulky disease, low LDH, and no involvement of the central nervous system or bone marrow have a good outlook with aggressive chemotherapy regimens. Unfortunately, this makes up the minority of patients. The larger group of patients with the opposite characteristics have done very poorly (i.e. $\leqslant$ '20 % survival) with commonly utilized chemotherapy regimens. The difference in the results for children and adults has not been clear. Proposed explanations include a difference in the dose intensity between regimens usually utilized for chil-dren and adults, or that the tumors that occur in children are in some way different and more sensitive to therapy. The results of a study using a vary dose intensive chemotherapy regimen just completed at Vanderbilt University, where 65 % of adult patients with extensive, small noncleaved cell lymphoma achieved prolonged remissions, suggest that the dose intensity explanation might apply at least for small noncleaved cell lymphoma [3].

AIDS related lymphoma

The recent epidemic of AIDS related to infection by the human immunodefi-ciency virus (HIV) has led to a striking increase in secondary lymphomas. Patients with AIDS related lymphoma can be divided into 2 groups from the point of view of therapy. Those patients in whom the lymphoma develops after the diagnosis of AIDS have an extremely poor outlook. Therapy is often asso-ciated with a worsening of opportunistic infection and seems to shorten these patient's life. In contrast, patients in whom the diagnosis of AIDS is made because of the development of lymphoma but with no opportunistic infections do seem to benefit from chemotherapy. While some patients will develop oppor-tunistic infections during treatment and have a poor outlook, others seem to have durable remissions induced by chemotherapy. There is evidence to sug-gest that the most intensive chemotherapy regimens might be less effective because of an increased risk of opportunistic infections [4].

Future therapeutic advances

The treatment for patients aggressive non-Hodgkin lymphoma continues to evolve. At the present time, it appears unlikely that a new combination of medicines is likely to make an important advance. However, the development of new chemotherapeutic agents might improve our therapeutic abilities considerably.

With the presently available agents, increasing dose intensity to overcome treatment resistance appears the most likely way to improve treatment outcome. Increased dose intensity can be accomplished by very high doses of drugs with amelioration of hematopoietic toxicity by bone marrow transplantation, or with the use of hematopoietic growth factors. Whether the increased dose intensity allowed by either of these maneuvers will be sufficient to strikingly increase the cure rate will be shown in the next several years. Several studies to address these issues are now underway.

Future treatments are likely to involve more specifically targeted therapies. These might include monoclonal antibodies labeled with radioactivity molecules or toxins directed against specific targets on tumor cells that are not present on normal cells. Trials using such agents are currently underway. Specifically targeted therapies could be aimed at molecules involved in drug resistance and not be cytotoxic in themselves. Such agents might improve the efficacy of currently available antilymphoma drugs. Studies utilizing calcium channel blockers to modify drug resistance in patients with lymphoma that have already been performed at the University of Arizona are examples of this approach [5].

References

1. Longo D (1989) Combined modality therapy for localized aggressive lymphoma : enough or too much ? J Clin Oncol 9 : 1179-1181
2. Armitage JO (1991) The place of third-generation regimens in the treatment of adult aggressive non-Hodgkin's lymphoma. Annals Oncol 2 : 37-41
3. McMaster ML, Greer JP, Greco FA, Johnson DH, Wolff SN, Hainsworth JD (1991) Effective treatment of small noncleaved cell lymphoma with high intensity, brief duration chemotherapy. J Clin Oncol (in press)
4. Levine AM (1990) Lymphoma in acquired immunodefficiency syndrome. Sem Oncol 17 : 104-112
5. Miller TP, Grogan TM, Dalton WS, Spier CM, Scheper RJ, Salmon SE (1991) P-glycoprotein expression in malignant lymphoma and reversal of cliical drug resistance with chemotherapy plus high-dose verapamil. J Clin Oncol 9 : 17-24

Third International Congress
on Neo-Adjuvant Chemotherapy

Under the auspices of :
**Ministère de la Solidarité, de la Santé et de la Protection Sociale,
Ministère de l'Éducation Nationale, de la Jeunesse et des Sports,
Ministère des Affaires Étrangères**

Organized with the sponsorship of :
American Cancer Society (ACS) - Association pour la Recherche sur le Cancer (ARC) - Centre Médico-Chirurgical de Bligny - Centre de Recherche Appliquée à la Chimiothérapie (CRAC) - Institut National de la Santé et de la Recherche Médicale (INSERM) - Ligue Nationale Française contre le Cancer (Comité de Paris) - Lion's Club Paris le Doyen - M.D. Anderson Cancer Center - Memorial Sloan Kettering Cancer Center - Union Internationale Contre le Cancer (UICC) - University of Chicago, the Pritzker School of medicine - Sydney University - The Prince Alfred Hospital.

Supported in part by grants of :
Allianz - Air France - Automobiles Peugeot - Banque Eurofin - Caisse d'Épargne Écureuil de Paris - Caisse Nationale des Télécommunications - L'Équité (Compagnie d'Assurances) - Fédération des Industries Mécaniques et Transformatrices des Métaux - La Garantie Médicale et Chirurgicale - Le Généraliste - Orkem - Pernod Ricard - Printemps - Union des Assurances de Paris (UAP) - Union de Banques à Paris (UBP) - Valeurs Actuelles - Vitalaire.

And with the financial support of :
Institut Servier I.R.I.S. - Laboratoires Asta-Sarget - Beaufour - Beecham - Bristol-Myers - Cordis - Eurocetus - Glaxo - Léderlé - Pfizer - Pharmacia - Pierre Fabre Oncologie - Roche - Roger Bellon - Roussel Uclaf - Takeda.

Achevé d'imprimer par Corlet, Imprimeur, S.A.
14110 Condé-sur-Noireau (France)
N° d'Éditeur : 296 - N° d'Imprimeur : 1760 - Dépôt légal : novembre 1991
Imprimé en C.E.E.

UROMITEXAN®   HOLOXAN®

UROMITEXAN · 400 - FORME ET PRESENTATION : Ampoules injectables (I V) de 4 ml boîte de 15 **COMPOSITION :** Mesna (DCI) ou mercapto ethane sulfonate de Na p ampoule 400 mg, p boîte 6 g - Edetate de sodium p ampoule 1 mg, p boîte 15 mg Excipient hydroxyde de Na (q s p pH 7,5), eau pour preparations injectables **PROPRIETES :** Antidote de l'acroleine, métabolite irritant pour la muqueuse vesicale, forme au cours de la biotransformation des oxazaphosphorines L'acroleine est bloquee sous forme d'un thio éther stable, soluble, rapidement et totalement elimine par l'organisme L efficacite antitumorale des oxazaphosphorines n'est pas modifiee par l'UROMITEXAN · 400 **SORT DU MEDICAMENT :** Après administration I V , le mesna est rapidement transforme dans le plasma en dimesna, lequel est absorbe par le rein et reduit a son niveau en mesna par les systemes thiol transférase et glutathion reductase Le mesna est rapidement elimine dans les urines sous forme active Sa demi-vie d'elimination est de l'ordre de 0.85 à 1,08 heure **INDICATIONS :** Prevention de la toxicite urinaire des oxazaphosphorines (cyclophosphamide, ifosfamide) **MISE EN GARDE :** Quelques cas d'encephalopathies, toujours spontanement reversibles a l'arrêt du traitement, ont ete decrits après utilisation conjointe d'ifosfamide et de mesna Leur imputabilite n'est actuellement pas etablie Une insuffisance renale est habituellement retrouvee comme facteur favorisant **PRECAUTIONS D'EMPLOI :** Utiliser de preference en perfusion intraveineuse après dilution extemporanee dans 100 ml d'une solution injectable de chlorure de sodium a 0,9 % **INCOMPATIBILITES MAJEURES :** Ne pas associer au platine et à ses derivés Il est necessaire de rincer la tubulure entre les deux produits **EFFETS INDESIRABLES :** Pas d'effets indesirables connus aux doses usuelles de 10 a 30 mg/kg par injection hormis la possibilite, chez certains sujets, d'une réaction inflammatoire locale de la paroi veineuse au point d'injection en cas d'administration intraveineuse directe (cf Precautions d'emploi) **MODE D'EMPLOI ET POSOLOGIE :** UROMITEXAN · 400 peut s'employer selon les mêmes modalites chez l'adulte et chez l'enfant La posologie est habituellement fixee a 60 % de la dose d'oxazaphosphorine (cyclophosphamide, ifosfamide) administree Le schema classique comporte l'administration, après dilution (cf Precautions d'emploi) d'un tiers de la dose des le debut de l'administration de l'oxazaphosphorine du second tiers 4 heures plus tard et du dernier tiers 4 heures plus tard (soit 8 heures apres la premiere administration) Actuellement certains auteurs utilisent UROMITEXAN · 400 en perfusion intraveineuse continue debutant 1/4 d'heure avant la perfusion chimiotherapique et se prolongeant 8 a 12 heures apres la fin de celle-ci, la dose totale de mesna atteignant - voire depassant - 100 % de la dose d'oxazaphosphorine utilisee Pour des doses superieures a 2 000 mg/m²/jour les risques potentiels de ce medicament ne sont pas connus **STABILITE :** - Apres ouverture de l'ampoule, le produit doit être utilise immediatement - Apres dilution la solution est stable au moins 6 heures **CONSERVATION :** Tenir a l'abri de la lumiere **LISTE II** A M M 327 399 7 (1984) Mis sur le marche [1986] UROMITEXAN 400 mg solution injectable I V ampoules de 4 ml (15) Prix public TTC **124,50 F** Modele reserve a l'hôpital UROMITEXAN 400 mg solution injectable I V ampoules de 4 ml (15) Remb Securite Sociale a 70 % - Agree aux collectivites Licence ASTA Pharma - fabricant Lab Lucien - 92700 COLOMBES

HOLOXAN · 1000 - FORMES ET PRESENTATIONS : • Solute injectable 1 flacon + 1 ampoule solvant 14 ml • Solute injectable 10 flacons (modele reserve a l'hôpital) **COMPOSITION** • Ifosfamide (DCI) p unite 1 g, p boîte 10 g • Ampoule eau pour preparation injectable p unite 14 ml **PROPRIETES :** Antineoplasique cytostatique alkylant L ifosfamide empêche la separation et la replication de l'A D N bicatenaire par alkylation et, de ce fait, inhibe les mitoses ou conduit a la constitution de cellules non viables Cette action rapide est cycledependante et respecte les cellules en Go **SORT DU MÉDICAMENT :** L'ifosfamide est inactif in vitro et doit être active au niveau du foie par oxydation microsomiale L'elimination est essentiellement urinaire **INDICATIONS :** Les resultats les plus demonstratifs ont ete obtenus dans les cancers des bronches, du sein, de l'ovaire, de la sphere O R L , des testicules et dans leurs metastases Sarcomes des tissus mous Sarcomes ostéogéniques **CONTRE-INDICATIONS :** • Insuffisance renale severe • Grossesse et allaitement **PRECAUTIONS D'EMPLOI :** • Surveiller regulierement le nombre des globules blancs, la numeration etant effectuee avant l'injection d'HOLOXAN · 1000 • Lors de l'emploi de doses elevees risque de cystite a eviter par une hydratation abondante du patient tout au long de l'administration du produit (3 a 4 litres/jour) ou par l'utilisation d'UROMITEXAN · 400 • L'alopécie, quand elle existe peut parfois être prevenue par la mise en place d'un garrot pneumatique a la racine des cheveux lors de l'injection ou par celle d'un casque refrigerant **EFFETS INDÉSIRABLES :** • Nausées ou vomissements possibles surtout en debut de traitement les prévenir ou les supprimer par les antiemetiques • Granulopénie moderee et thrombocytopenie inconstante • Cystite en cas de fortes doses (cf Precautions d'emploi) • Alopecie inconstante, transitoire et reversible **MODE D'EMPLOI ET POSOLOGIE :** La solution d'HOLOXAN· peut être reconstituee en prediluant la poudre dans les 14 ml de solvant L'utilisation se fait preferentiellement par voie I V directe ou dans la tubulure d'une perfusion (solution injectable isotonique de glucose ou de NaCl) ou dilue dans cette perfusion Pour eviter une irritation locale au moment de l'injection finale la concentration d'HOLOXAN· en solution ne doit pas exceder 4% HOLOXAN· 1000 est habituellement utilise par cycles courts comportant 1000 a 1500 mg/m²/jour voire plus durant 3 a 5 jours consecutifs les cycles sont repris toutes les 3 a 4 semaines L'association a d'autres antineoplasiques est possible HOLOXAN· 1000 peut être administre par voies I V I M (dans ces cas injecter lentement, toujours a distance des repas et chez un sujet allonge) D'autres voies (intra-arterielle locale, sous-cutanee, intra-lymphatique) peuvent être utilisees ou associees entre elles **STABILITE :** La solution diluee est isotonique et stable pendant 6 heures a temperature ordinaire **CONSERVATION :** Tenir a l'abri de la lumiere et a une temperature inferieure a 25° C Les solutions d'HOLOXAN· sont chimiquement stables En raison des considerations microbiologiques, les solutions doivent être utilisees apres leur preparation (ne pas conserver dans le refrigerateur au-dela de 24 heures) **LISTE I** A M M 318 954 1 (1975) Mis sur le marche [1976] HOLOXAN· 1000 solute injectable 1 flacon + 1 ampoule solvant 14 ml Prix public TTC **148,40 F** Modele reserve a l'hôpital HOLOXAN· 1000 solute injectable flacons (10) Remb Securite Sociale a 100 % - Agree aux collectivites Laboratoires SARGET Avenue J F Kennedy - 33700 MERIGNAC Licence ASTA Pharma - fabricant Lab Lucien - 92700 COLOMBES

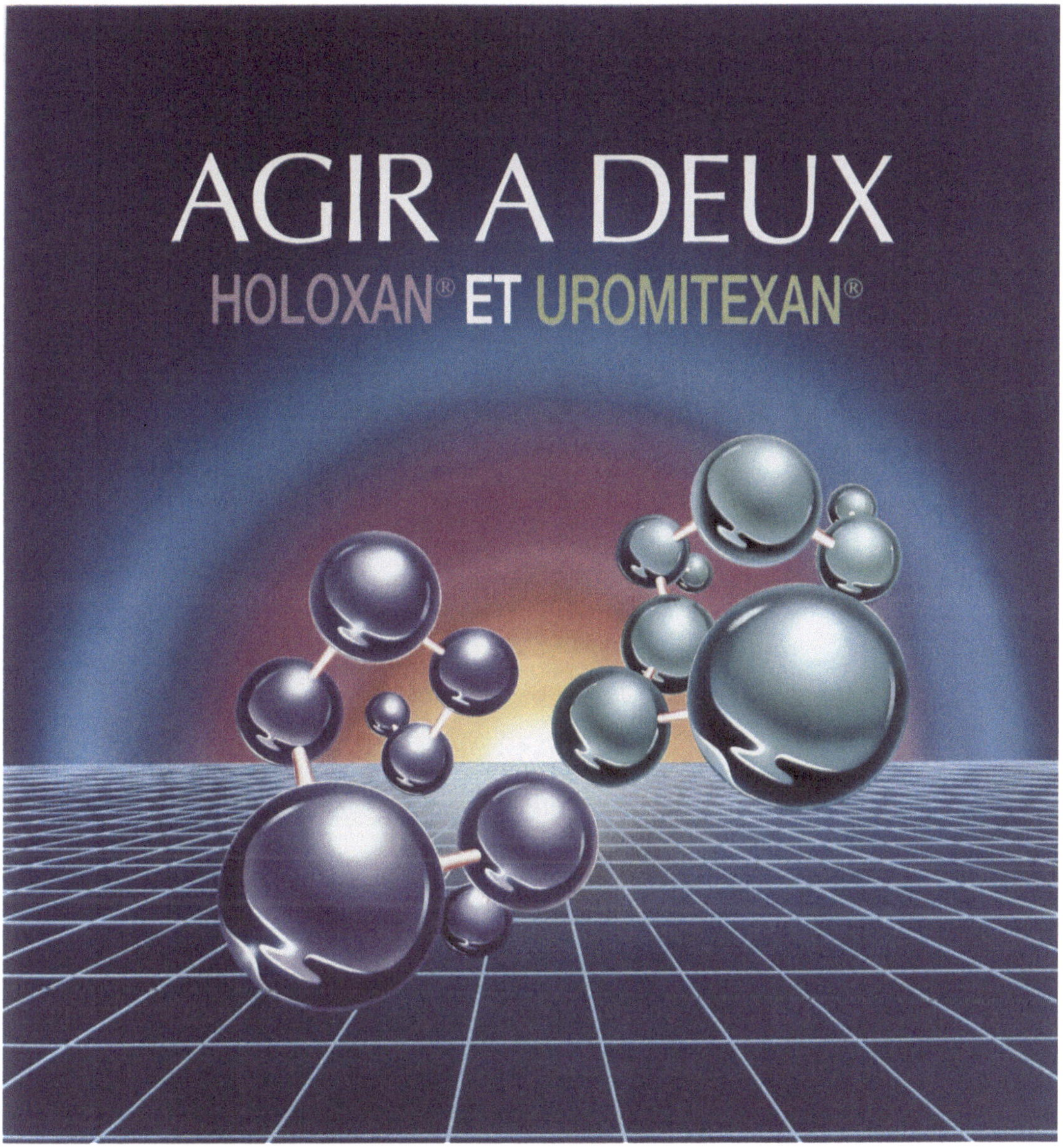

AGIR A DEUX
HOLOXAN® ET UROMITEXAN®

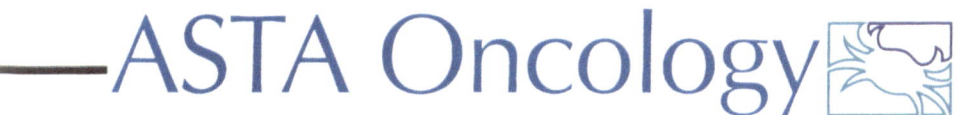

ASTA Oncology

Une division au service de l'oncologie

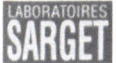

ASTA Oncology

LABORATOIRES SARGET AVENUE J. F. KENNEDY 33700 MERIGNAC